BASIC
PATHOLOGY

BASIC PATHOLOGY

An introduction to the mechanisms of disease

Sunil R. Lakhani
BSc, MBBS, MRCPath

Susan A. Dilly
BSc, MBBS, MRCPath

Caroline J. Finlayson
MBBS, MRCPath

**Department of Histopathology,
St. George's Hospital Medical School, London**

Edward Arnold

A member of the Hodder Headline Group

LONDON BOSTON MELBOURNE AUCKLAND

© 1993 Sunil R. Lakhani, Susan A. Dilly and Caroline J. Finlayson

First published in Great Britain 1993

British Library Cataloguing in Publication Data
Lakhani, Sunil R.
Basic Pathology: Introduction to the
Mechanisms of Disease
I. Title
616.07

ISBN 0-340-57192-6

Whilst the advice and information in this book is believed to be true and accurate at the date of going to press, neither the author nor the publisher can accept any legal responsibility or liability for any errors or omissions that may be made. In particular (but without limiting the generality of the preceding disclaimer) every effort has been made to check drug dosages; however, it is still possible that errors have been missed. Furthermore, dosage schedules are constantly being revised and new side effects recognised. For these reasons the reader is strongly urged to consult the drug companies' printed instructions before administering any of the drugs recommended in this book.

Typeset in 10/11 Palatino by Vivitext Creative Services, 65 Leonard Street, London EC2A 4QS
Printed and bound in Great Britain
for Edward Arnold, a division of Hodder Headline PLC, Mill Road, Dunton Green, Sevenoaks, Kent TN13 2YA by Butler & Tanner Ltd, Frome and London.

Preface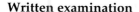

"What is the use of a book", thought Alice, "without pictures or conversations?"

– Lewis Carroll

Ask any artist and he will tell you that in drawing objects he cannot ignore the space between them. The picture exists as an entire composition and loses its meaning if only one area is viewed. To the musician, the pauses are as important as the notes. Yet when it comes to teaching, we forget this simple fact, consider our own speciality of unique importance and ignore connections with the rest of the undergraduate curriculum.

Our aim in this book is to create a tutorial on the mechanisms of disease over a background of history, science and clinical relevance. The target is to give students a sense of belonging to a movement – the movement from past to present and from laboratory to patient.

With this in mind, the book has been written so that the text on the left hand side of the page should be read fully and at leisure. This contains information about diseases as well as historical anecdotes and is supplemented by clinical scenarios. Examinations are an inevitable part of undergraduate life and so the right-hand side contains questions and lists to aid revision. The cartoons are intended both to illustrate facts and to raise a smile and give an idea of the relative importance of different topics. We draw attention to certain items in the margin and provide a logo system as follows:

Oral examiner
Short questions appropriate for MCQs, oral exams
or ward-round 'quiz'

Written examination
Subjects likely to appear in written exams

Small print
Amaze your friends!

Definitions
Saves you searching for the dictionary

The book is intended primarily for undergraduate medical students and we hope that it will amuse them enough to realise that basic pathology is not only important but fun. We believe that the book will also be useful for dental, human biology and some paramedical students and to those postgraduate students studying for pathology or surgical examinations.

SRL
SAD
CJF

LONDON
JANUARY 1993

Acknowledgement _____

The time from inspiration to the final product has been a long one and we would like to take this opportunity to thank the many people who have helped and encouraged us along the way.

Our particular thanks go to Prof. M. J. Davies, Prof. A. Dalgleish and Dr. M. Patton for finding time during their busy schedules to read chapters 2, 4 and 5 respectively and for giving us valuable comments to assist us in achieving a reasonable balance. We have also received considerable help and advice from a wide variety of scientific and clinical colleagues. Many have supplied us with photographs and special thanks is due to our Audio Visual Aid department.

We would also like to acknowledge the sources of the various pictures and quotations used in the book. Thanks are due to Macmillan London Ltd., The Publication Division (copyrights) HMSO, Harper Collins Publishers, Oxford University Press, Cordon Art B.V., Holland, Gryphon Editions Ltd., Oriel Press Ltd., The Journal of Clinical Pathology (BMJ) and the Wellcome Institute for the History of Medicine.

Mr Nick Dunton, Director of Health Science Publishing at Edward Arnold deserves a special mention as it was he who believed in us when we first approached him with our ideas. We would also like to thank Diane Leadbetter-Conway and her team, who have been responsible for the editing and production of the book. Finally, a note of thanks to our families for their encouragement and support.

S. R. Lakhani.

S. A. Dilly.

C. J. Finlayson.   London 1993.

Contents

Chapter 1

Inflammation, Healing and Repair

"No natural phenomenon can be adequately studied in itself alone, but to be understood must be considered as it stands connected with all nature."

– Sir Francis Bacon

What is inflammation? _____

Inflammation is a mechanism by which the body deals with an injury or insult. When living tissue is attacked, for example by physical, chemical or microbial agents, a series of local processes are initiated in order to contain the offensive agent, to neutralise its effect, to limit spread and hopefully to eradicate it. As part and parcel of this process, there is initiation of healing and repair of the injured tissue. Inflammation, healing and repair are like the black and white stripes of the zebra; in order truly to understand the zebra, one cannot study the stripes in isolation. In the same way, the processes of healing and repair have to be addressed in their relationship to the process of inflammation.

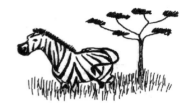

The circulatory system is of fundamental importance in the inflammatory response. In general terms, the offending agent, whatever it may be, causes a change in the microvasculature of the injured area leading to a massive outpouring of cells and fluid. This collection of cells and fluid is known as the **inflammatory exudate**, and within this exudate we find ingredients that are needed to combat the offending agent and to begin the process of healing and repair. However, this is only half the story. It is romantic to imagine an army being sent to deal with an invading force and to restore peace and tranquillity to the area. Life is not quite so simple; there is a price to be paid for war! The process of inflammation may have evolved to benefit mankind, but it can cause destruction and become more offensive than the original insult. The ugly side of it ranges from cosmetic problems, such as keloid scars, to life-threatening illnesses, like autoimmune diseases.

John Hunter, surgeon to St. George's Hospital from 1768 to 1793, was interested in inflammation and repair. He was an incredible man whose aim was the total understanding of mankind! Hunter was born in Scotland on 14th February 1728, the last of 10 children. He spent the first 20 years there and his childhood has been described as 'wasted and idle'. This is because he "… wanted to know all about the clouds and the grasses, and why the leaves changed colour in the autumn …". Hunter's inquisitiveness and fascination with nature stood him in good stead when he began to unravel the mysteries of the human body. His book, *A treatise on the Blood, Inflammation, and Gunshot Wounds*, is a monument to his thoroughness and powers of observation in delineating the processes of disease. Hunter was one of the first to ob-

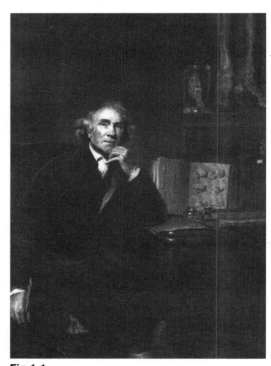

Fig 1.1
John Hunter (1728–1793).
(Courtesy of the Wellcome Institute for the History of Medicine).

serve that inflammation was not a disease but a response to tissue injury whose attempts at repair were sometimes more harmful than the original disease.

Many of Hunter's experiments are absolutely fascinating as well as crazy and amusing, but more of that later, so keep reading!

Anyone who has had a boil on their bum, or anywhere else for that matter, will be familiar with the four cardinal signs of inflammation: **rubor (redness)**, **calor (heat)**, **tumour (swelling)** and **dolor (pain)**. These were first described by a Roman physician, Cornelius Celsus, in the first century AD. To this a fifth sign was later added, **functio laesa (loss of function)**; however, this is not a necessary accompaniment of the inflammatory process.

So what is the pathophysiology behind these clinical signs?

Microvasculature

As mentioned previously, the microvasculature plays a central role in inflammation and the *redness* is caused by **vasodilatation**. This is important for increasing the flow of blood to the affected area and, hence, delivering cells and plasma-derived substances needed for combat. Vasodilatation also produces the *heat*. The *swelling* results from **increased permeability** of vessel walls leading to the outpouring of fluid and cells, the inflammatory exudate. In some circumstances, the swelling may cushion the affected part and lead to immobilisation (*loss of function*). The sign that is the most difficult to explain is *pain*. This probably arises from the combination of stretching of tissue by exudate and the action of some of the **chemical mediators** involved in inflammation.

We are indebted to Julius Cohnheim (1839–1884) for investigating the pathophysiology of inflammation. He was a German pathologist, a pupil and later assistant to the father of cellular pathology, Rudolf Virchow. He delineated the vascular changes of inflammation using living preparations of thin membranes, such as the mesentery, and demonstrated the vasodilatation and the subsequent exudation of fluid. But what are the underlying mechanisms of this process? In broad terms, there are two aspects to consider:

- chemical mediators
- cells of inflammation

The chemical mediators

In 1927, Sir Thomas Lewis identified **histamine**, present in tissue mast cells, as a mediator of acute inflammation. Since then a vast array of mediators have been identified, but not all have a proven role *in vivo*. They may be derived from the plasma, the participating inflammatory cells or from the damaged tissue itself.

". . .inflammation in itself is not to be considered as a disease, but as a salutary operation, consequent either to some violence or some disease. But this same operation can and does go vary; it is often carried much further even sound parts. . . .

Where it can alter the diseased mode of action, it likewise leads to a cure; but where it cannot accomplish that salutary purpose, as in cancer, scrofula, veneral disease, etc it does mischief."

– John Hunter

What are the cardinal features of inflammation?

1. Redness
2. Swelling
3. Heat
4. Pain
5. Loss of function

The **cell-derived products** include:

- vasoactive amines
- cytokines
- arachidonic acid derivatives
- platelet activating factor
- lysosomal enzymes
- growth factors
- oxygen-derived free radicals

The **plasma-derived mediators** include:

- kinin system
- coagulation and fibrinolytic system
- complement system

Some are important in the amplification of the inflammatory response; others play their role in the elimination of the offending agent. The mediators and their role in inflammation will be discussed in more detail later.

Cellular mediators

The principal **cells of inflammation** are the lymphocytes, plasma cells, macrophages and the polymorphonuclear leucocytes, which include neutrophils, eosinophils and basophils. A Russian microbiologist, Elias Metchnikoff, working at the Pasteur Institute in Paris in 1884, demonstrated that leucocytes **phagocytose** bacteria and concluded that the purpose of the inflammatory response was to bring phagocytic cells to the area to kill the organisms. Inflammatory cells descend on a focus of tissue damage in 'waves': the first cell type recruited is the neutrophil polymorph (an 'acute' inflammatory cell), which is followed by macrophages, lymphocytes and plasma cells ('chronic' inflammatory cells). Later, the tissue generates new blood vessels and fibrous scar tissue as reparative work begins.

Of course we know now that humoral agents (**antibodies**) are also important in the inflammatory response. Antibodies are protein molecules that are produced by the plasma cells in response to foreign molecules invading the body. The molecules that stimulate antibody production are called **antigens**. The production of antibody helps eliminate the antigen as well as forming part of the basis of immunity. The first contact with the antigen imparts some memory that is used to mount a more effective attack on subsequent contact with the antigen. Paul Ehrlich, who developed the humoral theory, shared the Nobel Prize with Metchnikoff in 1908.

Causes of inflammation

We have considered the reaction to tissue injury but what are the causes? Because infections are so common, there is a

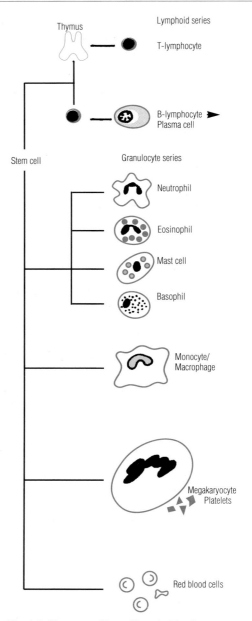

Fig 1.2 Haemopoeitic and lymphoid cell precursors

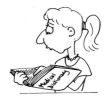

Phagocytosis is the process of engulfing foreign or injured material. Macrophages and polymorphs are phagocytic cells.

tendency to think that infection and inflammation are synonymous and it is easy to overlook other important causes. Causes of inflammation include:

- mechanical injuries
- bacteria, viruses, fungi, parasites
- ischaemia
- chemical injuries
- extremes of temperature
- radiation (e.g. ultraviolet light)
- immune mechanisms (e.g. autoimmune disease)

The common feature is that the agent first damages the patient's cells, initiating the fascinatingly complex process of inflammation. The patient with the boil on the bum, however, will be less impressed than we are with the inflammatory processes taking place. He may regard the fact that the injury has caused microvascular changes via mediators, leading to cellular and humoral factors accumulating at the site of injury as of less importance than the burning question, What will happen next?

There are a number of possibilities. The process may restore the tissue to its normal state, with nothing to suggest that anything had been amiss. Healing may take place but leave a scar. The injury and the inflammation may grumble on for a long time or the injury may completely overwhelm the body and lead to death. This last outcome is especially likely where inflammatory defences are deficient, such as in AIDS, cancer patients treated with cytotoxic drugs or patients receiving immunosuppresive drugs for auto-immune diseases or following organ transplantation. The final outcome depends on the interactions between the various processes involved in inflammation. Just as the zebra is neither black with white stripes nor white with black stripes, so it is the combination of the various inflammatory components that determines the texture of the whole.

Types of inflammation

Inflammation is divided into acute and chronic forms based on the duration and the predominant inflammatory cell type. Acute inflammation, generally, is of short duration, lasting from a few minutes to a few days and the cellular exudate is rich in neutrophil polymorphonuclear leucocytes. Chronic inflammation tends to be more variable, may last for months or years and the chief cells involved are lymphocytes, plasma cells and macrophages. The inflammatory process, whether acute or chronic, may be modified by a whole host of factors such as the cause of the damage, nutritional status, the competence of the immune system and intervention with antibiotics, 'anti-inflammatory drugs' or surgery.

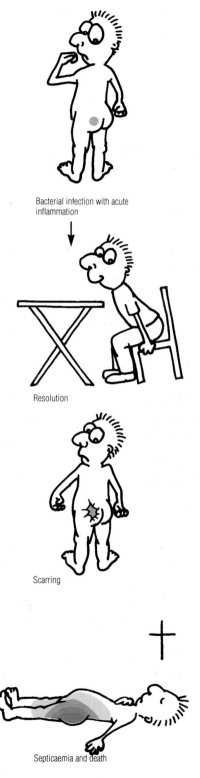

Bacterial infection with acute inflammation

Resolution

Scarring

Septicaemia and death

Fig 1.3 Possible outcomes of acute inflammation

Acute inflammation

Lobar pneumonia

A disease exemplifying acute inflammation is lobar pneumonia, named because the lung parenchyma is involved in continuity so that a whole lobe or lobes are affected by the process. *Streptococcus pneumoniae*, a Gram positive diplococcal bacterium, is the commonest cause of lobar pneumonia. It invades the lung leading to changes in the microvasculature and a massive outpouring of fluid into the alveolar spaces resulting in **congestion***(a)*. This fluid is rich in fibrin. Soon afterwards, neutrophils follow and the fibrin-rich fluid and cells spread from alveolus to alveolus via the pores of Kohn. The neutrophils attack the organisms and phagocytose them leading to the death of both organisms and many neutrophils. Not surprisingly, the alveoli are airless and the lung is now firm and red with the texture of liver; this stage is termed **'red hepatisation'***(b)*. As this process progresses, the macrophage is recruited not only to phagocytose dead neutrophils and bacteria but also to digest the fibrin mesh. The lung is still firm but the large inflammatory cell infiltrate and reduction in vasodilatation give it a grey colour and, hence, the term **'grey hepatisation'** *(c)*. The final outcome will depend on the competence of this system and whether the basic framework of the lung tissue is intact. Ideally, the alveoli will be cleared, re-aerated and **resolution** *(d)* will take place. If the alveolar framework has been destroyed or the exudate has not been cleared, **organisation** will occur leading to scar formation. The infection may persist in destroying lung tissue but become localised so that an **abscess** is formed. This is a collection of pus walled off by fibrous tissue. Alternatively it may spread to the rest of the lung, involve the pleura, cause an empyema, disseminate via the blood stream to other areas of the body or even lead to death.

Acute appendicitis

Another good example of acute inflammation is acute appendicitis. The classical symptoms of appendicitis are pain (first in the periumbilical region and then localising to the right iliac fossa), nausea, vomiting and fever. The point of maximum tenderness in the right iliac fossa is known as McBurney's point after an American surgeon Charles McBurney (1845–1913). His description appears in the *New York Medical Times* in 1889 and states that the pain is to "be determined by pressure of one finger, and the point lies 1^1/$_2$ in. from the anterior superior iliac spine on a straight line drawn from that process to the umbilicus". McBurney also described the muscle-splitting or grid-iron incision used for appendicectomy.

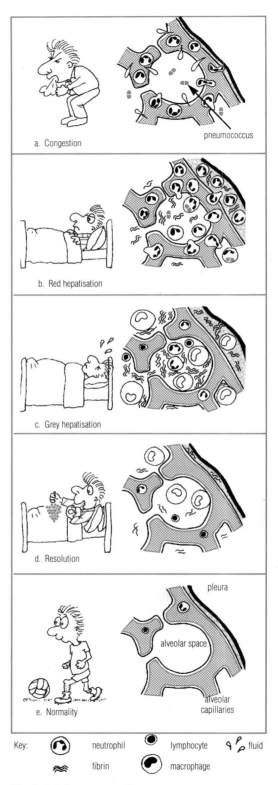

a. Congestion — pneumococcus

b. Red hepatisation

c. Grey hepatisation

d. Resolution

e. Normality — pleura, alveolar space, alveolar capillaries

Key: neutrophil lymphocyte fluid
fibrin macrophage

Fig 1.4 Lobar pneumonia

The initiating event of appendicitis is not always clear but may be obstruction of the lumen by a faecolith (hardened calcified faecal material) or collections of pinworms. The build up of pressure from the obstruction may affect the blood supply and lead to ischaemic injury of the appendiceal wall which is then invaded by bacteria normally present within the gut. This triggers the process of inflammation. Neutrophils migrate out of the damaged vessels and into the appendix wall, together with large amounts of fibrin which are deposited on the serosal surface. The inflammation may settle down, but more usually does not. If there is a delay in surgical intervention, destruction of the appendiceal wall may produce a perforation resulting in inflammatory and necrotic debris spilling into the peritoneal cavity. Here it sets up a widely disseminated inflammatory response over the entire peritoneal membrane (peritonitis). At this stage, the inflammatory response causes severe shock and is life-threatening.

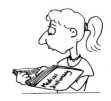

Empyema
An accumulation of pus within a body cavity

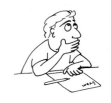

Now that we have the overall concept of inflammation and its clinical relevance, we must look more closely at the complex cellular and molecular events of this process. We shall first examine the changes in the microvasculature.

What is the predominant cell of acute inflammation?

Neutrophil polymorph

What are the predominant cells of chronic inflammation?

Lymphocytes
Macrophages
Plasma cells

Vascular changes

Many of the vascular events which follow injury were delineated by Julius Cohnheim, who was mentioned previously. His experiments with frog mesentery beautifully demonstrated that injury produced vasodilatation and increased blood flow, followed by slowing down of the blood flow, lining up of white cells along the vessel wall (**margination**) and the movement of these cells into the extravascular compartment (**diapedesis** or **emigration**). He observed that the flow of blood could almost cease in some vessels and suggested that this was due to loss of fluid because of increased permeability of the vessel wall.

Before we consider the causes of altered vascular permeability, it is worth revising the normal physiological factors that control the movement of fluid across a small vessel wall (see Fig. 1.5). Fluid flows away from areas of high hydrostatic pressure and towards areas of high osmotic pressure. Thus, fluid leaves from the arterial end of the capillary network and is reabsorbed at the venous end *(a)*, with any excess being removed via lymphatics. A rise in hydrostatic pressure within the vessel without changes in permeability will increase leakage of fluid out of the vessel but it will have no protein in it *(b)*. Normally, large molecules, such as albumin, do not leak out. However, if the permeability of the vessel wall increases, then fluid can move more readily and protein molecules may leak across. Movement of protein molecules will alter the osmotic

Summarise the events in inflammation

1. Changes in microvasculature
2. Exudate formation
   Fluid
   Cells
3. Either
   Resolution
   Scarring
   Chronic inflammation/abscess formation
   Spread
   Death

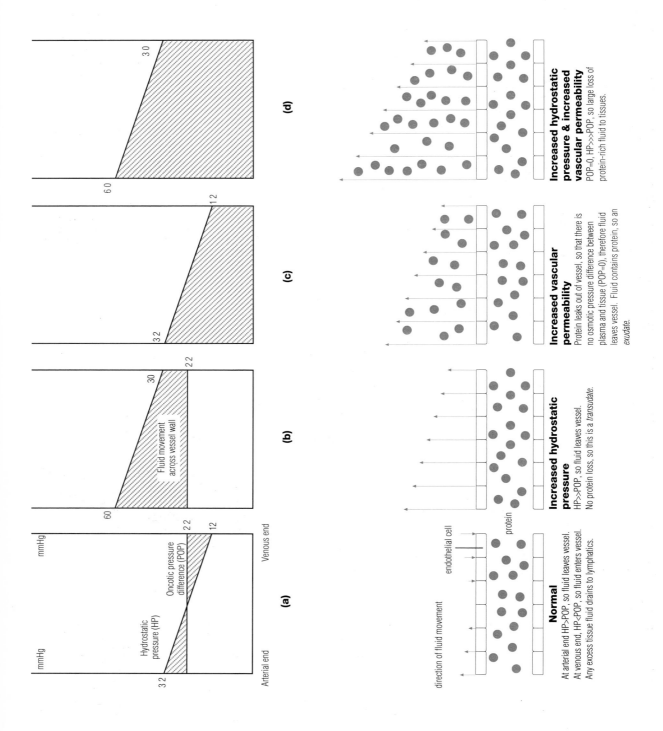

Fig 1.5 Factors affecting the movement of fluid across vessels

pressure gradient, such that less fluid is reabsorbed into the blood and tissue fluid will increase *(c)*. In areas of inflammation there is usually a rise in hydrostatic pressure and an increase in vascular permeability *(d)*.

This is an appropriate time to introduce a number of new words. An **exudate** is the fluid within the extravascular spaces which is rich in protein and hence has a specific gravity greater than 1.020. On the other hand, a **transudate** has a low protein content and specific gravity of less than 1.020. **Oedema** simply refers to the presence of excess fluid within the extravascular space and body cavities and may be an exudate or transudate. **Pus** can be thought of as a special kind of exudate, a **purulent exudate**. Besides the protein-rich fluid, it contains dead or dying bacteria and neutrophils. The consistency of the pus depends on the amount of digestion by neutrophil enzymes and the colour depends on the type of organism and the presence of neutrophil-derived myeloperoxidase, which imparts a yellow-green colour.

If we examine the fluid that forms during an inflammatory reaction, we find that it is an exudate. This means that large protein molecules have leaked out of the microvasculature. What is the mechanism of the increased permeability? Electron-microscopical studies suggest that there are two distinct 'pore' systems for the transport of molecules within normal endothelial cells. The large 'pore' system consists of pinocytic vesicles which form on the luminal side of the cell membrane by the cell membrane wrapping around the fluid, analogous with phagocytosis of larger particles (see later). The extracellular fluid containing large molecules is then transferred, inside these membrane-bound vesicles, to the extraluminal surface where they are discharged. The small 'pore' system is more controversial but is probably formed by the intercellular junctions. Most vessels are lined by this type of endothelium which is termed '**continuous**'. In endocrine organs, intestines and renal glomeruli, the endothelium is normally more permeable because it contains 'windows', hence the name **fenestrated endothelium**, while in the spleen, liver and bone marrow the endothelium is **discontinuous**.

What happens following injury has been elegantly demonstrated using simple experiments involving intravenous injection of indian ink. The ink will remain within the vascular compartment except in the liver and spleen where the discontinuous endothelium allows ink to escape. If a mild injury is produced (e.g. by using heat), the damaged area will turn black. Microscopical examination would reveal that the ink particles have crossed the endothelial layer and are trapped at the basement membrane. Guido Majno demonstrated that injection of a vasoactive substance, histamine, caused the endothelial cells of the small venules to contract, creating gaps through which the ink molecules could pass. In reality, the situation is more complicated as the vascular changes will depend on the severity of the insult.

What is oedema?

It is excess fluid within extravascular space or body cavities

What is the difference between Transudate and Exudate?

A transudate is fluid of low protein content and specific gravity of <1.020, hence an ultrafiltrate of blood. An exudate has a high protein content with a specific gravity >1.020. It also contains fibrinogen and will clot spontaneously

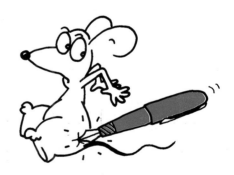

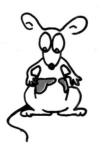

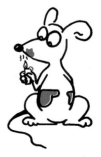

Three types of vascular response have been demonstrated, although they generally overlap in real situations:
- the immediate-transient response
- the immediate-persistent response
- the delayed-persistent response

The immediate-transient response

This occurs immediately following injury, reaches a peak after 5–10 minutes and ceases after 15–30 minutes. This response can be produced by histamine and other chemical mediators and is blocked by prior administration of antihistamines. The leakage occurs exclusively from small venules which develop gaps between the endothelial cells as the endothelial cells contract. This occurs following nettle stings or insect bites.

The immediate-persistent response

This results from severe injury such as burns, where there is direct damage to endothelial cells. The leak starts immediately and reaches a peak within an hour. As the endothelial cells are damaged and may even slough off, the leak will continue until the vessel has been blocked with thrombus or the vessel is repaired. Unlike the previous example, it can affect any type of vessel.

The delayed-persistent response

This is a very interesting type of response, familiar to anyone who has overindulged in a tropical holiday after a period under the clouds of England. There is an interval of up to 24 hours before the leak starts from both capillaries and venules. Small aggregates of platelets and endothelial cells are seen in some capillaries and it seems that the endothelial cells are damaged directly.

We shall next look at the cellular component of the inflammatory response.

Cellular events

The principal cells of the acute inflammatory response are the neutrophils and macrophages.

Following injury, the neutrophils migrate out of the vessels, the number recruited depending on the type of injury. For example, infections with bacteria attract more inflammatory cells than do purely physical injuries. After the neutrophils, there is a second wave of cells, the macrophages. The movement of neutrophils out of the vessels and their role in combat can be divided into discrete steps. These are:

- margination
- adhesion

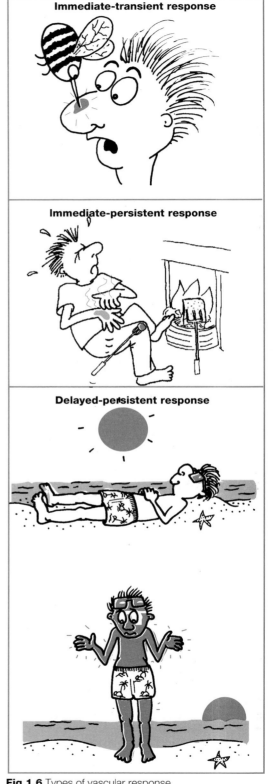

Fig 1.6 Types of vascular response

- emigration
- chemotaxis
- phagocytosis and degranulation

Margination and adhesion

When haemodynamic changes take place in the vasculature during inflammation, white cells fall out of the central axial flow and line themselves up along the wall (a little reminiscent of the school disco!). The cells then adhere to the endothelium although precisely how this occurs is still a mystery. It appears that there are specific complementary '**adhesion molecules**' which stick leucocytes to endothelial cells, and the number of these molecules on the cell surfaces is increased by inflammatory mediators. One pair of such molecules is ICAM-1 (intracellular adhesion molecule 1) on endothelial cells and LFA-1 (lymphocyte function antigen 1) on leucocytes, which bind together like a 'lock and key'. Resting cells express very few adhesion molecules but some inflammatory mediators increase expression of LFA-1 (e.g. complement fragments (C5a) and leukotrienes (LTB4)), while other mediators enhance ICAM-1 expression (e.g. interleukin-1 (IL-1) and bacterial endotoxin). This adhesion is of great importance and people with a genetic deficiency of these adhesion molecules suffer from repeated bacterial infections.

Our knowledge of adhesion molecules is expanding rapidly. Broadly, there are three families involved in inflammation, the **integrins**, the **immunoglobulin gene superfamily** and the **selectins**. Some (but not all) of their family members are listed in Table 1.1. Their expression changes during inflammation so that different types of cells adhere at different stages. Histamine or thrombin makes **P-selectin**, (contained in the Weibel–Palade bodies of the endothelial cells) move to the cell surface where it tethers inactive neutrophils. Histamine or thrombin also causes co-expression of **platelet activating factor** (PAF) on the endothelial surface which activates the neutrophils ready for emigration. Both of these molecules are expressed rapidly (within a few minutes) but transiently. The P-selectin acts as a **tethering** molecule for inactive cells which are then activated by the **signalling** molecule, PAF. It is likely that continued adherence and migration of cells over the following hours depends on other tethering molecules, such as **E-selectin**, co-expressed with signalling molecules, such as **IL-8**, which have delayed but prolonged expression stimulated by the cytokines, TNF (tumour necrosis factor) and IL-1.

Some of these molecules have been termed **addressins** because they act as address labels to allow cells to leave the circulation in a specific tissue. This is particularly important in the recirculation and 'homing' of lymphocytes which is discussed on page 24.

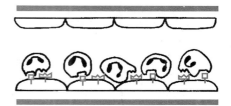

Neutrophils align along the side of the blood vessels, bound by adhesion molecules

Fig 1.7 Margination

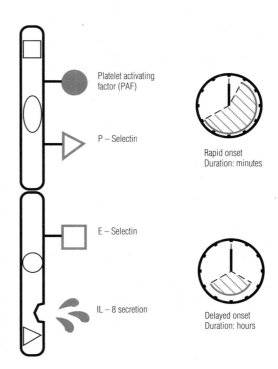

Platelet activating factor (PAF)

P – Selectin

Rapid onset
Duration: minutes

E – Selectin

IL – 8 secretion

Delayed onset
Duration: hours

Fig 1.8 Endothelial cell signalling mechanisms

Table 1.1 – Adhesion Molecules

Family	Adhesion molecule	Principally expressed on	Binds to	Notes
Integrins	LFA-1	T cells (esp memory cells)	ICAM-1 ICAM-2	LFA-1 = leucocyte function associated antigen 1, CD11a/CD18 VLA-4 = very late antigen 4
	VLA-4	Memory T cells	VCAM-1	MAC-1 = CD11b/CD18, Mo-1
				ICAM-1 = intercellular adhesion molecule-1, CD54
	MAC-1	Monocytes	ICAM-1	VCAM-1 = Vascular cell adhesion molecule-1
				E-selectin = ELAM-1 : Endothelial leucocyte adhesion molecule
Immuno-globulin gene superfamily	ICAM-1	Activated endothelial cells (+ other cells)	LFA-1 MAC-1	L-selectin = MREL-14, LAM-1, LEU-8, TQ-1, LECAM-1, DREG 5.6 P-selectin = CD62, GMP-140, PADGEM
	ICAM-2	Resting endothelial cells	LFA-1	CD15 is expressed on resting memory T cells, monocytes and PMNs
	VCAM-1	Activated endothelial cells	VLA-4	'Vascular addressins' are expressed on activated endothelial cells and HEV of lymph nodes
Selectins	E-selectin	Activated endothelial cells	CD15	P selectins bind to an unknown molecule expressed on PMNs, monocytes and lymphocytes
	L-selectin	Lymphocyte subsets, PMNs Monocytes	'vascular addressins'	HEV = high endothelial venues PMN = polymorphonuclear leucocyte
	P-selectin	Platelets, Activated endotheilial cells	?	

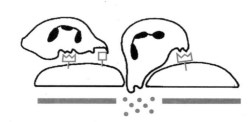

Fig 1.9 Emigration

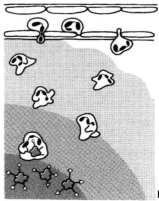

Fig 1.10 Chemotaxis

Emigration and chemotaxis

Once the cells have adhered to the endothelium, they form foot-like processes termed **pseudopodia** which push their way between the endothelial cells. Eventually, the leucocyte lies between the endothelial cell and the basement membrane where it releases a protease to digest the basement membrane which allows it to reach the extravascular space. Neutrophils, basophils, eosinophils, macrophages and lymphocytes all use this route. Red blood cells may also pass through the gaps, but only as passive passengers.

The cells are able to move towards a chemical signal; this specific movement is termed **chemotaxis**. (Note that this is different to **chemokinesis**, which is an increased and accelerated *random* movement.) The Boyden chamber is a popular system for demonstrating chemotaxis. It consists of two chambers separated by a micropore filter. The cells go into one chamber and the putative chemical mediator is placed in the other. If cells move from the first to the second chamber, then chemotaxis is demonstrated. The compounds that have been suggested as chemotactic agents include bacterial products, fragments of the complement system (e.g. C5a) and products of arachidonic acid metabolism (e.g. prostaglandins and leukotrienes).

How does it work? Well, like so many cellular stimuli, the first stage depends on the chemotactic agents binding to specific receptors on the leucocyte cell membrane. This leads to an increase in ionised calcium within the cytoplasm which promotes construction of the contractile elements, **actin** and **myosin**, responsible for movement. However, precisely how these interact to produce directional movement of the cell is not known.

Phagocytosis

Once the neutrophils and macrophages have arrived at the site of injury, they ingest the debris and bacteria, a process termed phagocytosis. This requires a number of distinct steps: the material has to be recognised as foreign or dead, it has to be engulfed and ingested and, finally, it has to be killed or degraded.

Not all of the processes by which neutrophils and macrophages differentiate between normal tissue and foreign or dead tissue are known; however, it is clear that bacteria coated with certain substances are ingested more readily. The factors which coat bacteria are called opsonins and the process is termed **opsonisation**. This is derived from the Greek word 'opson' meaning 'relish' (i.e. getting ready for eating). There are two major opsonins:

- immunoglobulin (IgG)
- C3b component of complement

In order for the neutrophils and macrophages to recognise these opsonins, there must be receptors on the cell surface. There are two such receptors, one for the Fc fragment of IgG

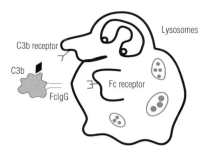

Pseudopodia extend toward opsonised particle

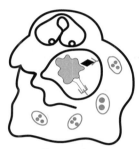

Phagosome forms

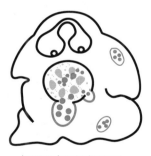

Lysosome fuses to phagosome and releases its digestive enzymes

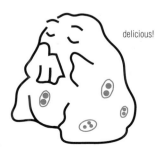

delicious!

Fig 1.11 Phagocytosis

(page 28) and the other for C3b (page 21). After the opsonised fragment attaches to the receptor, the cell puts out a pseudopodium. This extension of cell cytoplasm encircles the particle so that it becomes wrapped in what was originally cell surface membrane. This new intracytoplasmic membrane-bound sac is termed a **phagosome**. Another such sac, normally present in the cell and packed with destructive enzymes, is the **lysosome**. A lysosome fuses with the phagosome producing a **phagolysosome**. This allows the enzymes to have access to the engulfed particle and it is within this vesicle that the killing takes place. If some proteolytic enzymes leak out of the phagolysosome, as may occur if the lysosome fuses with the phagosome while the phagosome is still open to the cell surface, they may damage adjacent tissue – a phenomenon described, rather poetically, as 'regurgitation during feeding'

Mechanisms for bacterial killing

There are essentially two mechanisms for bacterial killing: oxygen-dependent and oxygen-independent.

The **oxygen-dependent system** relies on the **respiratory burst** that occurs during the process of phagocytosis. This is a burst of oxygen consumption accompanied by the production of oxygen metabolites. Oxygen is reduced to superoxide ion which is then converted to hydrogen peroxide (H_2O_2). This is not, however, the most powerful bactericidal chemical. Neutrophils contain an enzyme, myeloperoxidase, which converts H_2O_2 to HOCl (hypochlorous acid) in the presence of halide ions (e.g. chloride). This is a powerful oxidant active against bacteria, fungi, viruses, protozoa and helminths. This system is of clinical importance as its absence produces '**chronic granulomatous disease of childhood**', an inherited disease in which the neutrophils are able to ingest bacteria but unable to kill them. This is because the child lacks the enzyme NADPH oxidase, which leads to a failure of production of superoxide anion ($O_2{}^-$) and hydrogen peroxide.

There are a number of **oxygen-independent** mechanisms that are useful in microbial killing. These include:

- **lysozyme**, an enzyme which attacks the cell wall of some bacteria (especially Gram positive cocci)
- **lactoferrin**, an iron-binding protein that inhibits growth of bacteria
- **major basic protein** (MBP), which is a cationic protein found in eosinophils and is active principally against parasites
- **bactericidal permeability increasing protein** (BPI), which, as the name implies, causes changes in the permeability of the membranes of the microorganisms

Also the **low pH** found in the phagolysosomes, besides being bactericidal itself, enhances the conversion of H_2O_2 to superoxide. Unfortunately, the leucocyte is not successful in killing all organisms and some bacteria, such as the

Oxygen-dependent killing mechanisms

$$O_2 + e^- \rightarrow O_2{}^-$$

(superoxide anion)

$$O_2{}^- + O_2{}^- + 2H^+ \rightarrow O_2 + H_2O_2$$

(hydrogen peroxide)

$$H_2O_2 + Cl + H^+ <\text{-}> H_2O + HOCl$$

(hypochlorous acid)

mycobacterium which causes tuberculosis, can survive inside phagocytes, happily protected from antibacterial drugs and host defence mechanisms.

We shall now go on to consider the chemical mediators involved in inflammation.

Chemical mediators

Since Sir Thomas Lewis demonstrated the role of histamine in inflammation, an enormous number of possible mediators have been put forward. A true mediator must fulfil a number of criteria:

- it must produce symptoms of inflammation when given in physiological doses
- it must be present at the site of inflammation
- its inflammatory effect should be blocked by a specific antagonist

Some of the proposed mediators meet only some of the criteria and so remain putative rather than having an established role.

Cell-derived mediators

Arachidonic acid derivatives
These are the **prostaglandins** and the **leukotrienes**. Just like the clotting and fibrinolytic system, they play a part in thrombosis as well as in inflammation. They are best thought of as local hormones. They have a short range of action, are produced rapidly and degenerate spontaneously or are degraded by enzymes. Arachidonic acid, the parent molecule, is a 20-carbon polyunsaturated fatty acid that is derived either from the diet or from essential fatty acids. It is not found in a free state but is present esterified in the cell membrane phospholipid. The two pathways of arachidonic acid metabolism and its products are shown in Fig. 1.13, which also depicts some of the roles of the products in inflammation. Drugs such as corticosteroids, aspirin and indomethacin act to reduce inflammation by inhibiting the production of prostaglandins.

Cytokines, lymphokines and monokines
A large array of polypeptides is being identified and these act principally to regulate immune and haemopoetic cell proliferation and activity. In addition, they have effects in the inflammatory response. They are produced by many different cells in the body: those produced by lymphocytes are called **lymphokines** and those from macrophages are termed **monokines**. Two of the most important are **interleukin 1** (IL-1) and **tumour necrosis factor** (TNF). They have a variety of important effects as shown in Fig. 1.14.

List the important chemical mediators of inflammation

1. Arachidonic acid derivatives
2. Cytokines, lymphokines, monokines
3. Platelet Activating Factor
4. Vasoactive amines
5. Lysosomal contents
6. Growth factors
7. Kinin system
8. Clotting and fibronolytic system
9. Complement system

Fig 1.12   **Origin of important mediators of inflammation**

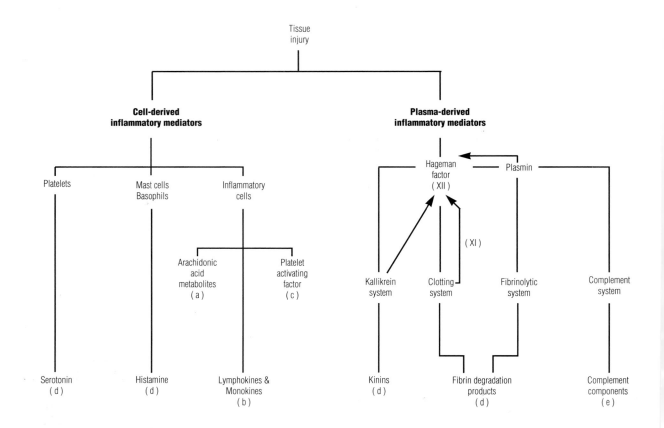

Letters in parentheses correspond
to reference tables and text

Fig 1.13   **Arachidonic acid derivatives (a)**

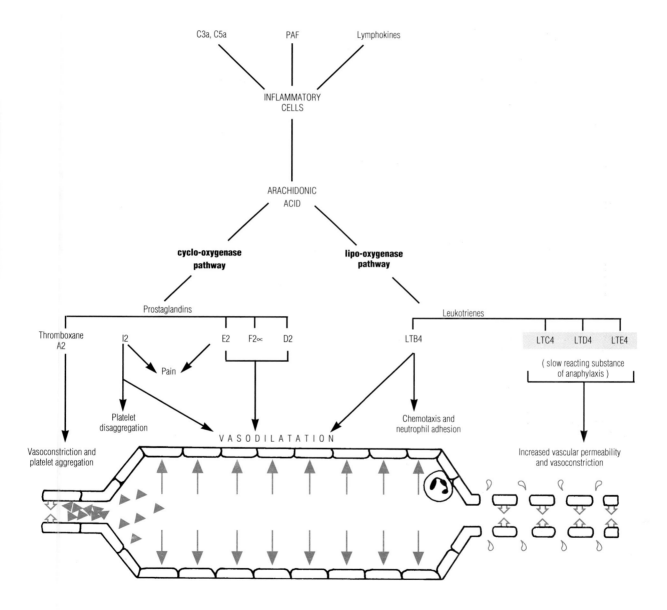

Fig 1.14

Cytokines in inflammation (b)

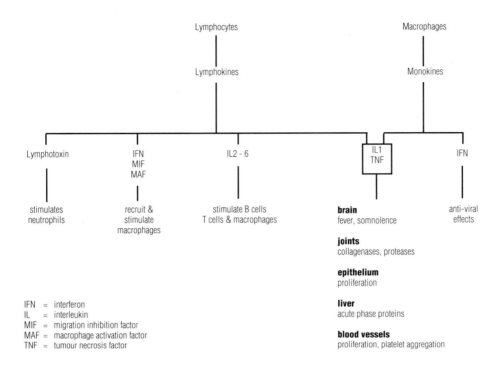

IFN = interferon
IL = interleukin
MIF = migration inhibition factor
MAF = macrophage activation factor
TNF = tumour necrosis factor

Fig 1.15

Platelet activating factor (c)

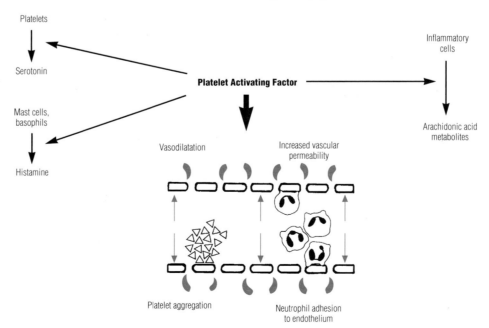

Fig 1.16

Actions of chemical mediators (d)

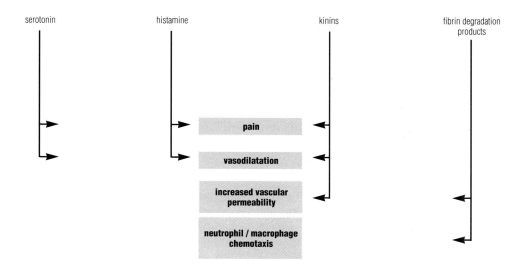

Fig 1.17

Complement system (e)

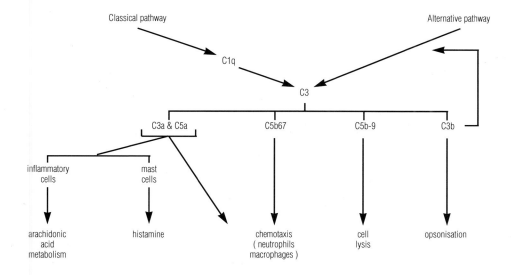

Platelet activating factor (PAF)

This is derived from antigen-stimulated IgE-sensitised basophils as well as neutrophils, macrophages and endothelial cells. In addition to activating platelets, it can cause vasodilatation, permeability changes, leucocyte adhesion, chemotaxis and stimulate the production of other mediators, in particular the arachidonic acid metabolites (Fig. 1.15).

Vasoactive amines

Histamine and serotonin (5-hydroxytryptamine) are stored in and released from mast cells, basophils and platelets. Their release causes vasodilatation and increases the permeability of venules. The action of histamine on vessels is mediated via H_1 receptors, while some of its other actions (e.g. bronchoconstriction) are effected via H2 receptors.

Many factors can lead to release of these substances, including IL-1 physical trauma, immunological reactions leading to formation of C3a and C5a and releasing factors produced by neutrophils, monocytes and platelets. The role of these amines is thought to be in the early phase of inflammation as it has been shown that antihistamines blocking H_1 receptors have no effect on the permeability that is present after 60 minutes.

Lysosomal contents

Lysosomal enzymes and accessory substances are present in neutrophils and monocytes, packaged in membrane-bound vesicles ('granules') to prevent them from damaging their own cell. There are two types of granules, the smaller *specific* and the larger *azurophilic*. These contain substances which increase vascular permeability and are chemotactic. The enzymes destroy many extracellular components including collagen, fibrin, elastin, cartilage and basement membrane, as well as producing intracellular killing in the phagolysosome as already described. If these processes were unopposed, there would be massive tissue destruction. So there are antiproteases within the serum and tissue fluids to neutralise these enzymes and thus regulate the extent of tissue damage. Does this seem a far-fetched idea, distant from clinical practice? Well not so!

A deficiency of one such antiprotease, α_1-**antitrypsin**, leads to unopposed action of elastase and hence destruction of elastic tissue, especially in the lungs and liver. Clinically, a patient with α_1-antitrypsin deficiency may suffer from emphysema of the lungs and liver cirrhosis.

Growth factors

Growth factors have a role in chemotaxis as well as inducing healing and repair of tissues and playing a part in the development of malignant tumours.

The principal growth factors are:

Lysosomal contents:

The specific granules contain:

Lactoferrin
Lysozyme
Alkaline phosphatase
Collagenase
Leucocyte adhesion molecule

The azurophilic granules contain:

Myeloperoxidase
Lysozyme
Cationic proteins
Acid hydrolases
Neutral proteases (elastase)

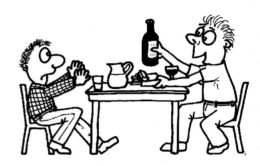

A patient with α-1-antitrypsin deficiency must avoid agents which damage the lungs or liver

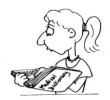

Emphysema
Abnormal permanent enlargement of the air spaces due to destruction of alveolar walls

Cirrhosis
Derived from the Greek meaning 'of yellow colour' because the patient (and internal organs) are jaundiced due to increased bilirubin. Cirrhosis is the end stage of chronic, diffuse liver damage leading to scarring and abnormal nodular architecture

- epidermal growth factor (EGF)
- platelet derived growth factor (PDGF)
- fibroblast growth factor (FGF)
- transforming growth factor (TGF)

Most of these can be produced by macrophages, which are numerous in areas of chronic inflammation. Not surprisingly, as with the antiproteases, there are inhibitors of growth factors and these include α-interferon and prostaglandin E_2.

Plasma-derived mediators

Kinin system
Bradykinin is the major active product of this system. It is a polypeptide which is one of the most powerful vasodilators known to man; it increases vascular permeability and also induces pain when injected into the skin. The kinin cascade is activated by Hageman factor and its relationship to the coagulation system is shown in Fig. 1.12. As with other cascades, this contains an amplification step because kallikrein itself acts to stimulate production of Hageman factor.

The Clotting and Fibrinolytic systems
This system is not only important in inflammation but is also central to blood clotting, which is discussed in Chapter 2 (Fig.2.5, page 65). It is the fibrinopeptides which act as chemical mediators in inflammation. These increase vascular permeability and are chemotactic for neutrophils. As in the kinin system, the cascade is activated by Hageman factor and includes an amplification loop so that plasmin stimulates Hageman factor. Plasmin is a multifunctional protease which also lyses fibrin clots to produce fibrin degradation products, which themselves induce permeability changes and also trigger the complement system by cleaving C3.

The Complement system
The system comprises a large number of proteins which are involved in increasing vascular permeability, chemotaxis, opsonisation and direct lysis of organisms.

The most important components concerned with the inflammatory reaction are:

- **C3a** and **C5a**: increasing vascular permeability and chemotaxis
- **C3b** and **C3bi**: opsonins
- **C5b–9**: membrane attack complex involved in cell lysis

Activation of this system occurs rapidly through the **classical pathway** initiated by antigen–antibody complexes, or more slowly through the **alternative pathway** (Fig. 1.17).

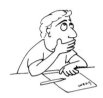

Discuss the effects of inflammatory mediators

1. Vasodilation
   prostaglandins

2. Vascular permeability
   vasoactive amines
   bradykinin
   leukotrienes

3. Chemotaxis
   C5a, C567
   leukotriene B4

4. Fever
   prostaglandins
   IL-1, TNF

5. Pain
   prostaglandins
   bradykinin

6. Tissue damage
   lysosomal enzymes

7. Amplification of reactions
   Hageman factor
   complement factors
   plasmin

To summarise the mechanisms operating in inflammation and their clinical relevance, we present a clinicopathological case study of lobar pneumonia.

Clinical

A 60 year old man presented to the casualty department complaining of a productive cough, fever, rigors and general malaise. The onset of symptoms was sudden and he had been perfectly well two days previously. He had no past medical history of note and he was not on any medication.

Systemic enquiry:
Respiratory system – he was coughing up rusty coloured sputum and also complained of chest pain on inspiration.

Allergies – nil known

Examination:
Temperature – 39.4°C (normal 37°C)
Pulse – 90/min regular (normal approx. 70/min)
Respiratory rate – 30/min (normal approx. 14/min)

Examination also revealed a dull percussion note in the right lower zone and auscultation confirmed decreased air entry and bronchial breathing. There was also a pleural rub over the affected area.

Investigations:
Full blood count – white cell count $18 \times 10^9/1$ (95% neutrophils)
(normal $4–11 \times 10^9/1$ with approx 65% neutrophils)

Chest X-ray — opaque right lower lobe

Sputum culture – *Streptococcus pneumoniae*

Diagnosis
Lobar pneumonia

Treatment
He was started on a course of penicillin. He did not have a history of allergy to this drug.

Pathology

The symptoms are due to local respiratory irritation from the inflammatory process and the fever is secondary to the production of pyrogens.

Inflammation causes vasodilatation, followed by margination and emigration of cells. Together with increased permeability, this leads to a purulent exudate within alveoli which is coughed up as sputum.
   The chest pain is due to friction between two inflamed pleural surfaces which are roughened and adherent due to the inflammatory exudate. This is also responsible for the pleural rub heard on auscultation.

Pyrogens cause a rise in body temperature by resetting the thermoregulatory centre in the hypothalamus. A rise in temperature will also increase the metabolic rate and therefore an increase in cardiac output. Decreased gas transfer plus the rise in temperature will lead to an increase in the respiratory rate.

The decreased air entry due to the inflammatory exudate within alveoli is responsible for the dull percussion note and the findings on auscultation.

Cytokines cause bone marrow stimulation and hence a leucocytosis.

Airless alveoli full of exudate appear white on X-ray.

This is the most common organism causing lobar pneumonia.

With effective treatment, there will be complete reversal of all the clinical and radiological signs as the exudate is cleared away from the alveoli.
   This ideal process may not occur and healing may take place by scarring. Lobar pneumonia differs from the more common bronchopneumonia in that the latter tends to be patchy and caused by a variety of organisms, e.g. Haemophilus influenzae.

The systemic effects of inflammation

Having considered lobar pneumonia, we have an idea of the *local* effects of inflammation. We have alluded to the fact that, at the same time, there are many *systemic* effects which may take place, such as fever, rigors, tachycardia, drop in blood pressure, loss of appetite, vomiting, skeletal weakness and aching. These are known collectively as **acute phase reactions**.

Fever is a regular accompaniment of inflammatory responses and occurs due to the 'resetting' of the thermoregulatory centre in the anterior hypothalamus. This probably produces a rise in temperature by constricting vessels in the skin, so reducing blood flow and limiting heat loss, and by promoting heat production in muscles by shivering. Biological substances that induce fever are called **pyrogens**. Many bacteria and viruses produce molecules that act as pyrogens and these are called **exogenous pyrogens**. **Endogenous pyrogens** are produced by the body and are listed opposite. It is thought that exogenous pyrogens stimulate leucocytes to release the endogenous pyrogen IL-1, which acts on the hypothalamus by raising local prostaglandin (PGE_2) levels. Aspirin is useful for lowering the temperature because it interferes with PGE_2 production.

Localised inflammatory responses lead to changes in plasma proteins due to alterations in liver metabolism. These proteins are called **acute phase proteins** and this change is thought to be mediated by IL-1, IL-6 and TNF. There is increased production of clotting factors and complement which is of importance because they are consumed during the inflammatory process. Transport proteins, such as haptoglobins, may be important in regulating the amount of amines and oxygen free radicals. Many other acute phase proteins, such as C-reactive protein and serum amyloid A, are produced but their role is not entirely clear. The acute phase reaction varies depending on the cause of inflammation. Viral infection is a poor inducer of acute phase proteins whereas bacterial infections produce a major response, probably by bacterial endotoxins acting indirectly through raised TNF-α levels. When investigating a patient, C-reactive protein is the most useful acute phase reactant to measure. If symptoms are equivocal, it may help to establish that there is organic disease rather than psychosomatic disease. In those patients with chronic diseases, a rise in the level may be an indicator of an acute exacerbation or of intercurrent infection.

The number of leucocytes in the peripheral blood increases in many forms of inflammation so that they are available to fight infection. It is assumed that cytokines act through colony stimulating factors to increase production and release of cells from the marrow. Again there are differences depending on the type of infection and this may be helpful in making a diagnosis. Bacterial infection provokes an increase in neutrophils, viral infections cause a rise in lymphocyte numbers and allergic reactions or

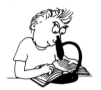

Endogenous pyrogens

Tumour necrosis factor
Interleukin-1
Noradrenaline
α-interferon
Prostaglandin E1
Prostaglandin E2

Acute phase protein response in disease

Major response in:
    Bacterial infection
    Rheumatoid arthritis
    Systemic vasculitis
    Trauma
    Malignancy
    Crohn's disease

Minor response in:
    Viral infection
    Connective tissue diseases e.g. systemic lupus
    erythematosus
    Ulcerative colitis

parasitic infections result in more eosinophils.

Trauma or stress of any kind also affects the hypo-thalamus–pituitary–adrenal axis resulting in the production of growth hormone, prolactin, ADH (antidiuretic hormone), ACTH (adrenocorticotrophic hormone) and adrenaline. These hormones are responsible for the breakdown of glycogen, changes in fatty acid metabolism and sodium–potassium transport. It is these metabolic changes that are responsible for the malaise, weakness, loss of appetite and other varied systemic effects observed during inflammation.

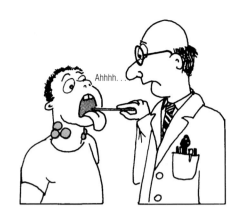

The lymphatic system in inflammation

Before we go on to discuss the other types of inflammatory response, we must consider the role of the lymphatic system in inflammation.

The lymphatic system comprises all of the collections of lymphoid tissue which are present throughout the body. Lymphocytes are produced and mature in the bone marrow and thymus. They migrate in the blood to populate and proliferate in the lymph nodes, the spleen and the lining of the gut and respiratory tract, the so-called mucosa-associated lymphoid tissue (MALT). The lymphatic system has a one-way circulation linked to, but separate from, the blood circulatory system. Generally, more fluid moves out of tissue capillaries than is returned, as we discussed when considering fluid flow across vessel walls in inflammation. This excess fluid is termed lymph and it drains into the lymphatic channels which are present in all tissues. In addition to the fluid, lymph also contains a variety of inflammatory cells, particularly lymphocytes and macrophages; the actual number of cells is very variable and increases if the tissue is inflamed. The lymphatic fluid filters through a chain of lymph nodes and, ultimately, most enters the blood via the thoracic duct at its junction with the left subclavian and internal jugular veins. Once immune cells are back in the blood, the cycle is repeated. This recirculation of lymphoid cells is important as it allows information about invading organisms to be shared with other areas of lymphoid cell production. A lymphocyte which has come from a specific area, such as the gut, recognises particular surface molecules on the endothelial cells of that area (**addressins**) that allow it to 'home' back to the same tissue.

Let us consider how this works in practice. Imagine that you have a severe sore throat making it painful to swallow. Fairly soon you will notice the lymph nodes enlarging, and even becoming painful, on either side of the sternomastoid muscle. If one of the nodes were to be excised for microscopical examination, it would show a number of changes.

First the sinusoids would appear more prominent (called **sinus histiocytosis**) because their lining cells, the macrophages, have an important job. The macrophages trap the organisms causing the sore throat (e.g. streptococci) to

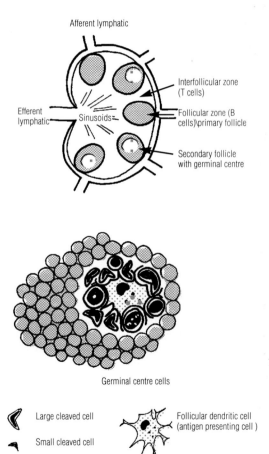

Fig 1.18 Lymph node

prevent dissemination into the blood. The macrophages have another vital role: that of initiating a specific immune response to the offending agent. This requires co-operation between B lymphocytes, T lymphocytes, macrophages and other antigen-presenting cells in the node.

. B lymphocytes are concentrated in the follicles of the node and can develop into plasma cells which produce antibodies against the invading organisms. This is particularly important in bacterial infections and the enlargement of the B cell areas is called **follicular hyperplasia**. If the sore throat is caused by a virus, which is more common, then the T cells are most important. These reside outside the follicles in the inter follicular zone which will enlarge.

The local lymph nodes trap the antigens in special cells which phagocytose antigens, process them and then display them on their cell surfaces. These are called **antigen-presenting cells** and they include **follicular dendritic cells** in the follicles, **dendritic reticulum cells** in the interfollicular zones and **macrophages** in a variety of areas. This method of antigen presentation activates specific lymphocytes and promotes the immune response.

Hopefully, this will contain the infection but, if it fails, the infection may reach the blood. Infection of the blood (or septicaemia) may also occur by tissue organisms directly entering blood vessels. The septicaemic patient is gravely ill with fevers, shivering attacks (rigors) and dangerous lowering of the blood pressure ('shock'). Now it is the turn of the spleen to trap organisms and promote immune cell proliferation. Its structure and functions are analogous to the lymph node with macrophages lining sinusoids and specific B and T cell areas; however, the fluid percolating through is blood rather than lymph.

Our knowledge of immunology has expanded enormously over the last 25 years so that a detailed account is outside the scope of this book. However, its principles and beginnings are too fascinating to omit.

Immunisation

It would be a crime to consider immunisation without pausing for a moment to think about its history and the man responsible for developing its use. The man is Edward Jenner (1749–1823), a pupil of John Hunter. Jenner lived with Hunter for the first two years after coming to London and the friendship they developed continued after Jenner left London to start General Practice in Berkeley, Gloucestershire. Jenner was profoundly influenced by Hunter's interest in natural history and in his methods of scientific investigation. To one of Jenner's questions, Hunter is said to have replied,

"... I think your solution is just; but why think? why not try the experiment?..."

Even before Jenner, it had been noticed that an attack of smallpox protected against further disease. It was known that the epidemics varied in severity and that it was best to contract a mild form of smallpox as this resulted in life-long

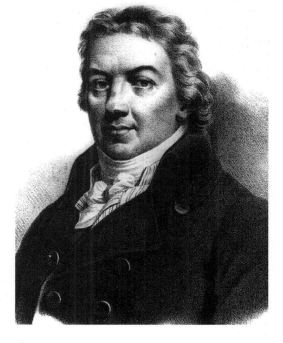

Fig 1.19 Edward Jenner (1749–1823). (Courtesy of the Wellcome Institute for the History of Medicine).

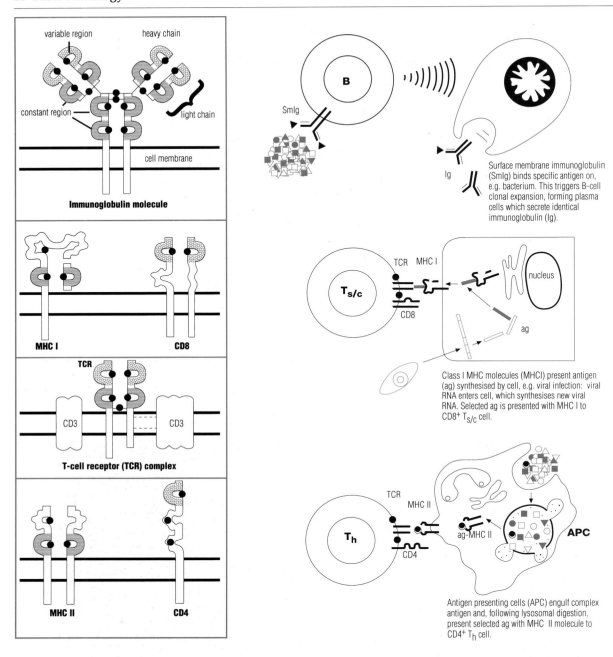

Surface membrane immunoglobulin (SmIg) binds specific antigen on, e.g. bacterium. This triggers B-cell clonal expansion, forming plasma cells which secrete identical immunoglobulin (Ig).

Class I MHC molecules (MHCI) present antigen (ag) synthesised by cell, e.g. viral infection: viral RNA enters cell, which synthesises new viral RNA. Selected ag is presented with MHC I to CD8$^+$ T$_{s/c}$ cell.

Antigen presenting cells (APC) engulf complex antigen and, following lysosomal digestion, present selected ag with MHC II molecule to CD4$^+$ T$_h$ cell.

Homologous regions shared by members of the immunoglobulin (Ig) gene superfamily include constant and variable regions, and other areas show structural divergence.

Key: • = disulphide bonds   T$_h$ = T helper cell   T$_{s/c}$ = T suppressor cytotoxic cells

Fig 1.20 The immunoglobulin gene superfamily

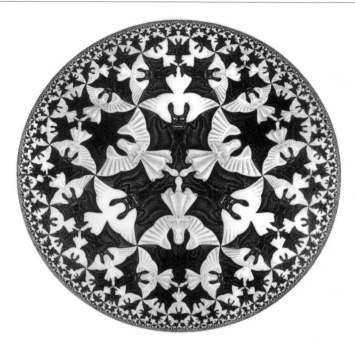

Escher's pictures, **Circle Limit IV** and **Encounter**, illustrate some concepts in molecular recogntion. For maximum effect, the pairs of molecules should have complementary shapes so that there is a close three dimensional fit. The two molecules may have no other similarities, as occurs in most antigen-antibody pairs; this is analogous to Escher's angels and devils. Alternatively, the pair of molecules may have structural homology and common genetic ancestry as do the immunoglobulin gene superfamily molecules. This may be likened to Escher's human figures in Encounter.

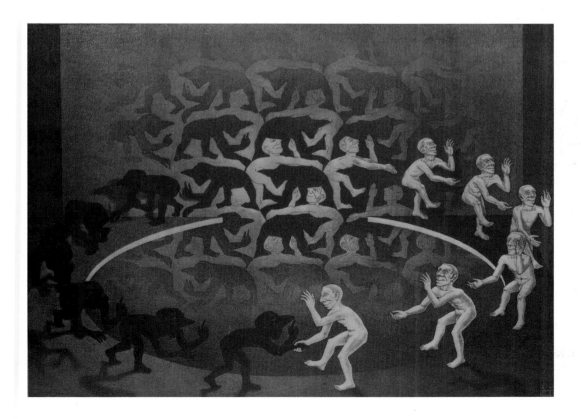

protection. This knowledge was widespread: in India, children were wrapped in clothing from patients with smallpox; in China, scabs from smallpox patients were ground and the powder was blown into the nostrils; in Turkey, female slaves were injected under the skin with dried preparations of pus from smallpox patients. Inoculated slaves fetched a high price while pock-marked slaves were worth nothing! Lady Mary Wortley Montagu, the wife of the British Ambassador in Constantinople, was aware of these techniques and she took the risk of having her own children inoculated. When she returned to England in 1718, she tried to convince her friend, the Prince of Wales, that he should do the same. He was worried about experimenting on the royal children but, when six orphan children were successfully immunised against smallpox, he consented and the royal children were inoculated. Medical ethics have made some advances since those days!

Jenner had noticed that cows suffered from a pustular disease resembling smallpox which he called 'variolae vaccinae' – cowpox. It was known that it could be transmitted to humans and that, apart from local symptoms, there were no ill effects. There was a widespread belief that those who had suffered from cowpox became immune to smallpox. The idea of using the cowpox virus to induce immunity to smallpox thrilled Jenner but, rather than jumping to conclusions, he followed Hunter's example and experimented. On 14th May 1796, Jenner inoculated a boy of eight named James Phipps with cowpox. The boy's illness took a predictable course and he recovered. On 1st July, he inoculated the boy with smallpox and no reaction occurred, either on this occasion or on a subsequent occasion a few months later. Jenner described this experiment to the Royal Society but it was rejected. He continued to make his observations and, in 1798, published his work entitled *An Inquiry into the Causes and Effects of the Variolae Vaccinae*. It was later realised that the immunity was not life-long but that it could be renewed by repeated inoculation. Hence inoculation with smallpox was replaced by inoculation with cowpox. The word '**vaccination**' came into use and smallpox is no longer a major killer.

We now know that, at the first encounter with an antigen, there is a proliferation of immunologically identical B cells, called a **clone**, together with memory cells. The clone will produce the antibody appropriate to the antigen. Initially, the antibody is of type IgM and later the clone switches to produce IgG. If the antigen is encountered again, the memory cells will stimulate clonal proliferation of the appropriate antibody-producing cells. This process is called **acquired immunity** and it may occur either as a result of encountering the antigen naturally or after artificial exposure as part of immunisation.

How does a B cell produce the correct antibody for a new antigen?

A B cell has no choice in the matter! Each B cell has the genetic code for a single antibody and it displays this

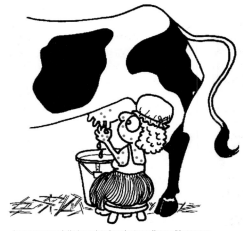

Jenner successfully inoculated against smallpox with cowpox

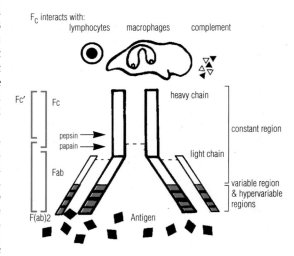

The constant parts of the heavy & light chains interact with other cells and mediators. The variable regions form 3-dimensional antigen recognition sites.

Digestion with pepsin cleaves the Ig molecule into Fc' & F(ab)2 fragments, whilst papain digestion produces Fc & Fab, due to the positions of the disulphide bonds (- - -).

Fig 1.21 Immunoglobulin molecule

antibody on its own cell surface. This means that only B cells with the correct antibody will bind to the new antigen and be stimulated to proliferate. It is really the antigen which chooses the B cell best equipped to fight it! Of course, this requires an enormous number of B cells with different genetic codes so that the body has a B cell equipped to fight any new foreign antigen. (There are at least 10^8 different immunoglobulin molecules in the serum.) Nature discovered a brilliant way of producing this variety of codes, which we shall describe in Chapter 5, and then used a similar approach for T cells. T cells do not produce antibody or have antibody on their surface but they recognise antigen through a T cell receptor combined with other surface molecules.

What does immunoglobulin do?

Most importantly, immunoglobulin recognises antigen through the **variable regions** on the molecule. After that, the **constant regions** initiate the biological functions, such as complement fixation and opsonisation, appropriate for the immunoglobulin class. Each immunoglobulin molecule is formed from two identical **heavy chains** and two identical **light chains** joined by interchain disulphide links. There are two types of light chain (**kappa** and **lambda**) and five types of heavy chain (**G, A, M, D, E**). The light chains can combine with any type of heavy chain and do not influence biological function whereas each heavy chain type supports different biological functions (table 1.2).

How is antigen recognised?

Although diagrams generally depict antibody molecules as simple 'bent dinner forks', they have a complex three-dimensional structure with many 'folds'. We have already mentioned that antigen binds to the variable region; however, this region has some areas which show enormous diversity and are called **hypervariable regions** whereas other areas are more constant and act as 'hinge' points. This means that the variable region folds to bring its hypervariable areas together to form a potential 'pocket' for antigen attachment. This has a shape dependent on the outer electron clouds of its atoms which determines the antigen *shape* that it recognises. The important point is that this interaction depends on the antigen and antibody having complementary profiles; no covalent bonding is involved, so the chemical composition is not crucial. The shapes don't have to be a perfect fit but a close fit gives the strongest binding.

T cell recognition of antigen is more complicated and only just beginning to be understood. T cells differ in their biological roles with some acting as **helper** cells, some as **cytotoxic** cells and some as **suppressor** cells. T cells can be further subdivided. The CD8$^+$ cells are a mixture of suppressor and cytotoxic cells. The CD4$^+$ cells can be split into suppressor/inducer and helper/inducers with the helper/inducers further divided into T$_H$1 and T$_H$2 cells (table 1.3). They have a variety of surface molecules, some of

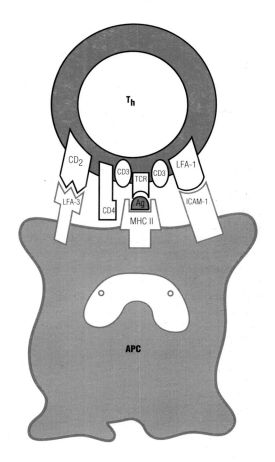

Fig 1.22 Surface receptor interactions between helper T cells (T$_h$) and antigen presenting cells (APC)

Table 1.2 Immunoglobulin types

	Complement fixation by		Macrophage/ polymorph binding	Mast cell/ basophil binding	Cross placenta	Function
	Classical pathway	Alternative pathway				
IgG	++	−	++	−	++	Combats microorganisms and toxins. Most abundant Ig in blood and extravascular fluid
IgA	−	+ −	+ −	−	−	Most important Ig for protecting mucosal surfaces. Combines with secretory component to avoid being digested
IgM	+	−	−	−	−	Important in early response to infection as it is a powerful agglutinator
IgD	−	−	−	−	−	?function. Present on the surface of some lymphocytes and may control lymphocyte activation/suppression
IgE	−	−	+ −	+ −	−	Involved in mast cell degranulation, thereby protecting body surfaces. Important in allergy and parasitic infections

Table 1.3 T lymphocyte subsets

	CD4$^+$			CD8$^+$	
	Suppressor/ Inducer	Helper/Inducer		Suppressor cells	Cytotoxic cells
		T$_H$1	T$_H$2		
Genetic restriction (MHC)	II	II	II	I	I
Suppressor activity	++ (provide help)	−	−	++	−
Cytotoxic activity	−	+	−	−	++
Help for Ig production	−	+	+++	−	−

T cells are important in protecting against infections, in graft rejection, in graft versus host disease, some hypersensitivity reactions and tumour immunity. Cytotoxic CD8$^+$ cells are crucial for Type IV hypersensitivity reactions while T$_H$2 cells are involved in Type I hypersensitivity.

which are common to many T cell types (e.g. CD3) while others are limited to the various subtypes (e.g. CD4, CD8). These molecules are involved in antigen recognition by combining with the T cell receptor. The **T cell receptor** (TCR) of the majority of T cells is composed of an alpha chain and a beta chain with constant and variable regions analogous to those of immunoglobulins. In fact, the similarities between the TCR and immunoglobulin structure go even deeper as the genetic mechanisms for producing the necessary enormous diversity are almost identical. Nature has found this approach so useful that a common structure, the **immunoglobulin homology unit**, is the basic building block for a range of molecules involved in cell–cell recognition, the so-called **immunoglobulin gene superfamily** (Fig. 1.20). An important feature of the Ig domain structure is that certain areas are complementary shapes (i.e. they will fit together), which is why major histocompatibility structures (MHC), also part of the immunoglobulin gene superfamily, are important in helping T cells recognise foreign antigens.

Each person has an (almost) unique set of MHC molecules which are present on most cells and are inherited. This is relevant to transplantation where it is best to have a good 'match' between the donor and the recipient to minimise the risk of rejection. An identical twin will provide an excellent match and some siblings are a good match, but most people's organs carry MHC antigens which will be identified by the recipient's immune system as foreign and the tissue will be rejected. T cell recognition intimately involves MHC molecules because T cells do not react with free, native antigens (that is the job for the immunoglobulin molecules) but bind to antigens which have been processed by special antigen presenting cells or macrophages and are then displayed on the cell surface alongside MHC molecules. Helper cells with CD4 included in the receptor complex recognise processed antigen combined with class II MHC molecules, whereas cytotoxic T cells with CD8 molecules bind to processed antigen on class I molecules. Once the antigen and MHC molecule are bound to the TCR and subset molecule, the cell is activated by a signal which passes via the CD3 molecule to the cell's interior. Class I molecules are expressed on virtually all nucleated cells while class II molecules are restricted to antigen presenting cells, macrophages and B cells but can be expressed on many other cell types, if they are stimulated with γ-interferon.

Tolerance and autoimmune disease

This ability of the body to mount an immune response against foreign antigens raises a very important question. How does the immune system distinguish between an antigen that is foreign and one that is normally present on the cells in the body? This is achieved by selection in the thymus during fetal life. Stem cells in the bone marrow produce prothymocytes which are attracted to the thymus by the chemotactic agent, thymotaxin. Here they mature

Table 1.4 B lymphocyte subsets

Surface marker	B1 cells	Conventional (B2) cells
IgM	++	–
IgD	–	++
CD11b } peritoneal cells	++	–
CD23	–	++

B1 cells are a small subset of B lymphocytes, originally recognised by their CD5 positivity. They are common in the pleural and peritoneal cavities but absent from adult bone marrow and lymph nodes. They often produce autoreactive antibody and are probably important in autoimmune diseases. Many cases of chronic lymphatic leukaemia are derived from B1 cells.

along various pathways (Fig. 1.24) producing cells which recognise 'self' antigens as well as foreign antigen but the self-reacting T cells are eliminated or inactivated.

This mechanism induces **tolerance** so that antigens that are exposed to the immune system during fetal life are not capable of eliciting a response in later life. Hence, nature has divised a neat system of differentiating self from non-self. Or has it?

Parts of the body that are not exposed to the immune system during fetal life can produce a response later on – lens protein and spermatozoa are just two examples. Even antigens exposed during foetal life may provoke immune activation much later in life leading to a group of disorders called **autoimmune diseases**. It is assumed that in auto-immune diseases either the self antigen is modified or a new exogenous antigen closely resembles the self antigen or some changes in the immune system bypass the need for helper cells.

Autoimmune diseases include many clinically important and potentially life-threatening conditions such as Hashimoto's thyroiditis (antibodies to thyroglobulin and thyroid epithelium), myasthenia gravis (antibodies to acetylcholine receptors of the neuromuscular junction), pernicious anaemia (antibodies to intrinsic factor and gastric parietal cells) and systemic lupus erythematosus (SLE) (numerous antibodies, especially antinuclear antibodies). As you can see, the first three are **organ specific** while SLE is **non-organ specific**. We will briefly describe SLE to illustrate the wide ranging effects of producing antibodies against self.

Systemic lupus erythematosus is a systemic disorder in which there is chronic, relapsing and remitting damage to the skin, joints, kidneys and almost any organ. Like most immune disorders, it has a higher incidence in women. In America it is also more common in Blacks and it tends to occur in the second and third decades. Patients may present with a characteristic 'butterfly' rash on the face, or with more subtle symptoms. Many present after their kidneys have been damaged beyond repair, i.e. chronic renal failure. The fundamental feature of the disease is inflammation of the small arterioles and arteries (i.e. a vasculitis), often related to the deposition of antigen–antibody complexes in the vessel walls. Involvement of the glomerular capillaries in the kidney produces a variety of types of glomerulo-nephritis. The other sites of involvement are joints (synovitis), heart (non-infectious endocarditis – named after Libman and Sacks – and pericarditis), lungs (pleuritis and effusions) and central nervous system (focal neurological symptoms due to vasculitis). The course of the illness is extremely variable and unpredictable and may range from mild skin involvement to severe renal disease leading to death.

Autoimmune disorders represent a failure of the control mechanisms of the immune system. The response is well controlled but the initiating event of antigen recognition is wrong. Hypersensitivity reactions are also a failure of

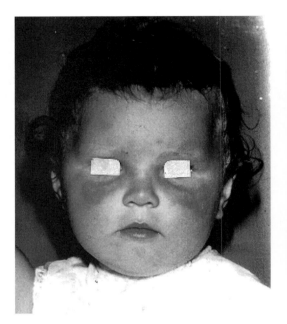

Fig 1.23 A child with the butterfly skin rash of SLE.

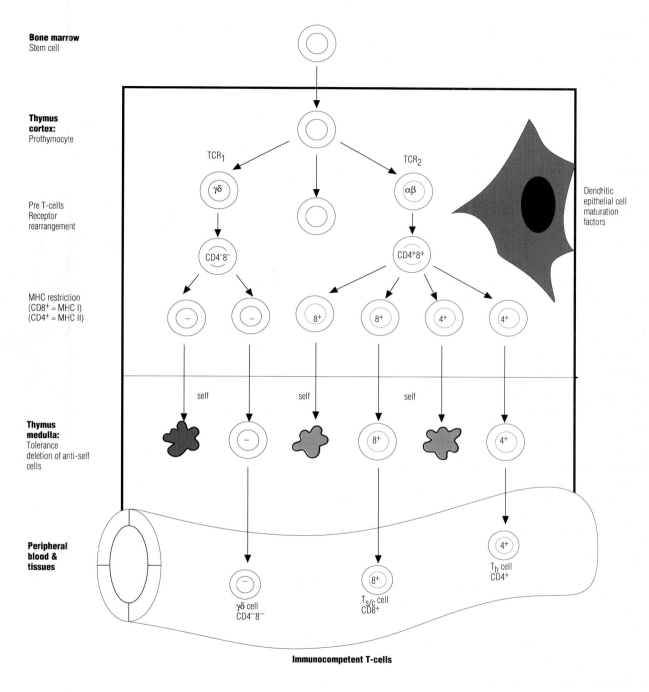

Bone marrow
Stem cell

Thymus cortex:
Prothymocyte

TCR$_1$ TCR$_2$

Pre T-cells
Receptor
rearrangement

γδ   αβ

Dendritic
epithelial cell
maturation
factors

CD4$^-$8$^-$ CD4$^+$8$^+$

MHC restriction
(CD8$^+$ = MHC I)
(CD4$^+$ = MHC II)

$-$ $-$ 8$^+$ 8$^+$ 4$^+$ 4$^+$

self   self   self

Thymus medulla:
Tolerance
deletion of anti-self
cells

$-$ 8$^+$ 4$^+$

Peripheral blood & tissues

4$^+$
T$_h$ cell
CD4$^+$

$-$
γδ cell
CD4$^-$8$^-$

8$^+$
T$_{s/c}$ cell
CD8$^+$

Immunocompetent T-cells

Prothymocytes proliferate in the thymic cortex and undergo rearrangement of the genes for the T cell receptor molecule. The pre-T cells express either the gamma (γ) and delta (δ) chains (TCR$_1$) or the alpha (α) and beta (β) chains (TCR$_2$). At the next stage of maturation, the TCR$_2$ cells exhibit surface CD4 and CD8 molecules while the TCR$_1$ cells are CD4 and CD8 negative. CD4$^+$ cells give rise to helper/inducer cells which function best in collaboration with Class II MHC molecules. This is termed MHC restriction. CD8$^+$ cells interact best with Class I MHC molecules and have suppressor/cytotoxic actions. Thymocytes that could attack "self" antigens are removed in the thymic medulla. γδT cells are a small subset of T cells with a large granular appearance. In humans, they are evenly distributed through the immune system and have cytotoxic activity.

Fig 1.24 T cell maturation

control but in this the antigen recognition proceeds normally but the response is exaggerated.

Hypersensitivity

Even today, there is public suspicion about some immunisation programmes because a tiny minority of children who are immunised suffer from adverse effects. The occurrence of these occasional idiosyncratic reactions should not deter one from protecting the vast majority of the population from serious disease. However, we should not believe that the immune system is all good; the immune mechanisms that exist to defend the host may also do harm. This phenomenon of damage caused by the immune system while trying to combat an injury is referred to as *hypersensitivity*. There are five main types of hypersensitivity reaction: types I–V.

Type I: Anaphylactic hypersensitivity

This operates in atopic allergies such as asthma, eczema, hay fever and reactions to certain food. An extrinsic allergen (e.g. grass pollen, house dust mite faeces, seafood) binds to IgE on the surface of mast cells in the mucosa of the bronchial tree, nose, gut or conjunctivae leading to release of chemical mediators. Generally, these act locally but they can also produce life-threatening systemic effects. Effects include constriction of smooth muscle in bronchi and bronchioles producing wheezing and dilatation, and increased permeability of capillaries resulting in increased nasal and bronchial secretions, red watery eyes, skin rashes and diarrhoea.

Type II: Antibody-dependent cytotoxic hypersensitivity

It is essential that any blood which is transfused into a patient is first cross-matched to ensure that the recipient does not possess antibodies to antigens on the donor red blood cells. This is because the donor red cells will become coated with antibody which may promote phagocytosis due to opsonisation through the Fc, or fix complement to produce cell membrane damage through C8 and C9 or phagocytosis through C3. Type II reactions are also involved in rhesus incompatibility (where rhesus antibodies from a Rh$^-$ mother cross the placenta to damage the RBCs of a Rh$^+$ baby), some autoimmune diseases (e.g. Hashimoto's thyroiditis and autoimmune haemolytic anaemia) and some drug reactions (e.g. chlorpromazine-induced haemolytic anaemia and quinidine-induced agranulocytosis). Natural killer cells, which are not restricted by HLA type, can kill through antibody-dependent cell-mediated cytotoxicity (ADCC) which may be important for killing large parasites or tumour cells.

Type III: Immune complex mediated hypersensitivity

Immune complexes can be soluble so that they circulate in the blood giving rise to **serum sickness** or they can be insoluble and precipitated where antigen first encounters antibody – the **Arthus reaction**. Soluble complexes tend to

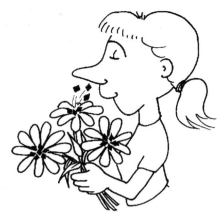

First exposure: nasal and bronchial mucosa exposed to pollen

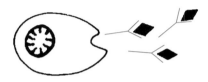

Soluble pollen antigen stimulates production of IgE antibodies

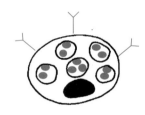

Fc component of IgE attaches to receptor on mucosal mast cell

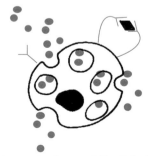

Second exposure to pollen: cross-linking of IgE molecules on mast cell stimulates release of primary and secondary inflammatory mediators

Fig 1.25 Type I hypersensitivity

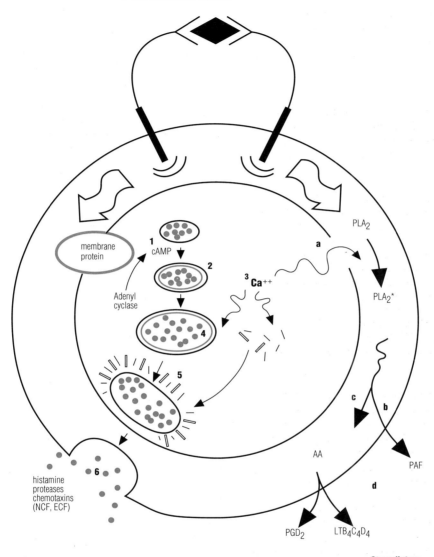

Cross-linkage of antigen starts energy-dependent release of primary and secondary mediators

1° mediators

1. ↑cAMP produced
2. Phosphorylation of perigranular protein
3. Ca^{++}-dependent enzymes initiate microtubule & microfilament assembly
4. Ca^{++} & water enter granule, which swells
5. Granule moved toward membrane by microtubules and filaments
6. Discharge of pre-formed mediators invokes inflammatory response in 5–30 mins, lasting approximately 1 hour

2° mediators

a. Ca^{++}-mediated activation of membrane phospholipase A_2 (PLA_2)
b. Platelet activating factor (PAF) formed
c. Arachidonic acid (AA) formed
d. AA metabolites and PAF produce sustained response starting 8–12 hours after stimulus, lasting 2–3 days

Fig 1.26 Mast cell activation

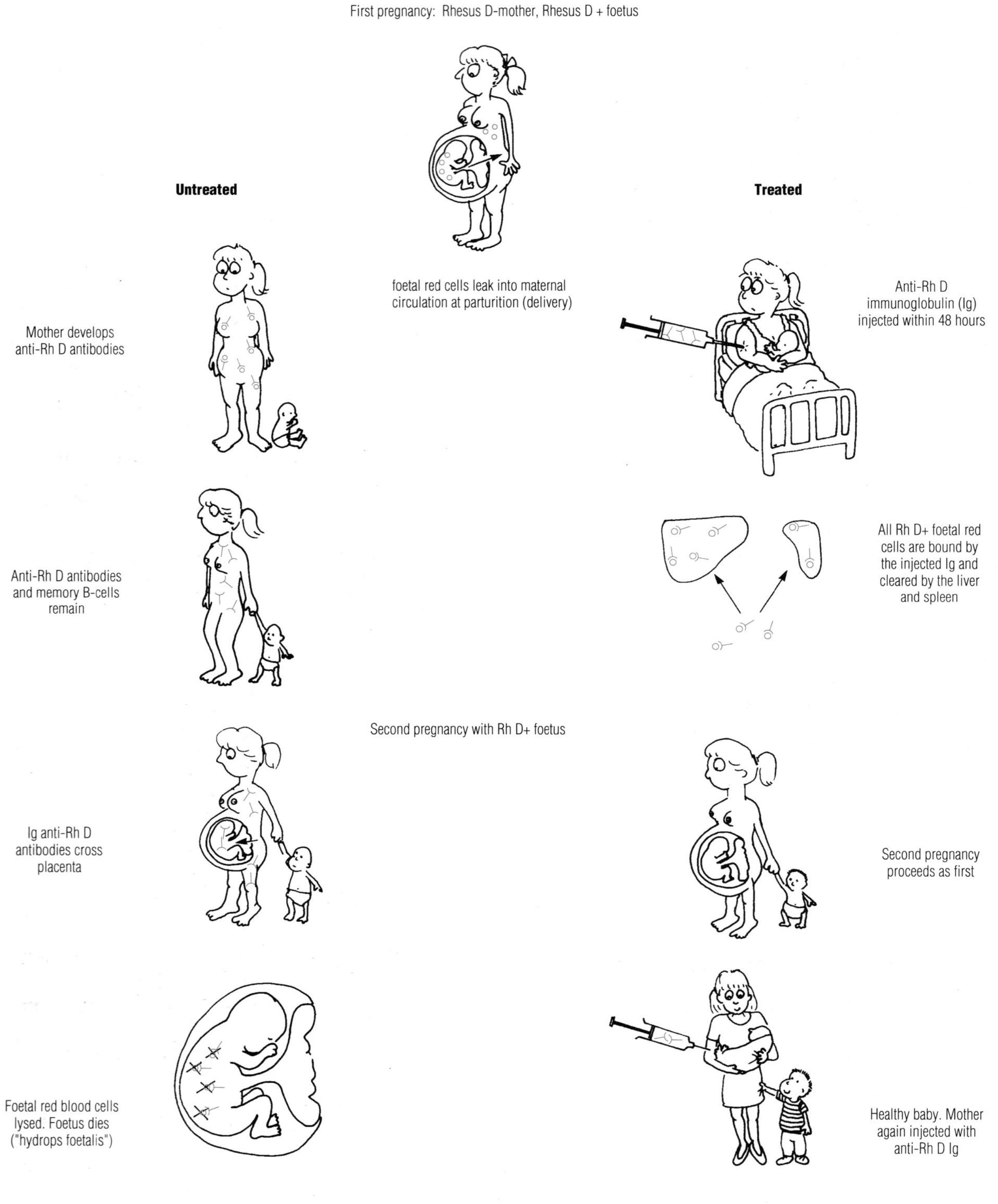

First pregnancy: Rhesus D-mother, Rhesus D + foetus

foetal red cells leak into maternal
circulation at parturition (delivery)

Untreated

Treated

Mother develops
anti-Rh D antibodies

Anti-Rh D
immunoglobulin (Ig)
injected within 48 hours

Anti-Rh D antibodies
and memory B-cells
remain

All Rh D+ foetal red
cells are bound by
the injected Ig and
cleared by the liver
and spleen

Second pregnancy with Rh D+ foetus

Ig anti-Rh D
antibodies cross
placenta

Second pregnancy
proceeds as first

Foetal red blood cells
lysed. Foetus dies
("hydrops foetalis")

Healthy baby. Mother
again injected with
anti-Rh D Ig

Fig 1.27 Type II hypersensitivity e.g. Rhesus incompatibility

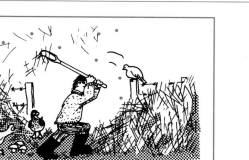

First exposure: inhalation of protein,
e.g. spores in mouldy hay

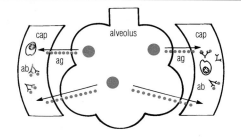

Sensitisation: soluble antigen (ag) diffuses into alveolar capillaries (cap),
provoking IgG antibody (ab) formation

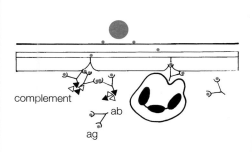

Second exposure: soluble ag swamped by circulating ab, forming ag–ab
complexes in capillary wall. FcIgG activates complement and neutrophils

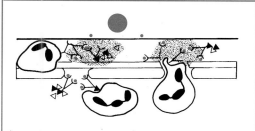

Release of inflammatory mediators causes tissue damage.
Increased vascular permeability allows IgG to seep into alveolar wall;
ag–ab complexes cause local tissue damage,
culminating in fibrosis and restrictive airways disease.

Fig 1.28 Type III hypersensitivity e.g. extrinsic allergic alveolitis

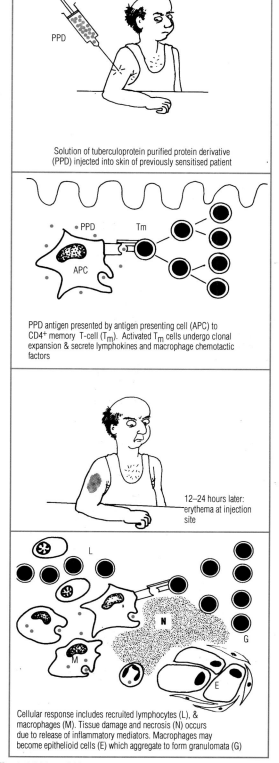

Solution of tuberculoprotein purified protein derivative
(PPD) injected into skin of previously sensitised patient

PPD antigen presented by antigen presenting cell (APC) to
CD4$^+$ memory T-cell (T$_m$). Activated T$_m$ cells undergo clonal
expansion & secrete lymphokines and macrophage chemotactic
factors

12–24 hours later:
erythema at injection
site

Cellular response includes recruited lymphocytes (L), &
macrophages (M). Tissue damage and necrosis (N) occurs
due to release of inflammatory mediators. Macrophages may
become epithelioid cells (E) which aggregate to form granulomata (G)

Fig 1.29 Type IV hypersensitivity e.g. Mantoux test reaction

form when there is *antigen* excess while insoluble complexes result from *antibody* excess. Both types of complex can activate macrophages, aggregate platelets and initiate the complement cascade. Circulating immune complexes can lodge in vessels of many organs to give a **vasculitis**, principally affecting the kidney (glomerulonephritis), skin and joints. The Arthus reaction is commonest in the lung when an exogenous antigen is inhaled and precipitated locally. The antigens are generally animal or plant proteins which cause **extrinsic allergic alveolitis** and are often associated with specific occupations (Table 1.5).

Type IV: Cell-mediated (delayed type) hypersensitivity

Unlike the other forms of hypersensitivity, which involve antibody, type IV requires T lymphocytes. Over several hours, these recruit and activate other T cells and macrophages to produce tissue damage and granulomata. It can occur as an allergic response to many viruses, fungi, bacteria and insect bites and is often responsible for contact dermatitis related to simple chemicals.

It is a common mistake to confuse hypersensitivity and immunity. Consider the **Mantoux test** used to confirm immunity against tuberculosis. The test relies on the type IV hypersensitivity reaction. When tuberculin protein is injected into the skin of a sensitised patient, it sets up a response which leads to the accumulation of macrophages and inflammatory exudate at that site. Depending on the degree of the hypersensitivity response, there may be little tissue damage or massive necrosis and even ulceration of the skin. This reaction, which is based on the presence of the hypersensitivity phenomenon, is used to reflect immunity to tuberculosis. Hypersensitivity and immunity are a little like Romeo and Juliet – they are not the same thing yet we cannot talk about one without the other.

Type V: Stimulatory hypersensitivity

In this type of hypersensitivity, antibodies stimulate non-immune cells to perform their normal function in an uncontrolled way. For example, thyroid cells normally produce thyroxine when stimulated by thyroid stimulating hormone (TSH) from the pituitary. However, in patients with Grave's disease, there is an antibody which binds to thyroid cells and mimics the action of TSH leading to excess thyroxine production (thyrotoxicosis).

This type of hypersensitivity was grouped with type II reactions in the original Gell and Coombs classification but more modern authors usually separate it because there is no cytotoxic effect.

The immune system versus the microbes

On page 13, we discussed phagocytosis and other mechanisms of bacterial killing. However, these mechanisms may fail and infection may persist to produce chronic or granulomatous inflammation. In the war between the immune system and microbes, what strategies are adopted to outwit the opponent?

Table 1.5 Some causes of Extrinsic Allergic Alveolitis (EAA)

Agent	Disease
Aspergillus fumigatus Thermophilic actinomycetes	Farmer's lung
Aspergillus versicolor	Dog house disease
Avian protein (?pigeon faecal protein)	Bird fancier's disease Pigeon fancier's lung
Cryptostroma corticale	Maple bark stripper's lung
Fox fur proteins	Furrier's lung
Penicillium casei	Cheese washer's lung
Wood dust	Wood worker's lung

Bacteria frequently develop capsules which make them harder to phagocytose. Some capsules are also less likely to activate complement and are resistant to the insertion of the C5b–9 membrane attack complex, which would cause bacterial cell lysis. Other surface molecules can act as a 'decoy' to inhibit complement or bind factors that promote degradation of complement. Bacterial endotoxins may also poison leucocytes. The microorganisms can avoid provoking an immune reaction by colonising the *external* mucosal surfaces (e.g. the gut lumen) or by hiding inside the host's cells (e.g. mycobacteria). Some parasites (e.g. ascaris) disguise themselves with surface proteins that resemble the host's or even bind the host's own proteins to their surface (e.g. schistosomiasis). Many microorganisms change their surface antigens (**antigenic drift** and **antigenic shift**) each time the host develops antibodies so that the acquired immunity is ineffective. Several viruses, trypanosomes and the malarial plasmodia do this, which makes it extremely difficult to produce successful vaccines. In addition, mycobacteria can block macrophage activation, scavenge oxygen free radicals, inhibit lysosome fusion and escape from phagosomes into the cytoplasm.

The immune system fights back by producing antibodies to neutralise any toxins, to opsonise capsule-bearing bugs and to spread complement evenly over the cell surface. Mucosal surfaces are protected by IgA, secreted by local plasma cells and transported via epithelial cells, which inhibits microbial adherence. IgE also acts at mucosal surfaces to initiate the release of mast cell factors which attract protective IgG, complement and polymorphs. The killing of intracellular bacteria, viruses and parasites is initiated by specific cell-mediated immunity (T cells) and often involves activated macrophages. Any free microbes are attacked by antibody.

Fortunately, the immune system usually wins, but sometimes chronic and granulomatous reactions are required.

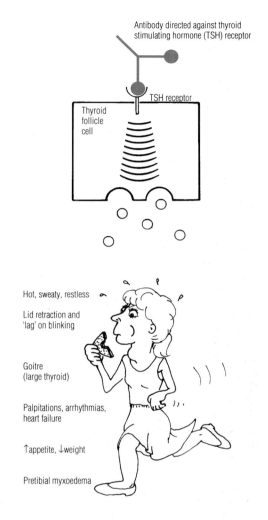

Some effects of excess circulating thyroid hormones

Fig 1.30 Type V hypersensitivity e.g. Graves disease

Chronic and granulomatous inflammation

Chronic inflammation differs from acute inflammation in a number of respects. Apart from the generally longer duration of the process, the main features of chronic inflammation are:

- mononuclear cell infiltrate composed of macrophages, lymphocytes and plasma cells
- tissue destruction
- granulation tissue formation, i.e. proliferation of fibroblasts and small blood vessels (this is not the same as a granuloma)
- fibrosis

Granulomatous inflammation is a special type of chronic inflammation, characterised by the presence of granulomata. A granuloma is a collection of macrophages frequently surrounded by a rim of lymphocytes. These macrophages are usually modified to become larger with more abundant pink cytoplasm and are referred to as 'epithelioid' cells.

Chronic inflammatory disorders are some of the most common, fascinating, devastating and mysterious diseases to affect mankind. They include tuberculosis, sarcoidosis, syphilis, leprosy, Crohn's disease, rheumatoid arthritis, systemic lupus erythematosus and the pneumoconioses. Despite the availability of treatment and some information on prevention, tuberculosis remains a significant worldwide problem. For this reason (and because it turns up in exams with frightening regularity!) we shall discuss this disorder first and then consider some of the other chronic inflammatory diseases.

Tuberculosis

The great German bacteriologist, Robert Koch, was the first to show that tuberculosis is an infective disease, a fact we take for granted now. Koch's original investigations (1876) were performed with anthrax which he demonstrated to be the cause of what was then known as 'splenic fever'. It was clear to Koch that, in order to implicate a particular organism as the cause of a disease, he must:

- demonstrate the organism in the lesions in all cases of that disease
- be able to isolate the organism and cultivate it in pure culture outside the host
- produce the same disease by injecting the pure culture into a healthy subject

These three criteria are known as **Koch's postulates**.

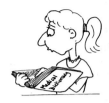

What is a granuloma?

A granuloma is a collection of macrophages. They are sometimes surrounded by a rim of lymphocytes

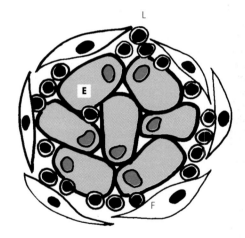

Group of epithelioid cells (E), with variable numbers of lymphocytes (L) and fibroblasts (F)

Other features of specific granulomatous conditions:
a. foreign material in foreign body type giant cells
b. parasites, foreign body type giant cells
c. tubercle bacilli, Langhan giant cells and caseous necrosis in tuberculosis
d. Asteroid & Schaumann bodies in sarcoidosis

Fig 1.31 Granuloma

On 24th March 1882, Koch announced the discovery of the tubercle bacillus to the Berlin Physiological Society. His work proved that 'pulmonary consumption' was not a disorder of nutrition but an infective disease that ran a chronic course. Although Koch is best remembered for his contribution to tuberculosis, he did not confine his interests to that disease. He discovered the cholera vibrio that had created havoc from India to Egypt, investigated bubonic plague in India, researched diseases caused by the tse-tse fly in East Africa and studied malaria in Java.

Tuberculosis is a world-wide problem and it is caused by *Mycobacterium tuberculosis,* sometimes called the 'Koch Bacillus'. Two strains infect humans: these are *M.tuberculosis* var. *hominis* and *M.tuberculosis* var. *bovis.* Bovine tuberculosis is passed from cattle to humans in milk so that it enters through the gastrointestinal tract to produce abdominal tuberculosis. It is uncommon in developed countries now that dairy herds are generally free of mycobacteria and milk is pasteurised. Infection with *M. hominis* is the common form and it produces pulmonary tuberculosis.

Tuberculosis is more common in the young and the very old and there are definite racial and ethnic differences in incidence. It is more common in Asians, American Indians, Africans, the Irish and Eskimos. It also flourishes in socially deprived areas, and poverty and malnutrition appear to be important predisposing factors. There is a higher incidence in males and in people suffering from alcoholism, chronic lung diseases and conditions causing immunosuppresion, e.g. cancer and AIDS. Patients with tuberculosis may present with a cough producing blood-stained sputum, or, more subtly, with night sweats, weight loss and vague symptoms of ill-health.

M. tuberculosis is a slender, rod-shaped organism, approximately 4 μm in length. It is not visible on haematoxylin and eosin stained sections but is stained using the Ziehl–Neelsen method. This reaction relies on the fact that, once stained, the organisms are resistant to decolorisation with acid and alcohol (hence acid and alcohol fast bacilli - AAFB). Mycobacteria grow very slowly in culture and may not be apparent for six weeks. Observing the bacilli in excised tissues will allow faster diagnosis and treatment, but they will not be seen in sections unless there are approximately 1 million bacteria per millilitre of tissue.

The pathogenesis of tuberculosis is reminiscent of a 'Romeo and Juliet phenomenon', the immunity and the hypersensitivity reaction. *M. tuberculosis* does not possess any toxins with which to harm its host; however, a number of cell membrane glycolipids and proteins act to provoke a hypersensitivity reaction and to help protect the bacteria against eradication. It is the hypersensitivity reaction that causes the tissue destruction that is so characteristic of this disease.

Primary tuberculosis

This occurs in individuals who have never been infected with *M. tuberculosis.*

What are Koch's postulates?

1. Demonstrate organisms in lesions of all cases

2. Isolate and cultivate pure cultures

3. Produce the disease by reinjecting into new subject.

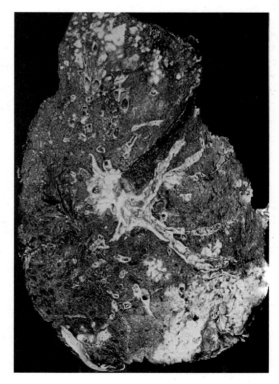

Fig 1.32 Cut surface of the lung showing white areas of caseation due to tuberculosis in the upper and lower lobes.

Inhalation of the organism produces a small lesion (approx. 1 cm in diameter), usually in the subpleural region in the lower part of the upper lobe or the upper part of the lower lobe. This is referred to as the **Ghon focus**. Lesions occur in these sites because the bacterium is a strict aerobe and prefers these well-oxygenated regions. When the tissue is first invaded by the mycobacteria, there is no hypersensitivity reaction, but an initial acute, non-specific, inflammatory response with neutrophils predominating. This is followed rapidly by an influx of macrophages which ingest the bacilli and present their antigens to T lymphocytes, leading to the proliferation of a clone of T cells and the emergence of specific hypersensitivity. The lymphocytes release lymphokines which attract more macrophages. These accumulate to form the characteristic granuloma, containing a mixture of macrophages, including epithelioid cells and Langhans-type giant cells. Tissue destruction leads to necrosis in the centre of the granuloma called **caseous necrosis** because, macroscopically, the necrotic area resembles cheesy material! Tubercle bacilli, either free or contained in macrophages, may drain to the regional lymph nodes and set up granulomatous inflammation, causing massive lymph node enlargement. The combination of the Ghon focus and the regional nodes is called the **primary complex**.

Thus, the development of hypersensitivity results in tissue destruction but also improves the body's resistance to the mycobacterium by promoting phagocytosis and reducing intracellular replication of bacilli. It is not known why the granulomatous response to mycobacteria produces caseation whereas most other granulomatous reactions do not. Another puzzle is why the attraction of macrophages in most inflammatory responses produces a dispersed infiltrate while in granulomatous reactions they form well-demarcated collections – granulomata.

To return to our patient with tuberculosis and a Ghon focus; the next phase is that, in the majority of cases, this primary complex will heal. There will be replacement of the caseous necrosis by a small fibrous scar and the lesion will be walled off. Calcification may also occur in these lesions. Despite this, the organisms may survive and lead to **reactivation infection** at a later date, especially if the host defences become lowered, as can occur with cancer.

There are, however, a number of alternative outcomes. If the hypersensitivity reaction is severe, it will lead to a florid inflammatory response and the patient may present with a systemic illness. If the caseous necrosis is extensive, the tissue destruction may erode major bronchi and allow air-borne spread of organisms to produce satellite lesions in either lung. Alternatively, tubercle bacilli may enter the blood stream. If they enter a small pulmonary arteriole, then the bacilli will lodge in lung tissue. However, if they enter a pulmonary vein the bacilli may disseminate throughout the systemic circulation. If this occurs, numerous small granulomas may be encountered in almost any organ including meninges, kidneys and adrenals. This type of

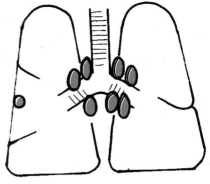

Ghon focus plus hilar lymph node enlargement (primary complex)

Fig 1.33 Primary tuberculosis

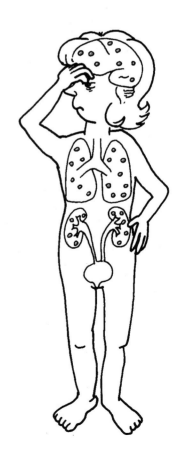

Fig 1.34 Miliary tuberculosis

disease is called **miliary** tuberculosis, so-called because the lesions look like millet seeds! Fortunately, systemic spread is not a common event in primary disease.

Secondary tuberculosis

Secondary, or postprimary, tuberculosis refers to infection occurring in a patient previously sensitised to the mycobacterium. Most of these cases are due to **reactivation** of latent mycobacteria following an asymptomatic primary infection. The latency period can vary tremendously and reactivation may not occur for many decades. Occasionally there is reinfection from an exogenous source.

Secondary infection tends to affect the subapical region of the upper lobe and, although the reasons for this are far from clear, it is believed to be due to the higher oxygen concentration in this part. (If you remember, tubercle bacilli are obligate aerobes.) This focus of reactivation is called the **Assman focus**. There are three possible outcomes of the secondary infection: healing, cavitation or spread. Due to the previous infection, the host will have some degree of immunity and, if this is sufficient, the infection will heal with **scarring** and subsequent **calcification**. Intervention with antituberculous drugs will also enhance and modify the healing process. If, on the other hand, the degree of hypersensitivity is high and/or the the organisms are particularly virulent, there may be considerable lung parenchymal tissue destruction and caseous necrosis, which can lead to the formation of a **cavity**. The infected caseous material may spread through destroyed tissue, or via bronchi to adjacent parts of the lung, and extend the local disease. The pleura may become involved, with the production of an effusion which can contain caseous and necrotic material, **tuberculous empyema**. Infected sputum may be swallowed, spreading the disease to the gastrointestinal tract. Systemic spread to produce miliary tuberculosis is more common in postprimary tuberculosis because tissue destruction is greater.

The natural history of the disease will depend on the host's immunity, hypersensitivity and factors such as nutritional status, associated disease and intervention with drugs. Tuberculosis is a treatable disease, yet, despite this, it remains a major problem in underdeveloped countries and there is a worrying trend towards the development of antibiotic-resistant strains in the developed countries.

Different types of mycobacteria cause two other clinically important diseases: leprosy and atypical mycobacterial infections.

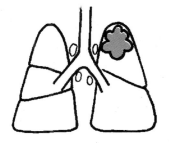

Assman focus: reactivation or post-primary infection

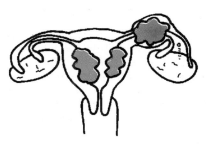

Blood-borne 2° tuberculosis in Fallopian tube or endometrium may cause infertility

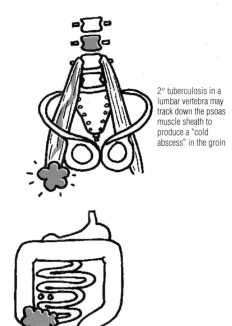

2° tuberculosis in a lumbar vertebra may track down the psoas muscle sheath to produce a "cold abscess" in the groin

Intestinal tuberculosis may be 1°, due to ingestion of milk infected by bovine tuberculosis, or 2° to swallowing infected sputum

Fig 1.35 Secondary tuberculosis

Leprosy

Leprosy, also called Hansen's disease after the discoverer of the organism, is caused by *Mycobacterium leprae*. It is stained using a modified Ziehl–Neelsen technique because it is more readily decolorised with acid than *M. tuberculosis*. It is an obligate intracellular organism and consequently has never been cultured in a cell-free medium. It can, however, be cultured in the footpad of the mouse and in the nine-banded armadillo!

Leprosy is a slowly progressive chronic disorder that principally affects the skin, testes, peripheral nerves and nasal mucosa, i.e. tissue that is generally cool. The major problems of the disease result from the involvement of nerves. For example, if a sensory nerve supplying a toe is destroyed, the toe becomes anaesthetic and may be injured repeatedly until it is damaged beyond repair. Leprosy is spread by droplet infection and, although the rate of transmission is low, it is endemic in many parts of the world and a staggering 10 million people are thought to be affected. Like tuberculosis, the host response to the infection involves cell-mediated immunity, i.e. T lymphocytes. The presence or relative absence of this cell-mediated immunity (and hypersensitivity) is responsible for the two well-recognised forms of the disease, tuberculoid and lepromatous leprosy. These represent the extreme ends of a spectrum and a large intermediate group also exists.

The **tuberculoid** form (also known as the TT form) is similar to tuberculosis with granuloma formation and very few bacilli. In the **lepromatous** form (also known as the LL form), there is a totally different response. The macrophages still phagocytose bacilli but, probably because of lack of stimulation by T cells, fail to kill them. The result is that, instead of proper granulomas, there are loose collections of lipid-laden macrophages containing numerous organisms. The lepromatous form is more extensive and destructive and more difficult to cure.

A very interesting feature of lepromatous leprosy is an increase in circulating immunoglobulins (hypergamma-globulinaemia). Although cell-mediated immunity is impaired, humoral immunity is not and antibodies to *M. leprae* are produced but are incapable of destroying the organisms. Instead they bind to the organisms to produce circulating antibody–antigen complexes which can deposit at various sites promoting complement activation and tissue damage (type III hypersensitivity reaction). Deposition in the vessels of the the skin leads to tender nodules called erythema nodosum leprosum, while deposition in the kidneys can produce a glomerulonephritis. Yet more examples of the side-effects of war!

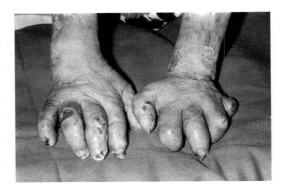

Fig 1.36 Hands demonstrating damage related to leprosy.

Atypical mycobacterial infections

These organisms have received publicity recently because they are common in AIDS cases. Atypical mycobacteria are found in the soil, water and animal faecal material and include *M. kansasii, M. avium–intracellulare* and *M. ulcerans*. They are normally of very low virulence and do not pose a significant threat. However, their opportunity to produce disease comes if a patient has chronic lung disease or is immunosuppressed – so these are termed **opportunistic infections**. Although these organisms are capable of inducing a granulomatous response, this is often lacking because of a deficient immune response by the patient. The problem with the atypical mycobacteria is that they are difficult to differentiate from *M. tuberculosis* and some do not respond to antituberculous therapy.

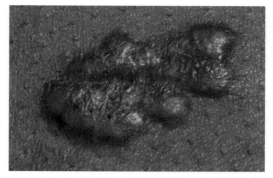

Fig 1.37 Raised skin lesion in sarcoidosis. Microscopy would show epithelioid granulomata.

Sarcoidosis

Sarcoidosis is a baffling systemic disease of unknown aetiology and is characterised by the presence of granulomas which, unlike tuberculosis, do not exhibit caseous necrosis and so are termed 'non-caseating granulomas'.

It is a systemic disorder of variable severity, hence it can present in numerous ways. Patients are often asymptomatic and diagnosis is only made postmortem. Almost every organ in the body may be affected, the commonest being lung, liver, spleen, skin and salivary glands with the heart, kidneys and central nervous system slightly less commonly affected. Most patients present with respiratory symptoms (shortness of breath, haemoptysis, chest pains) but some have a more rapid course with fever, erythema nodosum and polyarthritis. Patients may also present with signs and symptoms of hypercalcaemia and lytic bone lesions, especially in the phalanges, are strong supportive evidence for the disease.

There are many more examples of granulomatous inflammation which we have not considered and these form part of the differential diagnosis when a patient presents with manifestations of granulomatous disease. Examples are listed opposite.

A tissue biopsy may be essential to make the diagnosis of granulomatous disease and can be helpful in elucidating the cause. The only way to be certain of the cause is either to see it under the microscope, e.g. fungal hyphae, or to culture the organism. However, some macrophage variants are more common in specific conditions.

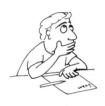

Discuss the causes of granulomatous inflammation

Bacterial
    tuberculosis
    syphilis
    leprosy

Fungal
    cryptococcus
    coccidioides

Protozoal
    pneumocystis
    toxoplasmosis

Parasitic
    schistosomiasis

Metals
    silicosis
    berylliosis

Unknown aetiology
    sarcoidosis

Foreign body reaction
    talc

Macrophages in specific disease

Epithelioid cells occur in all types of granulomatous disease. They have some resemblance to epithelial cells as they possess abundant pink cytoplasm, packed with endoplasmic reticulum, Golgi apparatus and vesicles. Thus the cells are well adapted to synthesise macrophage products, such as arachidonic acid metabolites, complement, coagulation factors and cytokines. However, they are less mobile and less proficient at phagocytosis than ordinary macrophages. The **multinucleate giant macrophages** principally form by fusion of epithelioid cells. Each may have 50 nuclei or more and it is the arrangement of these nuclei which distinguishes the types. The **Langhans giant cell** is typical of tuberculosis or sarcoid and has its nuclei arranged as a horse-shoe at the periphery. The **foreign-body giant cell**, predictably, is associated with foreign material which is sometimes identifiable in the cytoplasm. Its nuclei are randomly arranged throughout the cell.

These are the most important macrophage variants but, for completeness, we will mention two others. These are the **Warthin-Finkeldey** cell, pathognomonic of measles and characterised by the presence of eosinophilic nuclear and cytoplasmic inclusions, and **Touton giant cells**, which have a central cluster of nuclei surrounded by foamy lipid-laden cytoplasm. Touton cells occur in xanthomas, which are benign tumorous collections of lipid-laden macrophages in the skin.

The factors influencing granuloma formation are largely unknown but a variety of cytokines appear to be involved. Animal experiments suggest that IL-1 is important in the initiation of granulomata and that TNF is responsible for their maintainance. IL-2 has been shown to increase their size and IL-5 could attract eosinophils to the granulomata seen in parasitic disease. IL-6 is believed to have an important role in tuberculous granulomata.

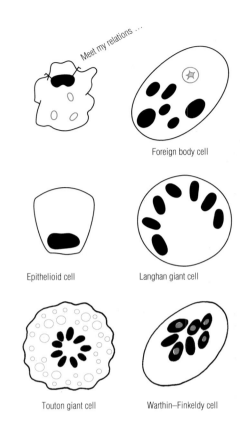

Meet my relations ...

Foreign body cell

Epithelioid cell

Langhan giant cell

Touton giant cell

Warthin–Finkeldy cell

Fig 1.38 Specific types of macrophages

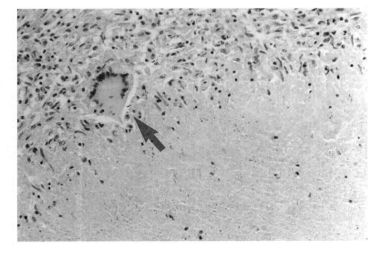

Fig 1.39 Photomicrograph of tuberculosis showing a Langhan's giant cell (arrow) at the edge of an area of caseous necrosis where cellular detail is lost.

To summarise chronic inflammation we will consider a clinicopathological discussion of syphilis.

Clinical

A 40 year old man presented to the genitourinary clinic complaining of a 'sore' on his penis. It had been present for approximately two weeks.

Past medical history:
He had had numerous sexual partners and had been treated in the past for gonorrhoea. He did not give a history of drug abuse.

Systemic enquiry:
He was in good health apart from the 'sore'. He had also noticed a lump in his right groin.

Examination:
He had an erythematous, painless ulcer on his penis, approx. 1.5 cm in diameter. It had an indurated base with a clean rim. There was no evidence of a secondary infection.

Investigations:
A smear taken from the ulcer was examined under dark-ground microscopy and revealed numerous spirochaetes.

A lymph node biopsy was consistent with the clinical diagnosis of syphilis.

VDRL (venereal disease reference laboratory), TPHA (treponemal haemagglutination assay) and FTA-Ab (fluorescent treponemal antibody) serological tests were also carried out and all were positive.
Investigations to look for other venereal diseases were negative.

Diagnosis:
Primary syphilis

Treatment
He was started on treatment with penicillin. The patient discharged himself without completing the course

Pathology

The 'sore' is called a chancre. This is usually present in the genital area, but in 10% of patients it is found in extragenital sites such as the lip.

Syphilis is a sexually transmitted disease and it is important to elicit a history of previous venereal infections. Other sexually transmitted diseases may be present concomitantly.

There is usually a regional lymphadenopathy in association with the chancre.

The chancre is full of organisms and it is possible to visualise these using dark-ground microscopy. Microscopically, the chancre shows many plasma cells, macrophages and lymphocytes with inflammation and destruction of blood vessels (obliterative endarteritis).

The lymph node may show non-specific follicular and T cell hyperplasia with increased plasma cells and occasional granulomata.

Serological tests are of two types: non-specific and specific.
VDRL is a non-specific test which is used for screening. The non-specific antibody is directed against a lipoidal antigen of human and mammalian tissues. This can be detected approx. one week after the development of the chancre.
The specific tests, TPHA and FTA-Ab, detect antibodies to the components of T. pallidum. The specific tests become positive in primary syphilis and remain positive irrespective of treatment or disease activity.

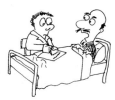

Clinical

Approximately three months later, the same man re-presented with a generalised rash. He also complained of aches and pains in his joints and of abdominal pain.

Examination:
This showed a maculo papular skin rash, pink to dusky red in colour, which also involved the mucous membranes. He had larger papular lesions in his perianal region which were elevated. The features were of genital warts. His joints were tender but he did not have any signs of active inflammation.
He was noted to have a generalised lymphadenopathy.

Investigations:
A smear taken from the genital warts revealed numerous spirochaetes on dark-ground microscopy.
Serological tests were again positive.
Biochemical tests also showed abnormal liver function tests with raised levels of liver enzymes.

Diagnosis:
Secondary syphilis

Treatment:
He was treated with a course of penicillin which on this occasion he completed. He made a full recovery. His contacts were also traced and offered treatment.

Pathology

The skin lesion, the rash, is similar to the chancre but contains fewer numbers of plasma cells.
Arthralgia is common in secondary syphilis and the abdominal pain is a result of hepatitis, as can be seen from the results of the liver function tests.

The genital warts are called 'condylomata lata' They have hyperplastic epithelium, many plasma cells and show obliterative endarteritis.
Spirochaetes are numerous.

The lymph nodes show similar features to primary syphilis.

The tests are in keeping with the diagnosis of syphilis and biochemistry results indicate a hepatitis.
A generalised bacteraemia can cause hepatitis, meningitis, iritis and periostitis. Arthritis can also occur but arthralgia (aching of joints) is more common than arthritis.

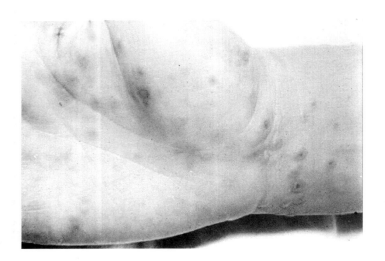

Fig 1.40 Wrist and palm of a patient with secondary syphilis showing the characteristic maculopapular rash.

Clinical

A 65 year old lady presented with chest pain and shortness of breath. This had started six months previously and in that time her exercise tolerance had decreased to half a mile. She had also noticed occasional palpitations.

Examination:
Cardiovascular system – collapsing (waterhammer) pulse and an early diastolic murmur at the left sternal edge. Apex beat was displaced to the left.

Respiratory system – there was evidence of pulmonary oedema and a small right pleural effusion

Abdominal examination – this revealed an enlarged liver with an irregular margin

Central nervous system: normal.

Investigations:
Chest X-ray – this showed a widened aortic root, cardiomegaly, pulmonary oedema and small bilateral pleural effusions

Liver biopsy : granulomatous inflammation

Serology – VDRL, TPHA and FTA-Ab positive

Diagnosis:
Tertiary syphilis

Treatment:-
Treatment is very difficult once there is widespread involvement. She died soon afterwards of cardiac failure. A postmortem was requested.

Pathology

The history of chest pain, shortness of breath and decreased exercise tolerance suggests severe cardiac disease

The examination suggests that she has severe aortic incompetence, these being the classical signs of regurgitation. In syphilis, the tunica media of the aorta is inflamed and weakened leading to aneurysm formation. Dilatation of the aortic ring leads to aortic incompetence.

Aortic incompetence leads to increased load on the left ventricle and eventually cardiac failure, pulmonary oedema and pleural effusions.

The enlarged liver is due to syphilitic involvement. This produces areas of necrosis with plump macrophages and fibroblasts pallisading around them; each of these is a type of granulomata called a syphilitic gumma. Extensive scarring results in gross distortion and this is called hepar lobatum.

Central nervous system involvement takes the form of meningovascular syphilis, tabes dorsalis and general paresis. She did not have neural involvement.

The results of the investigations confirm the clinical diagnosis of tertiary syphilis with gumma formation and cardiovascular involvement but without neurosyphilis.

Autopsy confirmed her aortic disease and aortic incompetence. She also had narrowing of her coronary ostia and left ventricular hypertrophy secondary to the regurgitation.
The liver showed multiple gummas with extensive scarring. In addition, she had gummas in the subcutaneous tissues and in her long bones.
The brain and spinal cord did not reveal any abnormalities.

Congenital syphilis

Treponema pallidum infection can be transmitted vertically from mother to child *in utero*. The organisms do not invade the placenta or foetus until about five months' gestation, hence they are a cause of late abortion, stillbirth or death soon after delivery. It is not a cause of early abortion.

The effects of congenital syphilis are very characteristic and include interstitial keratitis (inflammation of the stroma of the cornea), periostitis (inflammation of the periosteum of bone), saddle deformity of the nose due to the destruction of the vomer bone and Hutchinson's teeth. The teeth tend to be pointed or peg-shaped with a notched biting margin.
The sad fact about congenital syphilis is that it can occur up to five years after the mother has been infected, though the risk is highest soon after infection. It is a treatable disease and the fetus can be protected if adequate treatment is instituted early on in the pregnancy.

You may be interested to know that John Hunter is also remembered for inoculating himself with gonorrhoea pus – one experiment that is definitely not recommended! The signs and symptoms of gonorrhoea appeared quickly, and so did those of syphilis. Because he developed the symptoms of both syphilis and gonorrhoea, Hunter believed that they were the same disease. He was unlucky in having used pus from a patient who suffered from both diseases. He treated the diseases with local cautery, chemical burning and mercury. Until Alexander Fleming discovered penicillin, every medical student was aware that a night with Venus could mean a year with mercury!

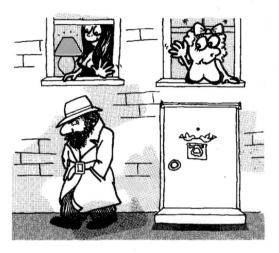

These days few scientists would choose to emulate John Hunter's auto-inoculation studies with gonorrhoea

Healing and Repair

When injury takes place and the process of inflammation is set in motion, the elements of repair and healing are also activated. For convenience we discuss these after acute and chronic inflammation, but the process actually begins early on.

If your patient, injured whilst at work as the target half of a circus knife-throwing act, asks how long it will be before he/she can take the bandages off and return to the arena, what must you consider before answering? Briefly, the processes that take place during and after the injury are:

- **removal** of dead and foreign material
- **regeneration** of injured tissue from cells of the same type
- **replacement** of damaged tissue by new connective tissue

Ideally, adequate tissue repair will occur within three weeks – we have already seen an example of this in lobar pneumonia. The infection causes an inflammatory response which leads to cells and debris accumulating in alveoli. When these are removed by the macrophages and the lymphatics, we again have normal intact alveoli which can participate in gas exchange. This process of restoring the tissue to pristine condition is called resolution. Resolution requires that the inflammatory process deals quickly with the insult, the tissue has not lost its basic scaffolding and any damaged specialised cells are capable of regeneration.

What happens if part of this system fails? In this case, other mechanisms must operate and, although healing may still take place, the result will not be perfect. If the exudate is not cleared, it will be organised; this means that there is an ingrowth of capillaries and fibroblasts, called **granulation tissue**, which leads to the production of fibrous connective tissue, i.e. a scar.

Cell capacity for regeneration

What happens when injury causes loss of normal tissue and leaves a defect, e.g. a cut in the skin? In this situation the end result depends on the size of the defect and the capacity of the tissue to regenerate. Not all tissues of the body have the same capacity to regenerate and cells can be divided into three major types: labile, stable and permanent.

The **labile** cells include epithelial and blood cells; these divide and proliferate throughout life and the cells have a set lifespan. **Stable** cells normally divide extremely slowly but can proliferate rapidly if required. If you remove half the liver, the cells will regenerate and return it to its original size! Other examples of stable cells are fibroblasts, vascular endothelial cells, smooth muscle cells, osteoblasts and renal tubular epithelial cells. **Permanent** cells cannot divide but may be capable of some individual cell repair if the nucleus and synthetic apparatus are intact. Examples include neurones and cardiac muscle cells. If a permanent cell is damaged but not destroyed, as in injury to a nerve axon, there may be regrowth of the damaged portion. However, if the whole cell is destroyed, it must be replaced by a small scar because its neighbouring cells are incapable of proliferating to replace it.

The size of the defect is very important as any destruction of the tissue scaffold will result in scarring. What is the tissue scaffold? The whole picture is not yet clear but the basement membrane is very important for well-organised tissue regeneration. The size of the defect may be extremely small, such as a sutured wound, or large, as in traumatic injuries. Healing in these instances is by primary and secondary **intention**, respectively.

Wound healing

Fig. 1.43 illustrates the healing of a skin wound. The damage to the small blood vessels causes haemorrhage which helps to 'glue' the edges together and provides the protective dry surface scab (*a*). First, neutrophils migrate from the vessels to the damaged area and epidermal cells proliferate at the

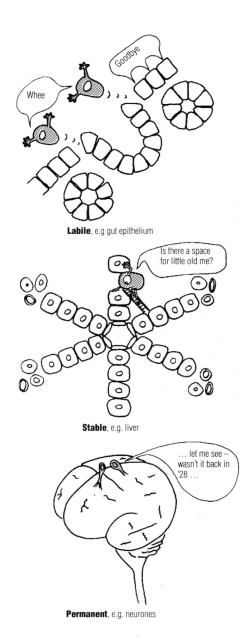

Labile, e.g gut epithelium

Stable, e.g. liver

Permanent, e.g. neurones

Fig 1.41 Cell capacity for regeneration

surface. Within 24–48 hours, the epidermal cells grow underneath the scab to form a thin but complete layer. Meanwhile, there is an influx of macrophages, proliferation of fibroblasts and ingrowth of many fine capillaries (granulation tissue) *(b)*. At this stage, there is a temporary matrix of type III collagen. Epithelial migration halts by contact inhibition and a definitive matrix (type I collagen) is laid down. The vessels and inflammatory cells reduce in number *(c)*. By day 5, bundles of collagen have been laid down across the damaged tissue to form a scar and the epidermis has returned to normal thickness *(d)*. Initially the scar is red, because of the increase in small vessels, but it will blanch over the next few weeks as the vessels regress and the collagen thickens. If the cut is fine and there is good wound apposition, the scar tissue is limited and the cosmetic result good, but how strong is the repair? Immediately after surgery, the wound has around 70% of the strength of normal skin but this is principally conferred by the sutures. When these are removed, after 7–10 days, the wound strength drops to 10% of normal – a point to emphasise to patients. Strength then increases rapidly over the next month to reach a maximum at around three months, when a well-healed scar will have 70–80% of the tensile strength of uninjured skin. Interestingly, the strength does not correlate with the amount of collagen but may be related to the type, with type I being stronger than the type III deposited early in the repair process.

Healing by primary and secondary intention

The figure opposite shows healing of a skin in which there is a sharp clean wound (primary intention) and one in which there is a large tissue defect (secondary intention). The processes are the same as described above but the sharp wound heals with little scarring whereas with large wound defects there is a more intense inflammatory reaction and a larger amount of granulation tissue. There is also contraction of the wound – an intriguing phenomenon, thought to be produced by myofibroblasts which, as the name implies, have features of both fibroblasts and smooth muscle cells.

Granulation tissue production is a fascinating process common to all forms of repair. Fibroblast growth factors (FGFs – see also later) stimulate the endothelial cells of capillaries and postcapillary venules to secrete proteases that digest the surrounding basement membrane. The endothelial cells then proliferate to produce a bud of cells protruding through the gap in the wall towards the source of the stimulus. At first the bud of endothelial cells is solid but eventually it canalises to allow the flow of blood, although quite how the circulatory loop is completed is not known.

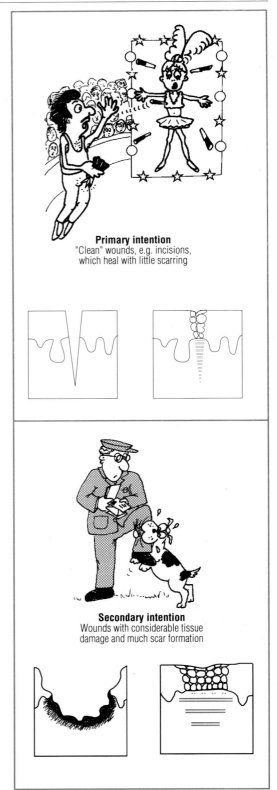

Primary intention
"Clean" wounds, e.g. incisions, which heal with little scarring

Secondary intention
Wounds with considerable tissue damage and much scar formation

Fig 1.42 Healing by primary and secondary intention

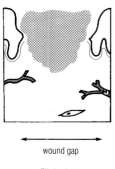 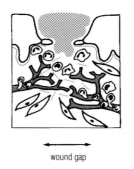 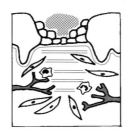 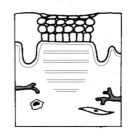

wound gap

wound gap

a. Fibrin clot

b. Day 1–2: cellular infiltrate, temporary matrix, wound contraction, epithelial migration, clot dissolution

Day 3–4: surface intact, new basement membrane, definitive matrix

Day 5: scar

Key:

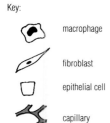

macrophage

fibroblast

epithelial cell

capillary

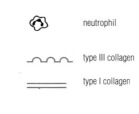

neutrophil

type III collagen

type I collagen

Fig 1.43 Wound healing e.g. large skin wound

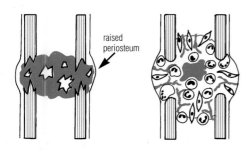 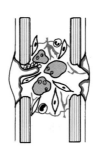 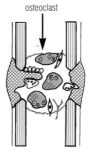 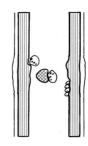

osteoclast

raised periosteum

Fibrin clot, bone fragments.

Inflammatory cell influx: debris removed. Fibroblast ingrowth. New blood vessels.

Provisional callus (osteoid & cartilage) → fibrocartilagenous callus.

Osseous callus: woven bone formation

Remodelling by osteoclasts and replacement of woven bone with lamellar bone

Fig 1.44 Bone healing

Most wounds, whether of skin or internal organs, will heal in this way but an interesting exception is bone. This breaks the rules and does not heal with a fibrous scar. Even if the 'scaffold' is completely distorted, as with a traumatic fracture, it will remodel to resemble the original structure and function. If it didn't the bone would remain flexible at the breakpoint.

Healing of bone

Fig 1.44 outlines the stages from fracture to healing and remodelling.

Following a fracture, there is bleeding from the damaged blood vessels so that blood and fibrin clot accumulate within the gap leading to elevation of the periosteum. Just as in soft tissues, this is organised by formation of granulation tissue and phagocytosis of debris and necrotic bone. It differs in that osteoid (non-calcified bone matrix) and cartilage appear after a few days and this is termed the '**provisional callus** or **procallus**'. Over the next week, the amount of fibrous tissue and number of bone spicules increase (**fibrocartilaginous callus**) and immobilise the fracture. The bone content continues to expand (**osseous callus**) and **remodelling** by osteoblasts and osteoclasts will occur according to the stresses acting on the bone. Initially, the collagen fibres in the osteoid are arranged in an irregular fashion, called **woven** bone. When the normal 'onion-skin' pattern has been restored, it is referred to as **lamellar** bone. Finally, as the internal callus is removed, marrow cells will return.

If the alignment is perfect, it may not be possible to see the site of the previous fracture, but if malaligned, complicated, infected or not properly immobilised, the end result is not perfect. Remodelling of bone is not confined to the healing of fractures. It occurs during normal growth and in pathological conditions unrelated to bone fractures, such as osteomalacia or Paget's disease.

The redoubtable Scot, John Hunter, investigated the healing of tendons. It is said that he ruptured his Achilles tendon while dancing, but since he did it at 4 a.m., this seems unlikely. By his own account, he did it while jumping, but why he was jumping at this hour is also a mystery! Either way, true to his nature, he did not let the opportunity go to waste and he observed the healing of his own tendon and later undertook experiments in dogs to show that they heal by formation of dense scar tissue.

Growth factors

Just as there is a wide range of chemical mediators co-ordinating inflammation, so there are innumerable factors controlling growth. These operate in normal growth, in benign and malignant tumours and in healing and repair. There are two complementary modes of action provided by **competence factors** and **progression factors**. As you will

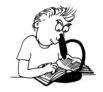

What are the factors involved in the control of growth?

Epidermal growth factor
Platelet-derived growth factor
Fibroblast growth factor
Transforming growth factor α, β
Interleukin-1
Tumour necrosis factor

recall from cell biology, proliferation involves a cell in **G1** phase synthesising chromosomal material (**S** phase) to reach **G2**. Mitosis (**M** phase) can then occur and the cell will either return to G1, to undergo further mitotic division, or enter the resting phase (**G0** phase). Progression factors act on competent cells to stimulate them to synthesise DNA. Competence factors act on cells in G0 or G1 to make them able to respond to progression factors; quite what this involves is not known. Many growth factors also act in inflammation.

Epidermal growth factor (EGF) acts as a progression factor for fibroblasts and epithelial cells. **Platelet-derived growth factor** (PDGF), not surprisingly, is stored and released from platelet alpha granules but can also be produced by macrophages, smooth muscle cells, endothelium and some tumour cells. It acts as a competence factor for macrophages, fibroblasts and smooth muscle cells. **Fibroblast growth factors** (FGFs) are a group of substances crucial for new blood vessel formation and are produced by activated macrophages. **Transforming growth factors** (TGF) are of two very different types. **TGF-α** is chemically and biologically very similar to EGF. However, **TGF-ß** acts as a growth inhibitor to some cells and deactivates macrophages. It promotes formation of fibrous tissue, as do **IL-1** and **TNF**.

Repair is really just a continuation of inflammation, so it is not surprising that the macrophage plays such a central role in both. In repair it is capable of phagocytosis, enzyme release and secretion of growth factors (PDGF, FGF, IL-1, TNF) and growth inhibitors (TGF- ß and prostaglandins).

Modifying factors

The scenario of healing and repair that we have described is an ideal one. There are several factors that can modify the response; we now go on to discuss these.

Blood supply
At the very beginning, we mentioned that the micro-vasculature is of fundamental importance to the inflammatory response. Similarly it is vital to healing. Without adequate perfusion, a small injury would lead to massive tissue destruction. It is the inadequate blood supply that may cause delay in wound healing in the elderly.

Infection and foreign material
The presence of infection or foreign material will delay healing by fuelling the process of inflammation. Infection in a fracture will delay union and healing. The foreign material does not have to be exogenous; the damaged tissue itself may act as 'foreign' material. Sutures are essential for limiting the size of the defect and holding the sides of the wound together; however, their presence stimulates continuing inflammation and provides an entry route for bacteria.

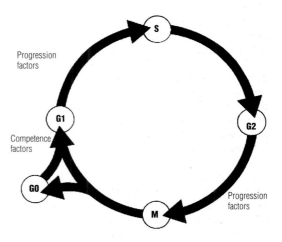

Fig 1.45 The growth cycle

Mobility

It is not difficult to imagine that if the ends of a broken bone are continually moved, they will not mend. The situation is not restricted to bone and applies in varying degrees to all tissues.

Nutrition

The role of nutritional factors in healing has been recognised for a long time. In parts of the world where malnutrition is widespread, impaired wound healing is a common phenomenon, probably exacerbated by infection. Vitamin C deficiency (scurvy) results in impaired synthesis of normal collagen as does a protein-poor diet. The trace element, zinc, is also important and deficiency may occur in patients with severe burns and those receiving long-term parenteral nutrition.

Steroids

It is well known that steroids damp down the inflammatory response and are of great use in diseases where the inflammatory response is causing more harm than good. In excess, however, they may have a deleterious effect.

Improving wound healing

The discussion of factors modifying wound healing emphasises that a clean, uninfected, immobile wound with the sides closely apposed in a healthy patient is most likely to heal quickly and neatly. There are several new approaches to wound healing which are under investigation. Wound healing may be improved by the local use of ultrasound or laser therapy, which are thought to increase vascular permeability. Synthetic growth factors, applied topically, may stimulate the healing of chronically ulcerated sites, such as venous leg ulcers in the elderly. Stubborn bone fractures may be persuaded to unite by the passage of electrical currents through the bone.

Before we finish, we should not forget the **complications of healing**. While a cleanly incised wound from an appendicectomy may only cause minor embarrassment to the vain, **scarring** resulting from severe burns may limit movement across joints due to **contractures**. A scar in the heart, following the death of muscle fibres from a myocardial infarction, may dilate to produce an **aneurysm**. This may become the site of thrombus formation and may also produce cardiac arrythmias, both of which may cause death. Repeated inflammation of the liver, because of alcohol ingestion or viral infection, may produce scar tissue that distorts the normal architecture and produces **cirrhosis**.

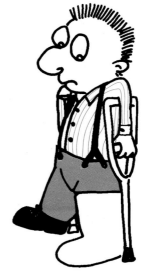

To achieve perfect alignment, the fracture site must be immobilised during repair

What factors modify the process of healing and repair?

Blood supply
Infection and foreign material
Mobility
Nutrition
Steroids

So we come to the end of this chapter which has considered the processes of inflammation and healing and looked at the mechanisms involved and their clinical relevance. It should be clear that the important thing is not to divide the phenomenon into different pieces, as in a jigsaw, but to think of them as interlacing connections. In any one situation, it is the unique combination of these connections that produces the final picture. The idea that it is the connections and not individual objects that is important is well recognised in atomic physics. As Heisenberg (of Heisenberg's uncertainty principle) said:

"[In modern physics], one has now divided the world not into different groups of objects but into different groups of connections ...,What can be distinguished is the kind of connection which is primarily important in a certain phenomenon... The world thus appears as a complicated tissue of events, in which connections of different kinds alternate or overlap or combine and thereby determine the texture of the whole."

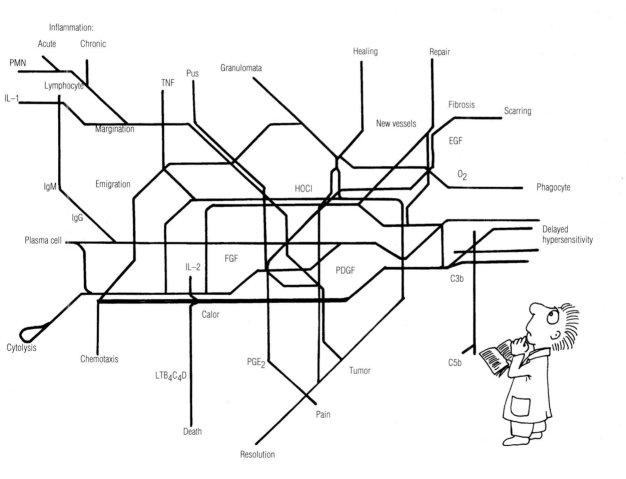

Further reading

K. Whaley & A.D. Burt. (1992). Inflammation, healing and repair. Ch 4. *Muir's Textbook of Pathology*. Ed. R.N.M MacSween & K. Whaley. 13th Edition. Edward Arnold. London.

R.S. Cotran, V. Kumar & S.L. Robbins. (1989). Inflammation and Repair. Ch 2. *Robbins Pathologic Basis of Disease*. 4th Edition. W.B. Saunders Company. Philadelphia.

M.J. Clemens. (1991). *Cytokines. The Medical Perspective Series*. BIOS Scientific Publishers. Oxford.

I.M. Roitt. (1991). *Essential Immunology*. 7th Edition. Blackwell Scientific Publications. Oxford.

P.C.L. Beverley. (1992). T Cells. Ch 4.5. *Oxford Textbook of Pathology*. Ed. J. McGee, P.G. Isaacson & N.A. Wright. Oxford University Press. Oxford.

M.R. Alison. (1992). Repair and regenerative responses. Ch 5.3 *Oxford Textbook of Pathology*. Ed. J. McGee, P.G. Isaacson & N.A. Wright. Oxford University Press. Oxford.

Chapter 2

Circulatory Disorders _____

"When I first applied my mind to observation from the many dissections of Living Creatures as they came to hand, that by that means I might find out the use of the motion of the Heart and things conducible in Creatures; I straightwayes found it a thing hard to be attained, and full of difficulty, so with *Fracastorius* I did almost believe, that the motion of the heart was known to God alone."

– William Harvey

General introduction

It is extraordinary to think that diseases whose effects are as diverse as those of gangrene, strokes, heart attacks and divers' 'bends' are all disorders of the same organ system. The general features of cardiovascular disease are almost the opposite of the cardinal features of inflammation – for 'calor, rubor, tumor and dolor' read 'coldness, pallor/cyanosis, pain and loss of sensation'. Why is this? The drop in temperature and change in colour are easily understood, since blood carries body heat from the core and dissipates it in the extremities and it is the red colour of the oxygenated haemoglobin pigment in the red blood cells which makes pale-skinned persons look pink. Anything decreasing blood flow to a finger or toe will decrease the tissue perfusion by warm blood, making it cold and pale. Any delay in delivery of red blood cells to the affected digit will mean that more of the haemoglobin will have given up its oxygen load, leaving blue-coloured deoxyhaemoglobin (**cyanosis**). **Pain** is a variable phenomenon, depending on the tissue affected and the type of injury. A 'heart attack' or myocardial infarction, caused by sudden blockage of a coronary artery, is usually associated with intense central chest pain, often radiating down the left arm, whilst a gradual 'furring up' of the arteries supplying the legs causes severe pain on walking, which disappears when the demand for oxygen by the leg muscles is removed by rest (**intermittent claudication**). By comparison, a 'stroke', in which the blood supply to part of the brain is suddenly interrupted, will generally cause weakness or paralysis, but no pain. **Loss of sensation** also varies according to the type of vascular disease and the tissue or organ affected; a stroke may destroy a sensory pathway to the brain, leading to a large area of numbness which may involve half the body, whilst blockage of the blood flow to a toe would cause numbness in just the area supplied by the vessel (due to ischaemic damage to the local sensory nerves).

You will have gathered from the preceding discussion that the term 'cardiovascular disease' encompasses a spectrum of symptoms and signs whose common denominator is the organ system involved. Cardiovascular diseases may be '**local**' or '**systemic**' and may gradually develop over months or years or strike suddenly and

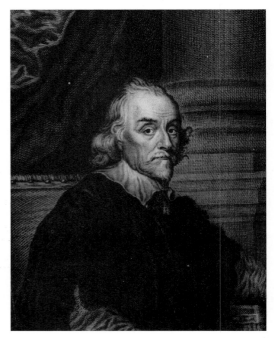

Fig 2.1 William Harvey (1578-1657) - Courtesy of the Wellcome Institute for the History of Medicine.

catastrophically. Perhaps the easiest way to look at these diseases is to relate them to a domestic plumbing system, the main components of which are the pipes and the pump. Pipes may gradually 'fur up' (**atherosclerosis)**, which may lead to a blockage (**thrombosis**). Sometimes small fragments may break off and be carried around the system until they lodge in a pipe with a diameter too small to let them through (**embolism**). Burst pipes (**haemorrhage**) are a nuisance and can be extremely damaging. Sometimes one can spot the area at risk, because the pipe may bulge alarmingly before it bursts (**aneurysm**). At least freezing in winter is not a common problem in the body (although 'frostbite' damages capillaries and causes gangrene). Pump failure for whatever reason is fairly disastrous (in the heart, this may be due to valve disease, myocardial infarction, infection, congenital abnormality, etc.).

Some solutions to these problems have been found; thus affected segments of piping can be replaced (arterial bypass grafts), pumps can be tinkered with (valve grafts) or replaced (heart transplants), high pressure causing strain on the system can be relieved (antihypertensive drugs) and sometimes it is possible to remove some of the 'scale' which furs up the pipes (reaming out of arteries using balloon catheters or, more recently, lasers). Of course these are usually only partial solutions and there is no doubt that prevention is the best medicine.

It would be unjust to discuss circulatory disorders without a brief mention of the historical figures involved. If you had been alive in the sixteenth century, you would have been taught that blood was produced by the liver and then carried in the veins to the organs where it was consumed; this was Galen's theory of the **regeneration** of the blood. The portion of blood from the liver which entered the right side of the heart divided into two streams. One route was through the pulmonary artery to bathe the lungs and the other route was across the heart through 'inter septal pores'. The left ventricle received this blood, which mixed with the 'pneuma' (air) coming to the heart through the pulmonary veins. The blood, fortified by the 'pneuma', was then ejected via the aorta towards the peripheral organs.

In 1628, this theory was challenged when Dr. William Harvey published his famous work, *De Motu Cordis*, describing the dual **circulation** of the blood; but even in the sixteenth century people were starting to doubt Galen's theory. There were several problems with the theory. Firstly, nobody had managed to identify 'inter-septal' pores so Michael Servetius, the Spanish theologian and physician, suggested that blood travelled from the right to the left ventricle by circulating through the lungs; an idea for which he died a martyr's death after being denounced by John Calvin for holding heretical opinions! Secondly, Galen's theory proposed a mixture of air and blood in the left side of the heart, which was a difficult concept to accept once the structure of the heart valves was established. Leonardo da Vinci had drawn these accurately but it was Andrea Caselapino who described the valves' actions correctly, in

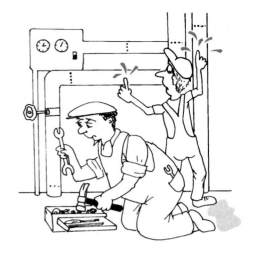

Definitions

Embolus; intravascular solid, liquid or gaseous mass carried in the blood from its origin to lodge in another site

Thrombus; solid mass of blood formed within the cardiovascular system involving the interaction of endothelial cells, platelets and the coagulation cascade

Blood clot; solid mass of blood formed by the action of the coagulation cascade

Infarct; localised area of ischaemic tissue necrosis generally caused by an impaired blood supply

Haematoma; extravascular accumulation of clotted blood

Haemorrhage; discharge of blood from the vascular compartment into the extravascular body spaces or to the exterior

Petechiae, purpura, ecchymoses; small haemorrhages

Hyperaemia; an increased volume of intra-vascular blood in an affected tissue which may result from increased flow (active hyperaemia) or reduced drainage (passive hyperaemia = congestion)

1571, and went on to use the term 'circulatio'. Thus Harvey, who studied in Padua from 1600 to 1602, would have been familiar with the Italians' ideas and was able to reach his own conclusions by 'standing on the shoulders of these giants'. Even Harvey was left with a problem: he could not demonstrate the connections between the arterial and venous sides of the circulation. The discovery of the capillaries had to wait for Marcello Malpighi's microscopical analysis of frog lung in 1661.

Thrombosis _____

To return to the present day, we shall first consider the problems of thrombosis.

Patients presenting with an **arterial thrombus** are generally middle-aged or elderly and may have circulatory problems due to atherosclerosis. Many will be smokers and some may suffer from diabetes. Their symptoms and signs will depend entirely on which vessel is affected. In contrast, a patient with **venous thrombosis** may be any age but generally will be rather immobile or forced to be immobile, such as after an operation. Such patients frequently complain of pain in a calf muscle and often swelling of the foot and ankle. (If you recall the discussion in Chapter 1 about flow of fluid in and out of capillaries, you can work out why the area is oedematous; it is because the hydrostatic pressure at the venous end of the capillaries is raised secondary to the obstructed venous flow.)

But why should such people suddenly develop a thrombus? Much is known now about normal haemostatic mechanisms but the most important factors influencing thrombus formation were described more than a century ago by Virchow.

Rudolf Ludwig Karl **Virchow** was born on 13th October 1821. As a child he excelled at school and his examination reports were rather monotonous as they contained only three terms: 'excellent', 'very good' and 'most satisfactory'! Virchow attended medical school in Berlin in 1839 and, even before the existence of platelets and clotting factors was known, had suggested that the development of a thrombus depended on:

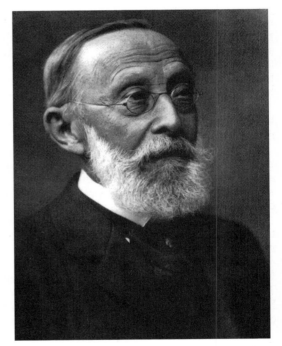

Fig 2.2 Rudolf Virchow (1821-1902) -— Courtesy of the Wellcome Institute for the History of Medicine.

● alteration to the constituents of the blood
● damage to the endothelial layer of the blood vessel
● changes in the normal flow of blood

These three factors are known as **Virchow's triad** and they are the clues which allow us to understand what has happened to our patients with venous and arterial thrombosis. But first we must revise the body's normal haemostatic mechanisms.

Normal haemostatic mechanisms

The normal haemostatic mechanisms must be capable of stopping blood from leaking through damaged vessels and also be finely controlled so that thrombus does not form under normal circumstances. There are three main components:

- platelets
- soluble blood proteins of the coagulation pathway
- vessel wall

Briefly, the sequence of events is as follows. Injury to the vessels causes an initial vasoconstriction which helps to slow the blood flow. The damaged endothelium of the vessel exposes the subendothelial connective tissue which attracts platelets and causes them to adhere to the damaged area to form the **primary haemostatic plug**. The adhesion of the platelets alters their physiology and causes them to release soluble factors which, together with tissue factors, results in the formation of **fibrin** via the coagulation pathway. The fibrin acts to stabilise the platelet plug and the process is termed **secondary haemostasis.**

If this was all that was involved in maintaining haemostasis, could we really survive the assault on our circulation? Of course not!

If the above system was set in motion with nothing to check its progress, soon the whole circulation would come to a standstill and become one big mass of thrombus. This is avoided by clearance, inhibition and inactivation of the coagulation factors as well as by digestion of fibrin.

Now if we return to Virchow's triad, we can consider both the normal physiology and pathology of each component in more detail.

Blood constituents in normal haemostasis

The most important blood constituents involved in normal haemostasis and thrombosis are platelets and the numerous components of the coagulation pathway.

Platelets

Platelets are small (2 μm diameter) cytoplasmic fragments produced by megakaryocytes in the bone marrow. They survive for 8–12 days in the peripheral circulation and contain a variety of granules (see later).

Their role in thrombosis can be divided into three phases:

- adhesion
- secretion
- aggregation

When the endothelium is damaged and collagen is exposed, the first event is **adhesion** of platelets. This is achieved via platelet surface membrane receptors:

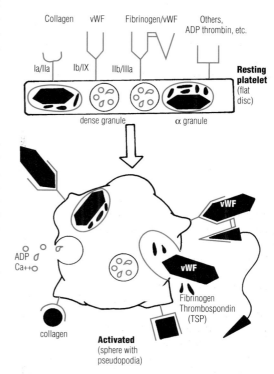

Fig 2.3 Platelets

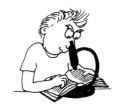

Platelet granules

α **granules**:

fibrinogen
von Willebrand factor
thrombospondin
platelet derived growth factor
fibronectin
platelet factor 4 (an anti-heparin)

dense granules

ADP/ATP
calcium
histamine
adrenaline
serotonin

- **gp Ia/IIa** which binds to collagen
- **gp Ib/IX** which binds to von Willebrand's factor (vWF or Factor VIII related antigen)
- **gp IIb/IIIa** which binds to fibrinogen and vWF

Following adhesion, the platelets release the contents of their granules. There are two main types of granules, the **alpha granules** and **dense bodies** whose contents are listed on the previous page. The most important secretory products are calcium, which is needed for the coagulation pathway, and adenosine diphosphate (ADP) and thromboxane A$_2$ which induce platelet aggregation. **Platelet aggregation** involves the gpIIb/IIIa receptor complex mentioned above. This is expressed after activation and is most important in binding fibrinogen which acts as a bridge to the adjacent platelet Fig. 2.4. Not surprisingly, there are 'loops' in this process to amplify the reaction. Most importantly, activated platelets express **platelet factor 3** which stimulates the intrinsic pathway of the coagulation cascade (see below) resulting in the production of thrombin. **Thrombin** acts to stimulate platelets and so enhances the reaction.

The platelet has another important facet to its character; that is its mechanical properties. An unstimulated platelet has a disc shape maintained by microtubules and actin and myosin filaments at the periphery. On activation, the platelet is transformed into a sphere with long pseudopods which spread over the damaged surface while, after aggregation, the filaments slide so that the platelet plug contracts to both stabilise and anchor it.

Coagulation Components
The components and pathway involved in coagulation are shown in Fig. 2.5. This is the same system as the one we mentioned in Chapter 1 when discussing inflammatory mediators. Then we were particularly interested in fibrin degradation products; now our interest focuses on **fibrin**, which is the final product of the pathway and acts to stabilise the plug of aggregated platelets.

The coagulation pathway has been divided traditionally into the extrinsic and intrinsic pathways, although a complex interplay occurs between them. The common pathway begins at factor X which acts on prothrombin to produce thrombin, which itself has a variety of actions but most importantly converts fibrinogen to fibrin. Generally each step in this cascade involves:

- activated enzyme
- substrate for a coagulation factor
- co-factor
- calcium ions (factor IV)
- phospholipid surface

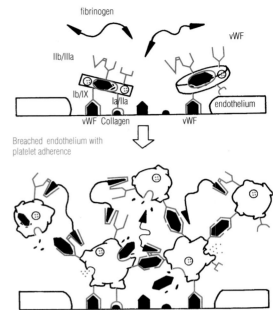

Breached endothelium with platelet adherence

Platelet activation and degranulation. Fibrin mesh forms.

Fig 2.4 Thrombosis

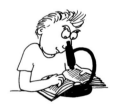

Rare diseases due to platelet abnormalities

von Willebrand's disease –
(lack of vW factor)

Bernard-Soulier syndrome –
(lack of gp Ib)

"Grey platelet" syndrome –
(lack of alpha granules)

Wiskott-Aldrich syndrome –
(lack of dense bodies)

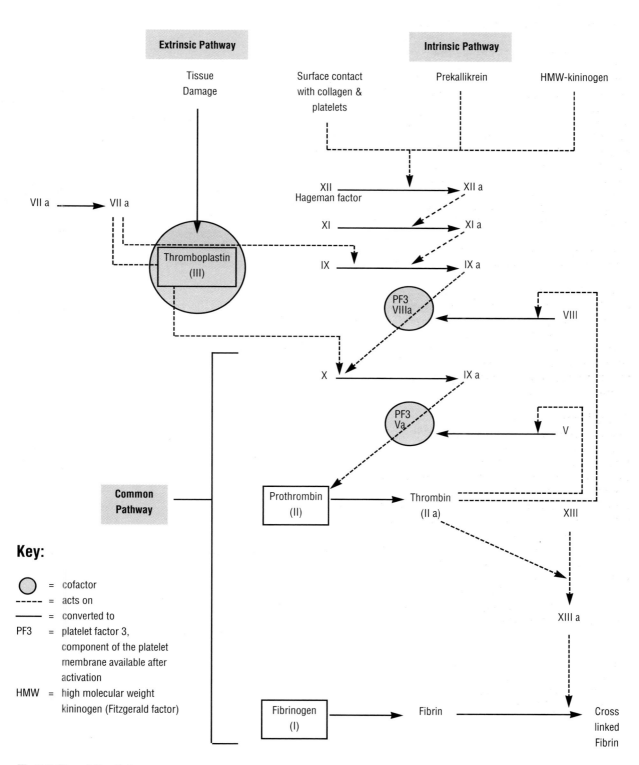

Fig 2.5 Coagulation Pathway

Some feedback loops are included in Fig. 2.5 but, for simplicity, the control mechanisms which inhibit or inactivate reactions have been omitted. These mechanisms include:

- depletion of local clotting factors
- clearance of activated clotting factors by the liver and mononuclear phagocyte system
- neutralisation of activated coagulation factors by forming a complex, e.g. antithrombin III, α_2-macroglobulin
- proteolytic degradation of active coagulation factors, e.g. protein C
- fibrinolysis – this is of major importance (see Fig. 2.6). The most important enzyme capable of digesting fibrin is plasmin. This is produced from plasminogen either by a factor XII-dependent pathway, by therapeutic agents such as streptokinase, or by tissue-derived plasminogen activators. Plasminogen activators (PA) fall into two classes:

- urokinase-like PA (uPA)
- tissue-type PA (tPA)

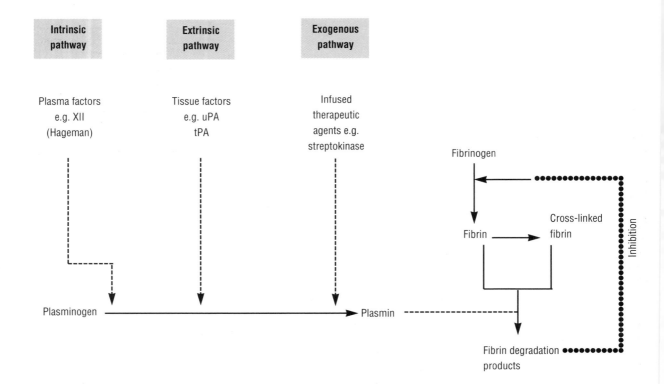

Fig 2.6 Fibrinolysis

They differ in that uPA activates plasminogen in the fluid phase whereas tPA (principally produced by endothelial cells) is active only when attached to fibrin. Conveniently, some plasminogen is bound to fibrin as a thrombus is formed and so is perfectly situated for conversion by the tPA to plasmin, which can then digest the thrombus. Compounds capable of breaking down thrombi have enormous therapeutic potential for restoring blood flow before significant myocardial or cerebral infarction has occurred.

Virchow point 1: Alteration in the constituents of the blood
Blood that clots more readily than usual is termed **hypercoaguable**. This may be caused by a variety of different mechanisms including:

- an increase in blood cells (polcythaemia)
- increased numbers of platelets
- increased amount or aggregation of plasma proteins (myeloma, cryoglobulinaemia)
- loss of the plasma fraction of the blood (severe burns)
- severe trauma
- disseminated cancer
- late pregnancy

Presumably hypercoaguability results from either an increase in activated coagulation proteins, an increased risk of platelet aggregation or a decrease in anti-thrombotic proteins; however, the actual sequence of events leading to this state are not clear at present. Some mechanisms have been elucidated such as deficiencies of protein C and hereditary lack of antithrombin III.

Endothelium

The fact that the vascular tree is lined by endothelium means that the endothelial surface must be resistant to thrombus formation. The endothelium is quite remarkable, for it is capable of initiating both thrombogenic and antithrombogenic stimuli (Fig 2.7). Normally these two groups of actions are finely balanced in favour of preventing thrombus formation. Damage to the endo-thelium, however, will tip the balance towards thrombosis. The endothelium also has another very important role which is to prevent the elements of blood from coming into contact with the subendothelial connective tissue, which is highly thrombogenic. This tissue normally comprises collagen, elastin, fibronectin and glycosaminoglycans. **Collagen** is by far the most important of these constituents and it activates the coagulation pathway as well as being a strong stimulator of platelet aggregation. In vessels affected by atheroma, not only is the endothelium more readily damaged but the subendothelial tissue consists of the components of atheroma which are extremely thrombogenic.

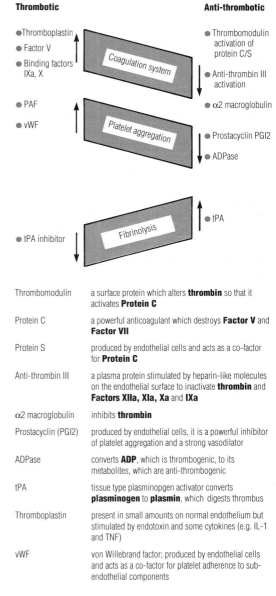

Thrombomodulin	a surface protein which alters **thrombin** so that it activates **Protein C**
Protein C	a powerful anticoagulant which destroys **Factor V** and **Factor VII**
Protein S	produced by endothelial cells and acts as a co-factor for **Protein C**
Anti-thrombin III	a plasma protein stimulated by heparin-like molecules on the endothelial surface to inactivate **thrombin** and **Factors XIIa, XIa, Xa** and **IXa**
α2 macroglobulin	inhibits **thrombin**
Prostacyclin (PGI2)	produced by endothelial cells, it is a powerful inhibitor of platelet aggregation and a strong vasodilator
ADPase	converts **ADP**, which is thrombogenic, to its metabolites, which are anti-thrombogenic
tPA	tissue type plasminopgen activator converts **plasminogen** to **plasmin**, which digests thrombus
Thromboplastin	present in small amounts on normal endothelium but stimulated by endotoxin and some cytokines (e.g. IL-1 and TNF)
vWF	von Willebrand factor; produced by endothelial cells and acts as a co-factor for platelet adherence to sub-endothelial components

Fig 2.7 Endothelial thrombotic/anti-thrombotic mechanisms

Virchow point 2: Damage to the endothelium
Endothelial damage is of most significance in **arterial thrombosis**. There may be obvious loss of endothelial cells or more subtle metabolic damage to the cells. Endothelial cells may be lost where an atheromatous plaque has ulcerated or when vessels are damaged by surgery, infection, immune-mediated damage (arteritis), indwelling vascular catheters or infusion of sclerosing chemicals in the treatment of varicose veins and haemorrhoids. Haemodynamic stress is believed to be important in producing metabolic damage to arterial endothelial cells in areas where there is turbulent flow or in patients with prolonged high blood pressure. Other potentially damaging agents include derivatives of cigarette smoke, bacterial toxins, immune complex deposition, transplant rejection and radiation.

In the heart, the endocardial surface is covered by endothelium which can be damaged in a myocardial infarction. Also the valve surface endothelium may be damaged by inflammatory endocarditis which promotes thrombus formation on valve leaflets resulting in altered function, a variety of heart murmurs and the danger of throwing emboli into the systemic circulation.

Clinically, the most important change is the endothelial damage related to atherosclerosis, which is discussed later in this chapter.

Blood Flow

Virchow point 3: Changes in the normal flow of blood
There are two principal ways in which the normal flow can be disturbed – the normal lamellar flow pattern can be altered (**turbulence**) or the speed may be reduced (**stasis**) – but both lead to similar changes.

During normal flow, red and white blood cells concentrate in the central, fast moving stream while platelets flow nearer to the periphery. The layer closest to the endothelium is usually devoid of cells and platelets but, if the blood flow slows down or turbulence produces local counter-currents, several factors increase the likelihood of thrombus formation:

- platelets come into contact with the endothelium
- turbulence may damage endothelial cells
- there is no inflow of fresh blood containing clotting factor inhibitors
- there is no clearance of blood containing activated coagulation factors

As you see, both turbulence and stasis operate in thrombosis but turbulence is more important in arteries whereas stasis is more important in veins.

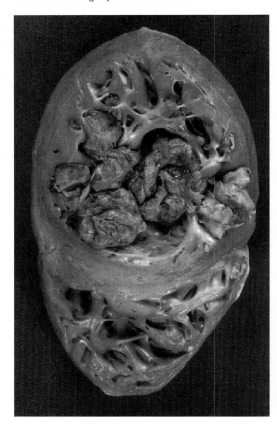

Fig 2.8 Apical section of heart with thrombus in left ventricle following myocardial infarction.

Discuss the factors influencing thrombus formation

Virchow's triad

Altered blood-
  ↑ cells
  ↑ platelets
  ↑ protein
  ↓ fluid

Altered wall-
  endothelial loss (atheroma)
  endothelial damage (smoking)

Altered flow-
  stasis
  turbulence

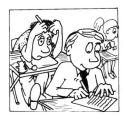

Arterial thrombosis

Turbulence of flow leading to thrombosis is of particular importance in the arterial side of the circulation. Turbulence tends to occur where arteries branch and over the irregular surface of an atheromatous plaque. It also occurs when cardiac valves have been damaged by inflammation, as may occur with rheumatic fever and infective endocarditis, or have been replaced by artificial valves.

Stasis is more likely to be of importance if the heart or arteries have been damaged. Abnormal dilatations of large vessels (aneurysms) will produce pockets of stagnant blood which will thrombose. Myocardial infarction may result in a localised area of damaged heart muscle, which does not move, or in an arrhythmia affecting the contraction of a whole chamber.

Venous thrombosis

Thrombus formation, related to stasis of blood, is more common in the venous circulation and particularly occurs in the legs or pelvic veins of immobile individuals. Why is stasis common in the leg vessels when the patient is immobilised? If you remember the physiology of venous return from the legs, you will recall that it is contraction of skeletal muscles which pushes blood along the veins and it is the presence of valves which ensures the direction of flow. Understanding this has influenced patient management. Patients are encouraged to move their legs regularly when confined to bed, leg muscles are stimulated to contract during long operations and it is no longer common to have patients bed-bound for weeks.

Thrombus formation often begins within the venous valve pockets. The initial cluster of platelets activates the clotting cascade to produce a small thrombus. A second phase of platelet aggregation then occurs to cover the original thrombus and promote a further wave of coagulation. This process is repeated again and again to extend the thrombus, so-called **propagation**. The resultant thrombus has alternate layers of platelets and a red cell/white cell/fibrin mixture which produces a rippled effect, termed '**lines of Zahn**'. The direction of the lines relates to the pattern of blood flow in the vessel.

Once a vessel is completely occluded by thrombus, blood flow ceases and the stagnant column of blood clots without the production of any 'lines of Zahn'. This is called '**consecutive**' clot and it is particularly dangerous because it is only adherent to the vessel wall through its attachment to the original focus of thrombus. This makes it especially likely to break off and embolise to another area (see later).

If the blood flow is slowed in the entire limb, then a very large consecutive clot is formed along the length of the limb's venous system. Alternatively, the consecutive clot only extends to the point where the next venous tributary enters the main vessel. Here the blood may be flowing at a reasonable speed, but the presence of activated clotting factors will promote the adherence of a layer of platelets which may result in a fresh wave of thrombosis from this

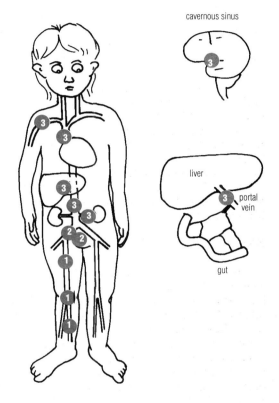

In order of frequency:	Associated factors
1. Leg veins	immobility, post-surgery and hyper-coagulability states
2. Pelvic veins	post-childbirth, puerperal sepsis, pelvic surgery and tumours
3. Others:	
inferior vena cava	extrinsic compression by tumour, extension from leg or iliac veins
renal vein	tumour extension from kidney
portal/hepatic veins	local sepsis, tumour compression
cavernous sinus	facial sepsis
superior vena cava	extrinsic compression by mediastinal tumour
axillary vein	trauma from rucksack, local surgery

Fig 2.9 Sites of venous thrombosis

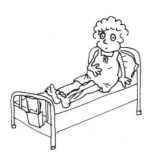

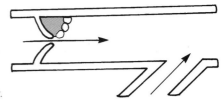

Decreased blood flow or increased coagulability
Thrombus forms in valve pocket. Platelets adhere to surface of thrombus.

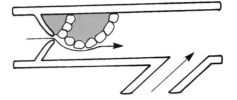

Platelet layer propagates further thrombus formation
"Lines of Zahn" formed by alternating red and white cell and platelet deposits, orientated along blood flow.
Fibrin contracts

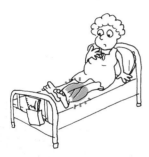

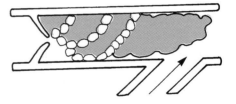

Once lumen occluded, 'consecutive' unstable, clot forms
No lines of Zahn, slow flow and no new platelets. Weakly attached to wall and easily dislodged.

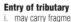

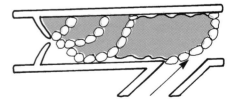

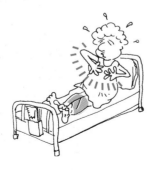

Entry of tributary
i. may carry fragments of thrombus into general circulation: embolisation
ii. may stabilize thrombus by re-attaching to wall

iii. permits further propagation

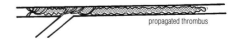

propagated thrombus

Fig 2.10 Venous thrombosis

point. The involvement of platelets, however, does mean that the clot will be anchored at the points where the tributaries enter and be slightly less likely to embolise. Arteries do not usually suffer from this potentially disastrous propagation of clot. These processes are illustrated in the Fig. 2.10.

It is also worth emphasising at this point that, like most phenomena in the body, the three major factors of Virchow's triad rarely work in isolation. In myocardial infarction, ischaemia damages the endothelial lining of the heart and the ischaemic myocardium fails to move normally, hence endothelial damage and local stasis contribute to thrombus formation within the ventricle. So, while it is imperative that one knows the basis for Virchow's triad, it is also important to remember that many factors interact to produce the final picture in a patient.

There are also a number of differences in the complications between arterial and venous thrombi and we deal with these next.

Natural history and complications of thrombosis

Once a thrombus has formed, what are the possible outcomes? As you know, the body possesses many effective systems for regulating thrombus formation during normal haemostasis. The ideal solution is that these systems halt the thrombotic process and remove the debris to leave a normal blood vessel. This process is termed **resolution**. If the thrombus cannot be removed, it may be **organised** or **recanalised**. Alternatively, it may be cast off into the circulation, i.e. it may **embolise**.

Resolution is thought to occur commonly in the small veins of the lower limb. Interestingly, venous intima contains more plasminogen activator than arterial intima, which may be the reason. Drugs with a thrombolytic action, such as streptokinase, can be given to patients early after thrombosis to promote dissolution of the clot and, hence, resolution. It is important that this drug is given within hours because the drug has much less effect on polymerised fibrin, which predominates later.

Organisation of a thrombus involves similar processes to the organisation of inflammation described in Chapter 1. When the thrombus has formed, polymorphs and macrophages begin to degrade and digest the fibrin and cell debris. Later, granulation tissue grows into the base of the thrombus so that the thrombus is converted into a mass of small vessels separated by connective tissue. These vessels originate from the vasa vasorum of the adventitia of the blood vessel and it is unlikely that the blood flowing through these is of much clinical importance (but see below for collateral circulation).

Compare and contrast arterial and venous thrombosis

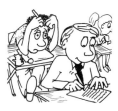

	Arterial	Venous
Patient risk factors	Presence of atheroma	Immobility
Major factors in pathogenesis	Turbulent flow Damaged endothelium	Stasis Hypercoagulable blood
Symptoms	Generally sudden onset	Generally slow onset
Complications	Infarction (small arteries) Arterial embolism (large arteries)	Pulmonary embolus

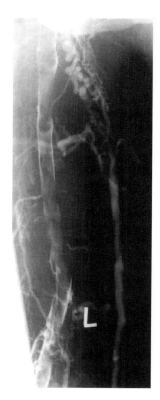

Fig 2.11 The femoral/popliteal vein (left in photo) is occluded by thrombus so that the contrast media only fills the edge of the vessel.

Resolution

Organisation

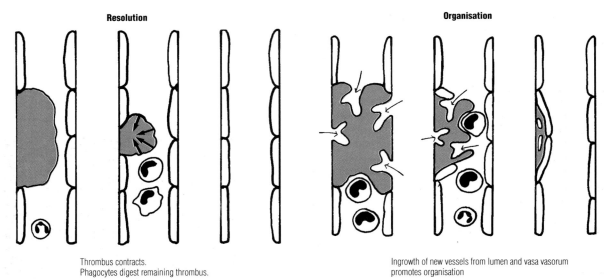

Thrombus contracts.
Phagocytes digest remaining thrombus.

Ingrowth of new vessels from lumen and vasa vasorum
promotes organisation

Luminal obliteration

Collateral circulation

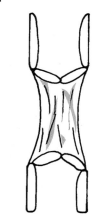

Failure to clear thrombus results in fibrous obliteration

Thrombus obliterates lumen and is replaced by a fibrous cord.
Collateral circulation opens up.

Recanalisation

Embolisation

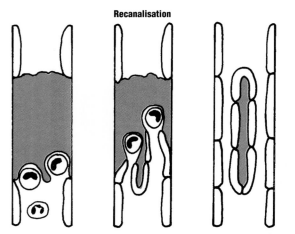

Phagocytes digest thrombus to produce channels that
become lined by endothelium

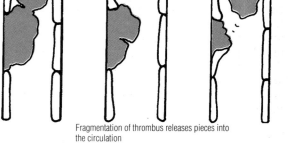

Fragmentation of thrombus releases pieces into
the circulation

Fig 2.12 Natural history and complications of thrombosis

Ultimately, the thrombus shrinks and is covered by endothelial or smooth muscle cells which produce platelet-derived growth factor (PDGF). As we shall see, this is of interest because of its potential role in the formation of atheromatous plaques (page 97).

Recanalisation is a term used by clinicians to indicate that there is useful flow through a previously occluded vessel. Obviously, if streptokinase treatment has been successful, the thrombus will be dissolved, the original intimal lining will still exist and the clinician will see flow on the arteriogram; he will call this recanalisation but we will not! A similar situation occurs if the clot retracts so that it is obstructing only part of the flow (2.12). The blood flow is, at least partially, restored but through the original lumen and not through new channels.

To a pathologist, recanalisation involves the production of *new* endothelial-lined channels which convey blood through the occlusive thrombus. This is thought to occur by the production of clefts within the thrombus, resulting from a combination of local digestion and shrinkage. The clefts extend through the clot and become lined by endothelial cells derived from the adjacent intima. This can produce several channels separated by loose connective tissue. The amount of flow through such a segment will depend on the number and size of the conduits but the vessel will not be 'as good as new'.

This is a convenient moment to digress and discuss the way in which the cardiovascular system tries to compensate for a reduced flow through a vessel. Just as you might try to avoid a traffic jam by driving through the back roads, so the blood will search for alternative routes. The availability of such routes depends on the local anatomy. In the venous circulation, there are specific anastomoses between the systemic and portal systems around the rectum, oesophagus and umbilicus; but the penetrating veins linking the deep and superficial lower limb venous plexuses are of more relevance to our patient with a deep vein thrombosis. Thus, if a segment of the deep veins is occluded, the blood will bypass it by moving into the superficial plexus.

The arterial system has some well-characterised alternative routes like the arterial roundabout of the circle of Willis and the dual arterial supply of the lung. However, most organs do not have a dual supply and must rely on collateral vessels opening up if the main supplying vessel is occluded. If we take the heart and coronary arteries as an example, then we can often see a collateral arterial circulation in a patient who has suffered a coronary artery thrombosis, as is demonstrated in Figs. 2.13, 2.14. The apparently new network of small vessels has always existed but, before the thrombus, little blood would flow through these channels because it was easier to flow down the larger artery. Now resistance to flow has increased in the main vessel, making the small channel route attractive and, hence, visible on arteriograms.

Where are these vessels? This is an area of great interest because, theoretically, any patient with a large network of

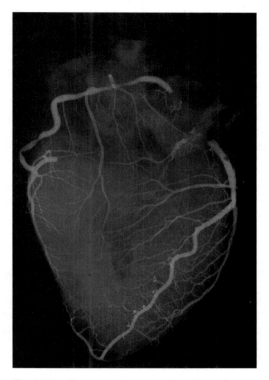

Fig 2.13 Coronary arteriogram showing main coronary arteries and numerous collateral vessels.

connecting vessels would have some protection from suffering a large myocardial infarction. There are three main possibilities which, in probable order of clinical importance, are:

● small arterioles within the myocardium
● side branches from the large coronary arteries
● vasa vasorum

John Hunter carried out an elegant experiment to demonstrate collateral circulation. He tied one of the carotid arteries in a stag from Richmond Park and observed the effect on the corresponding antler. The carotid pulse on that side disappeared and the antler went cold and stopped growing. Within a few weeks, however, the warmth returned and the antler started to grow again. Hunter demonstrated the collateral circulation by sacrificing the stag and injecting the carotid artery. Elegant as it was, such an experiment might not go down well nowadays!

We have noted that one of the complications of thrombosis is embolism and we will now go on to consider the different types of emboli and their complications.

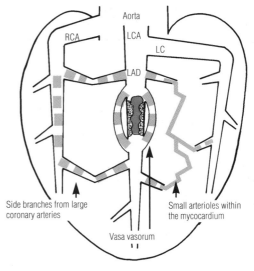

Key

LCA: left coronary artery

RCA: right coronary artery

LC: left circumflex

LAD: left anterior descending coronary artery

Fig 2.14 Collateral circulation

Embolism

An embolus is solid, liquid or gaseous material which is carried in the blood from one area of the circulatory system to another area. The majority of emboli arise from thrombi and, thus, there is a tendency to use the term **thromboembolism** as synonymous with embolism. This is not strictly true as there are many other, though admittedly rarer, causes of emboli. These include:

● fragments of atheromatous plaques
● bone marrow
● fat
● air or nitrogen
● amniotic fluid
● tumour
● foreign material, e.g. intravenous catheter

Since the majority of the emboli come from thrombi, we shall start our discussion with this particular type.

Where emboli lodge depends on their size, origin and the relevant cardiovascular anatomy. Those that arise in the venous system can travel through the right side of the heart to end up in the pulmonary circulation. Those that arise in the left side of the circulation will block systemic arteries and the clinical effect will depend on the organ involved, be it brain, kidneys, spleen or the periphery of limbs.

Emboli to the lungs from venous thrombosis represents an important preventable cause of morbidity in hospitalised patients and we shall consider this first.

Pulmonary embolism

The lungs are very interesting organs because they have a dual blood supply. Not only does the lung receive deoxygenated blood via the pulmonary arteries but also oxygenated blood from bronchial arteries feeding directly from the aorta. Hence, the lungs have an established collateral arterial circulation. This means that occlusion of a branch of the pulmonary artery rarely causes infarction of the lung parenchyma and, because the alveolar walls are intact, resolution is possible. The effects of a pulmonary embolus will depend on three factors:

- the size of the occluded vessel
- the number of emboli
- the adequacy of the bronchial blood supply

The size of the occluded vessel
If a **large embolus occludes a main pulmonary artery** or even sits astride the bifurcation of the pulmonary trunk, a so-called **saddle embolus**, the patient's blood pressure will suddenly drop and there may even be instant death. If the patient survives and reaches the hospital, it may be possible to lyse the embolus using medical therapy or remove it surgically (embolectomy). It is tempting to postulate that the circulatory collapse is due to acute strain put on the right heart by sudden obstruction to the outflow tract. However, this cannot be the whole story because patients tolerate ligation of the pulmonary artery during removal of a lung at surgery. Probably the left ventricular outflow drops because the left atrial filling has been reduced.

Around 95% of emboli originate in the ileofemoral venous system with a small number coming from the pelvic veins, calf muscle veins and superficial veins of the legs. Obviously, the diameter of these emboli will correspond with the diameter of the vessel of origin, which is less than the size of the major pulmonary arteries. So how does an embolus block a vessel larger than itself? It becomes coiled.

Not infrequently, a long single embolus may fragment in the circulation to produce numerous small emboli. These may reach the small pulmonary arteries as a 'shower' to occlude several vessels at the same time, producing similar sudden, severe clinical effects to a single large embolus.

If a **medium-sized pulmonary artery** becomes blocked, this may produce no clinical effect because the bronchial circulation is able to supply the lung parenchyma. Generally there will be local haemorrhage but no damage to the framework of the lung and so complete resolution can occur. If the haemorrhage is small, the patient may be asymptomatic but, if large, the patient may have some shortness of breath or haemoptysis.

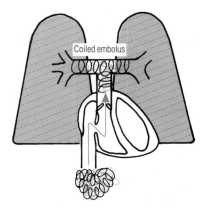

Large P.E.

Large embolus coils within major pulmonary artery. "Saddle" embolus blocks both pulmonary arteries. This produces circulatory collapse.

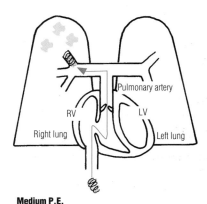

Medium P.E.

Dual blood supply protects lung from effects of pulmonary arterial obstruction.

Fig 2.15a Pulmonary Embolism

If the **small peripheral pulmonary arteries** are involved, there may be infarction because the area is beyond the territory of the bronchial collateral supply so the pulmonary arteries are, in effect, end arteries. Generally the area affected will be quite small but may produce symptoms, especially if there are multiple emboli.

The number of emboli

Multiple emboli may be thrown into the lungs as a single event or there may be successive embolic episodes. The first situation occurs when a single large embolus fragments into smaller emboli before reaching the lungs. The second scenario happens when initially only part of the thrombus breaks off but, hours or days later, a second piece follows. If a patient survives the initial pulmonary embolus, there is a 30% risk of suffering from a further embolus. This makes it extremely important that the patient receives prompt and effective anticoagulant therapy to reduce the risk. However, the anticoagulant therapy will not remove the existing embolus; that requires fibrinolytic treatment as described earlier. Sometimes a patient will remain in 'shock' despite complete lysis of the embolus and this is possibly due to intense vasoconstriction of the peripheral pulmonary vessels.

The adequacy of the bronchial blood supply

If a patient suffers from heart failure or has pre-existing pulmonary disease, the bronchial blood supply will be impaired and emboli lodging in medium-sized pulmonary arteries will result in infarction. Since the blockage is relatively proximal, the infarct will be large, extending as a cone with the apex at the blocked vessel and the base on the pleura. Initially, the area will be firm and purple because of the haemorrhage and congestion, but later it will be replaced by pale fibrous tissue and the area will shrink. Infarcts are most common in the lower lobes of the lungs and are multiple in 50% of cases.

These patients tend to get chest pain related to inflammation of adjacent pleura and shortness of breath due both to a reduction in lung volume and humoral and neural factors leading to vasoconstriction and bronchoconstriction (see page 82).

A typical clinical scenario is that of an elderly patient in hospital who has cardiac failure and a fractured neck of femur following a fall. The combination of recumbency, cardiac failure and postoperative dehydration combine to create an ideal situation for the formation of a deep vein thrombosis in the leg veins. A moderate-sized embolus, over a background of an inadequate collateral supply due to cardiac failure, results in significant ischaemia of the lung parenchyma and infarction.

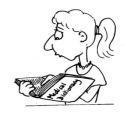

Dyspnoea; sensation of shortness of breath. When associated with cardiac failure, it may be due to pulmonary oedema interfering with gaseous exchange and lung stretch reflexes. If worse on lying flat, it is called orthopnoea

Haemoptysis; coughing up blood from the respiratory tract

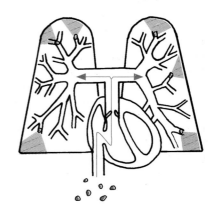

Multiple emboli combined with poor bronchial blood supply

Leads to pulmonary infarction

Bronchial artery supply not shown.

Fig. 2.15b Pulmonary Embolism

The fate of the embolus

In some ways this is similar to that of a thrombus. Ideally it will be lysed by the fibrinolytic system to restore patency of the vessel. If not, organisation takes place and the mass will be incorporated into the wall with possible recanalisation of the vessel. Spontaneous lysis is often very good so it is important to support the patient to allow 'nature' to do the healing.

If there are multiple emboli or repeated episodes of embolisation and organisation, the pulmonary vessel wall will thicken, resulting in a rise in pulmonary arterial pressure. This in turn means an increased work load for the right ventricle, which tries to compensate by becoming thicker (hypertrophy). Eventually, the right ventricle may not be able to compensate and cardiac failure will ensue. Right ventricular enlargement due to pulmonary disease is called **cor pulmonale**.

Systemic Embolism

Systemic emboli travel in the circulation and the majority originate in the left side of the heart from thrombi forming on areas of myocardial infarction. Other causes are listed opposite and include fragments of atheromatous plaques which result from fissuring or ulceration of a plaque which releases its fibrin, lipid and cholesterol mixture into the circulation.

Arterial emboli nearly always cause infarction. Emboli to the lower limbs may produce gangrene of a few toes or of the entire limb. Cerebral emboli cause death or infarction unless the embolus lodges in an area which receives adequate collateral supply through the circle of Willis. Other commonly affected sites are the upper limb and the gut, kidney and spleen. A special type of systemic embolus is the infected material from vegetations on the heart valves in **infective endocarditis**. These produce septic infarcts and large abscesses in the affected tissues.

Other types of emboli

The other types of emboli generally enter veins rather than arteries because veins have thinner walls and a lower pressure. Therefore, most are venous emboli which lodge in the lungs.

Bone marrow emboli

Bone marrow emboli are occasionally seen in histological sections of lungs at autopsy. This is especially likely if the patient has suffered major trauma, such as a road traffic accident, but can even occur with the 'trauma' of attempted cardiac resuscitation, particularly in elderly people whose costal cartilages have ossified. Anything which fractures bone can release bone and bone marrow into the venous circulation with resultant pulmonary emboli but the clinical significance of this type of embolisation is unclear.

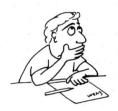

List the common sources of thromboemboli

Heart
left ventricle secondary to myocardial infarction
left atrium secondary to fibrillation
rheumatic heart disease
cardiomyopathy
infective endocarditis
valve prosthesis

Vessels
ulcerated arteriosclerotic plaques
aortic aneurysm
arterial prosthesis
paradoxical embolus; venous thrombi which pass through a right to left congenital cardiac anomaly

Fat emboli

Fat from the marrow cavities of long bones or from soft tissue also can enter the circulation as a result of severe trauma. However, they even form without any trauma (as listed opposite) and so alternative mechanisms must operate. Fortunately, although fat globules are found in the lungs of most victims of severe trauma, less than 5% will suffer from the 'fat embolism syndrome', which is characterised by respiratory problems and mental deterioration 24–72 hours after the injury. The syndrome is unlikely to result merely from mechanical blockage of vessels but probably involves **chemical injury** to the small vessels of the lungs, producing pulmonary oedema and activation of the **coagulation pathway** to cause disseminated intravascular coagulation (DIC). However, the exact mediators have not been identified. The origin of the fat in the non-trauma cases may be chylomicrons and fatty acids in the circulation coalescing to form droplets: the **emulsion instability theory**.

What are the causes of fat embolism?

severe trauma
diabetes mellitus
sickle cell disease
pancreatitis
hyperlipidaemias

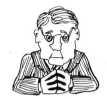

Air and nitrogen emboli

Large quantities of air within the circulation can act as emboli by forming a frothy mass which can block vessels or become trapped in the right heart chambers to impede its pumping. Air can either enter the circulation from the atmosphere or it can be produced within the circulation by alteration of pressure.

Severe trauma to the thorax may open large vessels allowing air to be sucked in during inspiration, or air may be forced into the uterine vessels during badly performed abortions or deliveries. Fortunately small quantities of air, as may be introduced during venesection, dissolve in the plasma and it probably takes about 100 ml to produce problems. A special type of air embolism occurs in deep sea divers. Normally insoluble gases, such as nitrogen or helium in the diver's breathing mixture, will dissolve in the blood and tissues at the high pressures which occur deep beneath the sea surface. As the diver surfaces, the pressure is reduced and the gas begins to come out of solution as minute bubbles. If the reduction of pressure is rapid then these bubbles form emboli which are particularly likely to lodge in the skeletal and cerebral circulation. The **acute form of decompression sickness** or 'bends' involves pain around joints and in skeletal muscle, respiratory distress and, sometimes, coma and death. In the early stages, it can be treated by putting the victim in a 'decompression' chamber where the high pressure will redissolve the bubbles and allow a slow, controlled decompression. The **chronic form** or **Caisson disease** produces multiple areas of ischaemic necrosis in the long bones.

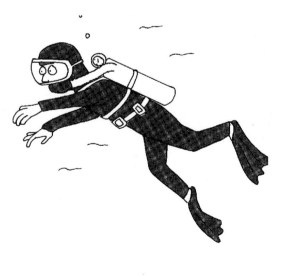

Amniotic fluid emboli

This is an uncommon, but life-threatening, form of embolisation. Basically, amniotic fluid is forced into the circulation due to tearing of the placental membranes and rupture of the uterine or cervical veins. These emboli are a mixture of fluid, fat, hair, mucus, meconium and squamous cells from the fetus and they most commonly lodge in the mother's alveolar capillaries. Clinically, there is sudden onset of respiratory failure often followed by cerebral convulsions and coma. There is also excessive bleeding as a result of DIC and the consumption of clotting factors. Over 80% of patients developing amniotic fluid emboli will die. The exact mechanism is still unclear but it is not simply due to blockage of the pulmonary vasculature; it is postulated that some factor, such as $PGF_{2\alpha}$ in the amniotic fluid may be involved.

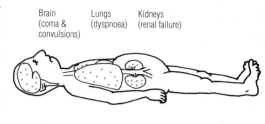

Brain (coma & convulsions) Lungs (dyspnoea) Kidneys (renal failure)

Most important affected sites

Tumour emboli

Embolisation of tumour is an important mechanism of tumour spread but it is unlikely to have any immediate cardiovascular effects. The mechanisms involved in this process will be discussed in Chapter 4.

Disseminated intravascular coagulation

This is a convenient moment to discuss DIC. We have just mentioned amniotic fluid embolism and we are about to move on to 'shock' – both conditions which can produce DIC. Furthermore, DIC results from a loss of control in the clotting and fibrinolytic systems, which should still be fresh in your memory!

There is no typical clinical presentation because any organ may be affected and the major problem may be excessive clotting, which blocks numerous vessels, or inadequate clotting resulting in haemorrhage. As a general rule, **sudden-onset DIC** presents with bleeding problems, is particularly associated with obstetrical complications and may resolve once the obstetric situation improves. In contrast, **chronic DIC** is commoner in patients with carcinomatosis and the thrombotic manifestations dominate.

Small thrombi form anywhere and produce microinfarcts. In the brain this may result in convulsions and coma, lung damage produces dyspnoea and cyanosis and renal changes cause oliguria and acute renal failure. Fibrin deposition not only produces thrombi but also results in a haemolytic anaemia as the red cells fragment whilst squeezing through the narrowed vasculature (**microangiopathic haemolytic anaemia**).

The fundamental problem is that there is excessive activation of coagulation which ultimately is complicated by consumption of the coagulation factors and overactivity of the fibrinolytic system. Clotting activation occurs through the extrinsic pathway, initiated by tissue thromboplastin, and the intrinsic pathway, commencing with activated factor XII. However, it must be remembered that clotting activation will also stimulate the fibrinolytic pathways, particularly through the factor XII path, and fibrin

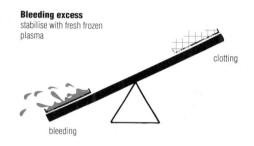
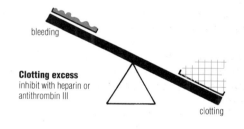
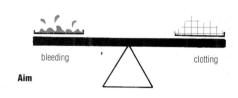

Bleeding excess stabilise with fresh frozen plasma

Clotting excess inhibit with heparin or antithrombin III

Aim

Fig 2.16 Disseminated intravascular coagulation (DIC)

degradation products inhibit fibrin production. These latter mechanisms will predominate in haemorrhagic DIC.

Many of the diseases mentioned produce DIC via the extrinsic pathway. For example, the placenta is believed to release tissue thromboplastin in obstetrical problems, mucus from some adenocarcinomas can activate factor X and bacterial endotoxins can prompt the release of thromboplastic substances contained in endothelial and inflammatory cells. However, nothing involving bacterial endotoxins is simple! They can also activate the intrinsic pathway directly through factor XII and indirectly by damaging endothelial cells. They even inhibit the anticoagulant activity of protein C.

Not surprisingly, the prognosis is very variable and the management extremely difficult because one is trying to balance a see-saw which is out of control. If you inhibit the clotting system too much with heparin or antithrombin III, the patient will bleed, but any bleeding tendency may require fresh frozen plasma which may contribute to microthrombus formation.

We shall now move on to discuss 'shock', which can produce DIC and may result from many causes, including massive embolism.

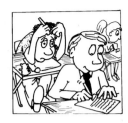

What are the major causes of DIC?

Infection
gram negative organisms
meningococci

Obstetrical complication
preeclamptic toxaemia
placental abruption
amniotic fluid embolism

Malignant tumours
pancreas
prostate
lung

Massive tissue damage
trauma
burns

Which organs are commonly affected by DIC?

kidneys
brain
heart
lungs
adrenals
liver
spleen

Shock

Shock is a wonderful word! It means such different things to medical and lay people. How often we hear news reports that someone has been taken to hospital suffering from shock after witnessing some tragic event. No doubt that person is surprised and possibly emotionally disturbed but they are not in a state of **circulatory collapse**, which is what a doctor regards as shock.

The 'shocked' patient is desperately ill and requires intensive treatment both to correct the condition which has produced the circulatory collapse and also to cope with the widespread ischaemic damage resulting from shock. By definition, the patient will have hypoperfusion of many tissues. His blood pressure may be low but need not be, as he may either have compensated by increasing peripheral vasoconstriction to keep the pressure normal or he may have had a high blood pressure which has now dropped. There may be pallor, cold extremities, sweating and a tachycardia; the first two signs are due to poor perfusion and the other two result from the attempt to compensate, which includes the release of adrenaline.

What has happened to precipitate this disastrous state? Well, logically, there will be a sudden generalised poor perfusion if the pump fails or if there is insufficient blood, so-called **cardiogenic** and **hypovolaemic** shock. Abrupt heart failure may result from myocardial infarction, arrhythmias and cardiac tamponade while hypovolaemic shock follows fluid loss due to haemorrhage, severe burns, diarrhoea or vomiting. Shock following pulmonary embolism mimics cardiogenic shock but the heart is normal and the reduced output is because the left atrial filling has dropped. A rather special but clinically very important form of shock is 'septic shock' due to overwhelming infection, especially those caused by Gram negative bacteria which have endotoxic lipopolysaccharides. Here the pathogenesis is complicated because of the varied effects of the bacterial products on endothelial cells, platelets and leucocytes which leads to a veritable web of interactions resulting in DIC and reduced blood volume because of vasodilatation and increased vascular permeability.

Whatever the cause, the effect at tissue level is similar with a reduced delivery of oxygen and nutrients so that the normal functions of cells are disturbed. The details of reversible and irreversible cell injury will be discussed in Chapter 3, so here we will concentrate on the clinical effects. The most important organs for immediate survival are the heart and brain, so the body has mechanisms for shunting blood from other tissues to protect these two organs. Frequently the kidneys and lungs will be underperfused and sufficiently damaged to be the immediate cause of death.

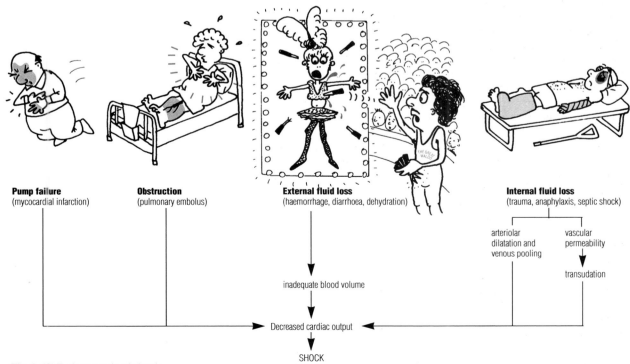

Fig 2.17 Pathogenesis of shock

Vascular changes

Bronchial changes

Release of serotonin and
thromboxane by platelets

Major vessel
obstruction and
vasoconstriction

Bronchoconstriction

Major pulmonary embolus

Hypoxia

Right heart strain
and reduced left
atrial filling

Heart failure

SHOCK

Fig 2.18 Pathogenesis of shock in pulmonary embolism

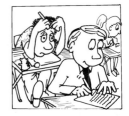

**Describe the damage that may occur in the organs of
a patient with shock.**

kidney	acute tubular necrosis
lung	ARDS
heart	ischaemic damage
brain	watershed infarcts
liver	fatty change/ necrosis
adrenal	focal haemorrhagic necrosis
pancreas	pancreatitis
stomach	erosive gastritis
duodenum	ulceration
small & large bowel	haemorrhagic gastroenteropathy/infarction

**What are the most important mediators of vascular
dilatation and increased permeability in septic
shock?**
histamine
thromboxane
serotonin
prostaglandins
leukotrienes
TNFα
IL-1α
C3a & C5a

Renal damage

Impaired renal blood flow results in **acute tubular necrosis**, a major cause of acute renal failure. This is not apparent immediately in a 'shocked' patient but will become evident once their 'shocked' state is under control and there is no circulatory reason for poor urine output. Then the patient will be noted to have oliguria (urine output of 40–400 ml/day; normal = 1500 ml/day), salt and water overload, a high plasma potassium and urea, and a metabolic acidosis. At this stage a renal biopsy would show numerous foci of tubular epithelial cell loss, affecting any area of the nephron, and epithelial 'casts', i.e. dead epithelial cells present in the tubular lumens. Grossly, the kidneys are large, swollen and congested, often with a pale cortex adjacent to a hyperaemic outer medulla due to blood pooling.

The important clinical point is that the patient with acute tubular necrosis can make a complete recovery provided that their renal problems are adequately handled (e.g. by dialysis) and that the cause of the shock can be rectified. After a few days, the tubular epithelium will regenerate and the urine volume will increase, often to above normal values because the tubules are unable to concentrate the urine, and there may be excessive loss of water, sodium and potassium – the so-called diuretic phase. Slowly the tubular epithelium returns to normal and reasonable renal function is restored.

Cardiac damage

The cause of the shock may lie within the heart (cardiogenic shock) but additional damage may then be produced by the hypoperfusion. There may be petechial haemorrhages or infarcts on the endocardial and epicardial surfaces, particularly of the left side of the heart. Zonal lesions may be apparent microscopically and consist of opaque transverse bands in a myocyte close to an intercalated disc, with distortion of myofilaments and Z bands. These are also seen following catecholamine administration and the use of a heart bypass pump during surgery.

Brain damage

Damage to the brain may be mild or devastating. The neurones are most vulnerable to ischaemia, particularly the large Purkinje cells of the cerebellum and the pyramidal cells in the hippocampus. A short episode of hypoperfusion may not cause any irreversible neuronal damage, or the number of neurones damaged may be too few to produce any clinical effect beyond temporary confusion. However, prolonged ischaemia will result in infarction which most commonly affects the 'watershed' areas at the junctional zones between the main arterial territories (see Fig. 2.19). This may result in severe permanent cerebral damage or coma and death.

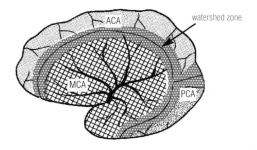

Lateral aspect of (L) cerebral hemisphere

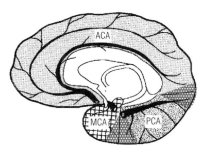

Medial aspect of (R) cerebral hemisphere

Key:
MCA Middle cerebral artery
ACA Anterior cerebral artery
PCA Posterior cerebral artery

Fig 2.19 Cerebral arterial supply – the watershed zones

Adult respiratory distress syndrome

The lungs are fairly resistant to short periods of ischaemia but, if prolonged, the patient may develop '**shock lung**' or '**adult respiratory distress syndrome**' (ARDS). This can be life-threatening as it is difficult to maintain adequate ventilation, even with a mechanical ventilator. For oxygen to reach the alveolar blood, air must move in and out of the lungs and be able to diffuse across the alveolar septae. In 'shock lung' there is severe oedema affecting peribronchial connective tissue and alveolar septae and spaces. This both reduces the lung compliance and impairs alveolar diffusion; that means double trouble and a mortality rate of around 50%.

The probable sequence of events (see Fig. 2.21) is that the 'shock' causes the release of mediators, such as activated complement (C5a), leukotriene B4 and platelet activating factor, which promote leucocyte aggregation and activation in the lung. The neutrophils produce arachidonic acid metabolites, such as thromboxane, which cause pulmonary vasoconstriction, oxygen-derived free radicals which injure the endothelial and epithelial cells, and lysosomal enzymes which digest local structural proteins.

The damaged alveolar capillary *endothelial* cells are leaky, which leads to interstitial alveolar oedema and fibrin exudation. The damaged alveolar *epithelial* cells, particularly the type I pneumocytes, desquamate to form the characteristic hyaline membranes in combination with surfactant and protein-rich oedema fluid (see *Fig. 2.20*). These are the same as the hyaline membranes in neonatal hyaline membrane disease and in both situations indicate severe epithelial injury with lack of surfactant. The lack of surfactant leads to collapse of alveolar air spaces (atelectasis) and so further reduces compliance and gas transfer.

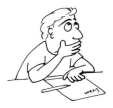

List some causes of ARDS

shock
diffuse pulmonary infection especially viral
oxygen toxicity
inhalation of toxins or organic solvents
aspiration pneumonitis
paraquat
cardiac surgery involving extra-corporeal pumps

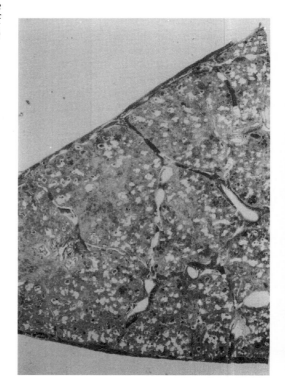

Fig 2.20 A section of lung from a patient with ARDS demonstrating the reduction in air spaces as alveoli fill with oedema and hyaline membranes.

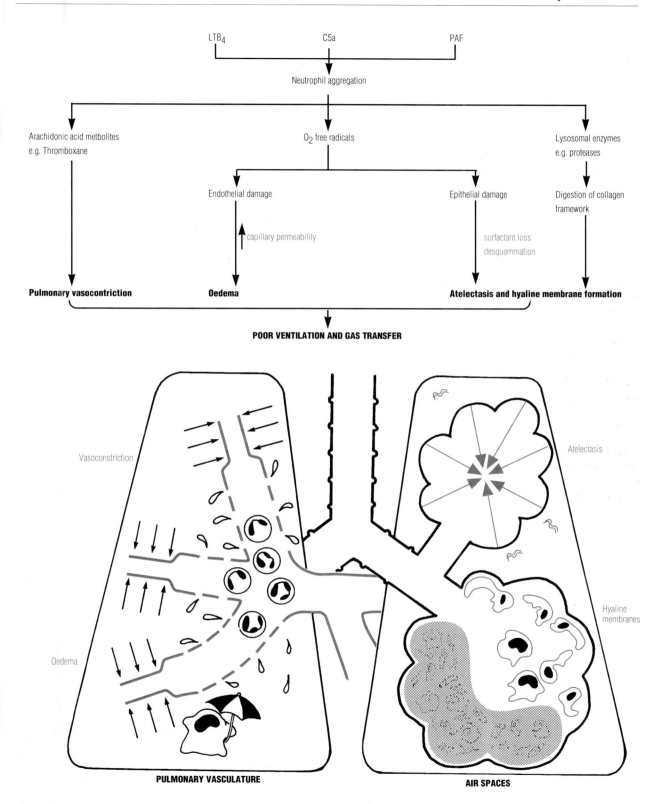

Fig 2.21 Adult respiratory distress syndrome (ARDS)

Arteriosclerosis

The first half of this chapter has concentrated on thrombosis, embolism and shock, all conditions which may suddenly affect healthy people of any age. Now we will move on to the major cardiovascular problems of later life, namely arteriosclerosis, hypertension, myocardial infarction and aneurysms. These are overwhelming causes of morbidity and mortality in developed countries but they are not an inevitable consequence of aging and so it is of great importance to try to identify the causative and risk agents.

The arteriopath

Let us briefly consider a possible clinical picture in a patient debilitated by vascular problems. A 48 year old man complains of blurring of his vision. He is known to suffer from diabetes which is a complex metabolic disorder characterised by hyperglycaemia (raised blood glucose). At the age of 14 years, he presented with the typical diabetic symptoms of tiredness, weight loss, polyuria (increased urine production) and polydypsia (increased thirst). The blood glucose was raised, glucose was found in his urine and he has been on insulin therapy since that time.

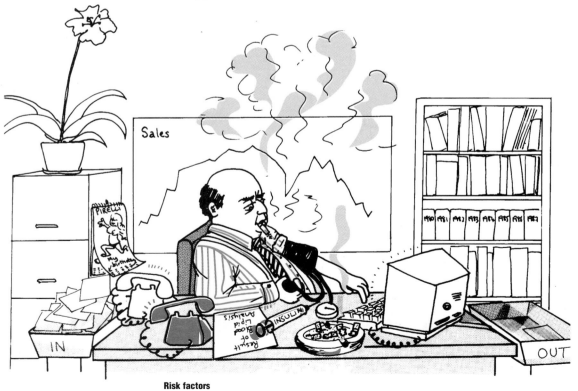

Fig 2.22 The arteriopath

Risk factors
- age
- sex (male)
- obesity
- smoking
- diabetes
- lack of exercise
- hypertension
- hyperlipidaemia
- "Type A" personality (impatient workaholic)

His present complaint of blurred vision started three months ago. On questioning, he also complained of shortness of breath, especially on exertion, and cramps in his calf muscles on exercise. On examination, he was found to have a raised blood pressure, a mild degree of cardiac failure with pulmonary oedema, small haemorrhages and small blood vessel proliferation in his retina and systolic bruits in his neck (abnormal sounds, heard through the stethoscope, caused by turbulent blood flow). His blood tests showed a small rise in urea and creatinine indicating a degree of renal impairment.

This unfortunate man is an 'arteriopath', i.e. he has widespread disease related to arterial pathology. The arterial pathology comes under the general heading of **arteriosclerosis**, commonly referred to as 'hardening of the arteries', although this does not relate to a specific pathologically recognised entity. His large and medium-sized arteries are likely to be narrowed by fibrolipid **atherosclerotic** lesions (see next section) and his small arteries and arterioles will show the proliferative or hyaline changes of **arteriolosclerosis**. Atherosclerosis is principally a disease of the intima and may result in narrowing of the vessel, obstruction or thrombosis. Arteriolosclerosis, on the other hand, affects the media with a resultant increase in wall thickness and decreased elasticity which may lead to hypertension.

Let's look at his symptoms to see if we can suggest a cause for each problem.

- His long-standing diabetes makes him much more likely to develop atherosclerosis than non-diabetic people of the same age.
- Fibrolipid atheromatous plaques in his coronary arteries will reduce the perfusion of the cardiac muscle resulting in chronic ischaemia which damages the heart muscle so that it pumps less efficiently. Because the left side of the heart generally fails first this will result in pulmonary oedema.
- Atheroma in the carotid arteries produces the bruit heard on auscultation and may lead to cerebral infarction.
- The combination of poor cardiac function and atheromatous plaques in the abdominal aorta and femoral vessels will explain the pain and cramp in his calf muscle, which is secondary to poor perfusion.
- Hyaline arteriolosclerosis will affect small renal vessels leading to glomerular damage which will induce hypertension through a complicated mechanism involving the hormones renin and angiotensin. This exacerbates the atheroma and worsens the cardiac failure.
- The cause of his blurred vision may be of vascular origin as the retina is frequently damaged by small haemorrhages, microaneurysms and new vessel formation, although diabetes can produce a host of other ocular changes.

The next stage in understanding this man's disease is to consider the actual appearance of his vessels.

What does the vessel look like?

The lesion of atherosclerosis is not one specific entity but a spectrum of arterial changes including:

- atheromatous fibrolipid plaques
- fatty streaks
- intimal cushion lesions

Inevitably there is controversy over whether the different lesions are stages in the evolution of an atheromatous plaque and we shall review the evidence when describing each lesion. From the clinical point of view, it is the atheromatous fibrolipid plaque which is to blame for producing occlusive vascular disease.

Atheromatous plaque

The **atheromatous plaque**, which is also referred to as a fibrous or fibrolipid plaque, is raised above the surrounding intima and protrudes into the lumen. It is whitish-yellow in colour and varies in size from 0.5 to 1.5 cm and may even become bigger if adjacent plaques coalesce. On slicing, the plaque is composed of a **fibrous cap** covering a soft yellow lipid centre, which reminded the early pathologists of porridge or gruel and so was termed **atheroma**. The intima is greatly thickened by the fibrofatty deposition and the media may be thinned due to a loss of smooth muscle cells resulting in both a loss of elasticity and a weakening of the wall. Generally the fibrous cap is composed of smooth muscle cells, collagen, elastin and proteoglycans. Beneath this there is a more cellular region of macrophages, T lymphocytes and smooth muscle cells covering the soft gruel-like mass of lipid, cellular debris, cholesterol clefts, plasma proteins and lipid-laden cells (foam cells) derived from macrophages and smooth muscle cells. At the edges of the lesion, there may be new vessel formation.

These plaques are more common in the aorta, femoral, carotid and coronary arteries where they may produce clinical problems by causing partial or complete occlusion, thrombosis, embolism or aneurysm formation (see later). Areas of turbulent flow are worst affected so that lesions often occur around the ostia of vessels. Interestingly, the abdominal aorta is more liable to atheroma than the thoracic aorta but the explanation for this is unknown.

Fatty streak

Fatty streaks, like atheromatous plaques, occur in large muscular and elastic arteries but differ in that they are commonest in the region of the aortic ring and the thoracic aorta. They do not affect blood flow but could represent a precursor lesion for atheromatous plaques. They first appear as tiny, round or oval flat yellow dots which become arranged in rows and finally coalesce to form a streak. The earliest streak is composed of just lipid-laden macrophages and T cells without any smooth muscle proliferation or extracellular lipid. Later, extracellular lipid and smooth muscle cells are found together with collagen, elastin and

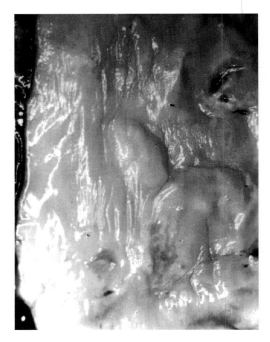

Fig 2.23 Abdominal aorta showing the irregular surface produced by atheromatous plaques

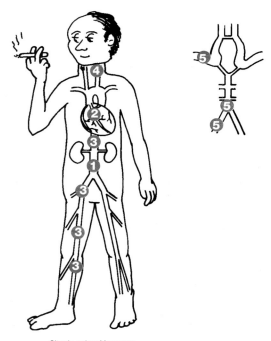

Sites in order of frequency:
1. Abdominal aorta
2. Proximal coronary arteries
3. Descending thoracic aorta, femoral and popliteal arteries
4. Internal carotid artery
5. Vertebral/basilar/middle cerebral arteries

Fig 2.24 Distribution of atheroma

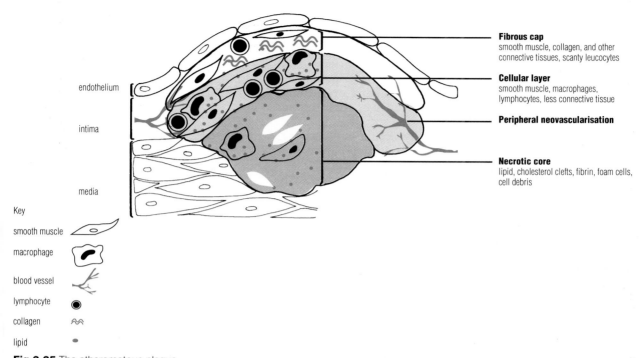

Fibrous cap
smooth muscle, collagen, and other connective tissues, scanty leucocytes

Cellular layer
smooth muscle, macrophages, lymphocytes, less connective tissue

Peripheral neovascularisation

Necrotic core
lipid, cholesterol clefts, fibrin, foam cells, cell debris

endothelium

intima

media

Key

smooth muscle

macrophage

blood vessel

lymphocyte

collagen

lipid

Fig 2.25 The atheromatous plaque

proteoglycans. Thus, the components are similar to those of an atheromatous plaque but there is far less fat and no necrotic centre. However, some people would only use the term 'fatty streak' for the earliest stage with the other forms representing a progression towards a fibrolipid plaque.

The aortic surface area covered by streaks increases up to the third decade but then declines as atheromatous plaques occupy the intima. Interestingly, they occur proximal to branch points and ostia in areas of low haemodynamic stress and so are not correctly sited to be forerunners of fibrolipid plaques. The population distribution is also very different, with fibrolipid plaques more common in males in developed countries whereas fatty streaks are found from a very early age and are independent of sex, race or geography.

Intimal cushion lesions

An **intimal cushion** is a white thickening at a branching point or ostium due to an increase in extracellular matrix and smooth muscle cells. There is almost no lipid and the suggestion that this is a precursor lesion for fibrolipid plaques is based on the similarity in their distribution and the presence of smooth muscle proliferation. Even in early infancy, smooth muscle cells have entered the intima raising the possibility that man is predestined to atheroma if suitable additional factors are present later.

Hyaline and hyperplastic arteriolosclerosis

Hyaline and hyperplastic arteriolosclerotic changes are very different to atheromatous damage. They only affect small vessels, do not have any increase in lipid and primarily affect the media, whereas atheroma is initially an **intimal** problem. Both are very important because of their strong association with hypertension.

Hyaline arteriolosclerosis generally occurs in elderly or diabetic patients and involves the deposition of homogeneous, pink material which thickens the media, resulting in a narrowed vessel. This material is probably a combination of increased extracellular matrix, produced by smooth muscle cells, and plasma components which have leaked through a damaged endothelium.

Hyperplastic arteriolosclerosis is found in patients who have a rather sudden or severe prolonged increase in blood pressure. The media of the vessel wall is thickened by a concentric proliferation of smooth muscle cells and an increase in basement membrane material. In the worst cases (malignant hypertension), there may be fibrinoid necrosis of the vessel walls.

Monckeberg's medial calcific stenosis

Another, but less important, form of arteriosclerosis is Monckeberg's medial calcific stenosis. This involves calcification of the media of muscular arteries and frequently occurs in the lower limb arteries of elderly people in association with atherosclerosis, but can occur in any organ. It is not thought to have much clinical significance but it delights, and sometimes confuses, radiologists. The cause is unknown but it is probably a degenerative change complicated by dystrophic calcification.

Risk factors for atherosclerosis

Now that we have a mental image of the appearance and distribution of atherosclerosis, we shall consider the risk factors which are believed to be important.

Age
Deaths from ischaemic heart disease increase with advancing age. However, populations of a similar age need not have the same amount of atheroma which suggests that it is not an inevitable degenerative process but may indicate the exposure time required for some causative agent. Interestingly, initial involvement by atheroma affects different vessels at different ages. Thus, small aortic lesions appear in the first decade, coronary artery lesions in the second decade and cerebral arterial lesions in the third decade.

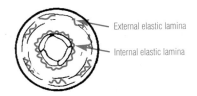

Normal artery

External elastic lamina
Internal elastic lamina

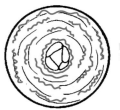

Hyaline arteriolosclerosis

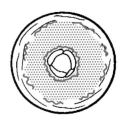

Reduplication of elastic laminae

Hyperplastic arteriolosclerosis

Sex

The death rate from ischaemic heart disease is higher in males than in females up to the age of 75 years, after which the incidence is similar. Myocardial infarction is extremely rare in premenopausal women suggesting that endocrine differences may be important and that the effect of oestrogens on lipid metabolism is a possible mechanism.

Smoking

Smoking one packet of cigarettes a day increases the likelihood of having a myocardial infarction by 300%. Traditionally more men than women have smoked but, as women have taken up the habit, their risk has risen. Fortunately, giving up smoking reduces the risk fairly quickly which means it is likely that smoking does not only promote atheroma but may also influence other factors, such as local thrombotic tendencies due to altered platelet function, which are necessary to convert clinically quiescent atheroma into an occlusive episode. An abstinence of one to two years reduces the risk of myocardial infarction to 'only' twice that of non-smokers. So-called 'safer' cigarettes, which have a lower tar and nicotine content, reduce the risk of bronchial carcinoma but do not appear to reduce the risk of coronary heart disease. How smoking damages vessels is not known but suggestions include increased free radical activity, raised carbon monoxide levels or a direct effect of nicotine.

Hypertension

Hypertension significantly increases the risk of ischaemic heart disease and 'strokes'. The diastolic blood pressure level is considered more important than the systolic level and a diastolic pressure consistently greater than 95 mmHg is deemed harmful. Drug treatment to reduce the blood pressure decreases the risk in patients with moderate to severe hypertension but it is unclear whether it benefits patients with mild hypertension. Most of the evidence suggesting the role of hypertension as a risk factor involves complex multifactorial analysis of large studies which, although the proper method for assessing the evidence, is not as easy to grasp as some simpler observations. Evidence of the direct role of hypertension in producing atheroma comes from two examples of congenital abnormalities of the cardiovascular system. Patients with congenital narrowing of part of the aorta (**coarctation**) develop atheroma in the proximal hypertensive segment but not in the distal region, where the pressure is lower. The other example is the rare abnormality of having one coronary artery originating from the low pressure pulmonary artery. The coronary artery linked to the aorta develops atheromatous changes with age but the artery linked to the pulmonary supply remains atheroma free.

What are risk factors for atherosclerosis?

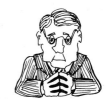

age
sex
smoking
hypertension
hyperlipidaemia
diabetes

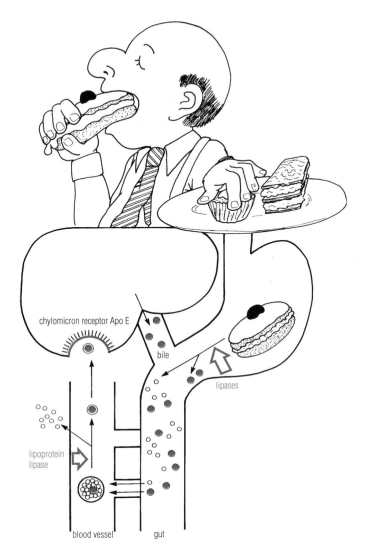

Fig. 2.26 Exogenous cholesterol pathway

Cholesterol enters the gut in the diet or in bile. Cholesterol and triglycerides are absorbed from the gut to be transported in the blood as chylomicrons. Triglycerides are delivered to a variety of tissues. The cholesterol is delivered to the liver when the chylomicron remnant is endocytosed via a receptor which recognises apoprotein E on its surface. Some cholesterol may be secreted in bile; the rest enters the endogenous cholesterol pathway.

Table 2.1 Hyperlipoproteinaemias

Type	Increased lipoprotein class	Primary defect
1	Chylomicrons	Deficiency of lipoprotein lipase
2a	LDL	Deficiency of LDL receptor
2b	LDL and VLDL	Unknown
3	Chylomicron remnants and IDL	Abnormal apoprotein E
4	VLDL	Unknown
5	VLDL and chylomicrons	Unknown and familial apoprotein CII deficiency

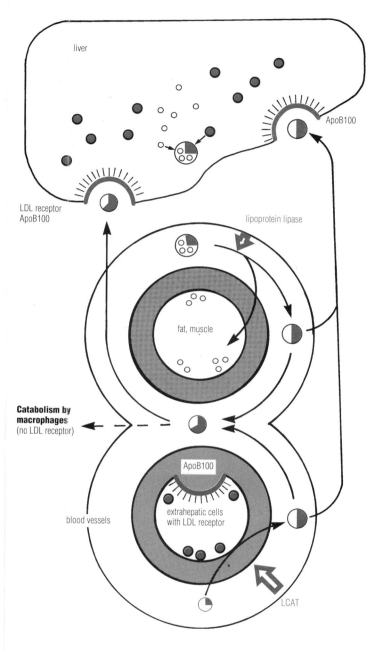

liver

ApoB100

LDL receptor
ApoB100

lipoprotein lipase

fat, muscle

**Catabolism by
macrophages**
(no LDL receptor)

ApoB100

extrahepatic cells
with LDL receptor

blood vessels

LCAT

Fig. 2.27 Endogenous cholesterol pathway

Cholesterol is secreted in very low density lipoproteins (VLDL), which are broken down by lipoprotein lipase in the endothelium of the capillaries in fat and muscle to release triglycerides and form intermediate density lipoproteins (IDL). Some IDL are absorbed by the liver via the LDL receptor, which recognises apoprotein B100; the remainder are metabolised to low density lipoproteins (LDL). LDL are taken up by the numerous extrahepatic tissues which bear the LDL receptor, and the remainder is either taken up by the liver or catabolised by macrophages. High density lipoproteins (HDL), also secreted by the liver, remove cholesterol from the tissues. This is catalysed by plasma lecithin-cholesterol acyltransferase (LCAT). IDL and LDL are formed by a series of metabolic steps

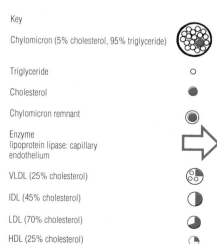

Key

Chylomicron (5% cholesterol, 95% triglyceride)

Triglyceride

Cholesterol

Chylomicron remnant

Enzyme
lipoprotein lipase: capillary
endothelium

VLDL (25% cholesterol)

IDL (45% cholesterol)

LDL (70% cholesterol)

HDL (25% cholesterol)

Fig 2.27 Endogenous cholesterol pathway

Hyperlipidaemia

Evidence for the role of fats in atheroma comes from a variety of sources. One approach is to analyse the contents of atheromatous plaques, another is to review retrospective population data to look for correlations between diet and clinical vascular disease. The experimentalist will look for animal models and the interventionalist will attempt to modify patients' diets in prospective studies. Hopefully, the combined information will lead to a common theory which can be used to provide advice or medication to reduce an individual patient's risk of atherosclerosis. The literature on the role of lipids in atherosclerosis would fill a library so we shall just highlight some of the more important points.

The analytical evidence
- Atheromatous lesions contain far more lipid than the adjacent intima.
- Atheromatous plaques are rich in cholesterol and cholesterol esters (65–80%), derived from blood lipoproteins.
- The major fatty acid in fibrolipid plaques is linoleic acid compared with oleic acid in juvenile fatty streaks.
- In normal arterial tissue, low density lipoproteins (LDL) from the plasma are preferentially retained compared with other plasma components.

$$\frac{\text{LDL in intima}}{\text{LDL in plasma}} : \frac{\text{albumin in intima}}{\text{albumin in plasma}} = 7:1$$

The experimental evidence
- Intimal lesions can be produced in some animals by increasing the plasma concentration of certain lipids through drug or diet manipulation.
- Smooth muscle cells accumulate cholesterol (LDL) and this is increased if there is endothelial damage.
- Immune stimulation (e.g. by injection of foreign protein) enhances the development of atheroma in rabbits *provided* that they are on high cholesterol diets.

Retrospective studies
- In populations with a high incidence of atherosclerosis, there are high plasma concentrations of certain lipids (LDL rich in cholesterol appear most harmful, very low density lipoproteins (VLDL) do some harm but high density lipoproteins (HDL) appear cardioprotective).
- In families with genetic disorders causing severe hypercholesterolaemia (see Table 2.1), there is severe early atherosclerosis.
- In groups with acquired hypercholesterolaemia (e.g. hypothyroidism and nephrotic syndrome), atherosclerosis is increased

Fig 2.28 Formation of the atheromatous plaque: "reaction to injury" theory

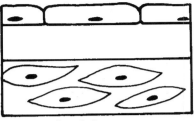

Normal artery

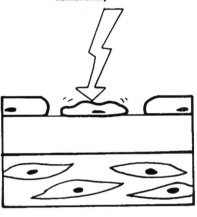

Endothelial damage
by toxic agents

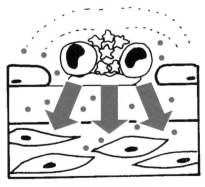

Platelet and leucocyte aggregation
PDGF and other growth factors released.
Chemotactic stimuli to other leucocytes.
Lipid insudation

Prospective studies
- Cardiovascular mortality can be reduced in *selected* patients with *hypercholesterolaemia* by lowering the plasma cholesterol with diet or drugs (e.g. cholestyramine).
- Plasma cholesterol levels can be lowered by reducing the dietary intake of cholesterol and *saturated* fats.

Diabetes

The risk of a myocardial infarction in a diabetic patient is twice that of a non-diabetic patient and, as our clinical scenario illustrated, their arterial disease is widespread

Other possible risk factors

- Lack of regular exercise
- Obesity
- High carbohydrate intake
- Oral contraceptives
- 'Type A' personality
- Hyperuricaemia and gout

How is the atheromatous plaque produced?

Now that we know who is most likely to suffer from atherosclerosis, we need to look at the theories of how atheroma is produced and to assess how well these theories explain the occurrence, distribution, known risk factors and experimental evidence.

There are two main theories: the 'reaction to injury' theory and the 'monoclonal hypothesis'. The former has its origin deep within the history books as it incorporates the ideas of Virchow, Duguid and Rokitansky.

Reaction to injury theory

Virchow believed that leakage of plasma proteins and lipid from the blood to the subendothelial tissue stimulated intimal cell proliferation. He regarded the cell proliferation as a form of low grade inflammation and termed it the 'imbibition hypothesis'; later often called the 'insudation' or 'infiltration' hypothesis. Rokitansky is credited with the 'encrustation' theory which suggested that thrombi forming on damaged endothelium could become organised to form a plaque. The modern 'reaction to injury' theory was proposed by Ross and Glomset in 1976. Essentially they suggest that some change or damage to the vascular endothelium causes increased permeability to proteins and lipid and also leads to the aggregation of platelets and monocytes. These leucocytes release various enzymes and growth factors which promote smooth muscle cell proliferation Monocytes migrate from the blood into the subendothelial layers, where they become macrophages and ingest the lipid. A short, sharp injury can be completely repaired but chronic repeated injury leads to the formation of an atheromatous plaque.

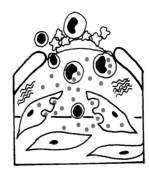

Leucocyte influx
Macrophages ingest lipid and become "foam cells".
Smooth muscle cells migrate from media to:
1. ingest lipid, becoming "foam cells"
2. secrete extracelleular matrix

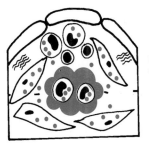

Uncomplicated atheromatous plaque

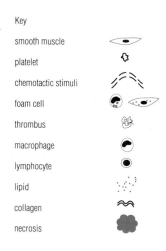

Complicated atheroma
ulceration and thrombus formation

Key

smooth muscle	
platelet	
chemotactic stimuli	
foam cell	
thrombus	
macrophage	
lymphocyte	
lipid	
collagen	
necrosis	

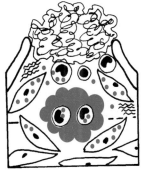

The monoclonal hypothesis

This theory proposes that the primary event in plaque formation is the proliferation of smooth muscle and that any endothelial changes are secondary. The stimulus for smooth muscle proliferation could be an unknown genetic or acquired abnormality of growth control. Acquired abnormalities might occur due to raised levels of lipids in the intima in hyperlipidaemic states, or exogenous agents such as viruses or the hydrocarbons in cigarette smoke. The exact mechanism remains unknown. This theory rests solely on the fact that in some plaques, all of the smooth muscle cells seem to have been derived from a single cell, i.e. they are monoclonal, and hence it is thought of as a type of 'tumour' formation. In other words, atheromatous plaques are benign tumours which result from the stimulatory effects of lipids, proteins or hydrocarbons.

Of course a hypothesis is only an idea about how things might work, it is essential to see what evidence there is in its support. Let's look at the various steps necessary in the 'reaction to injury theory'; this suggested that there was first an endothelial change which lead to increased permeability and aggregation of leucocytes.

Endothelial cell damage is known to be produced by a variety of factors such as haemodynamic forces, hyperlipidaemia, cigarette smoke, immune mechanisms, certain viral antigens, irradiation and various mutagens. We have already mentioned that atherosclerotic lesions commonly occur in areas of turbulent blood flow so **haemodynamic forces** damaging the endothelium would make sense. Hyperlipidaemia and cigarette smoke induced endothelial damage would provide a mechanism to explain the increased risk of atheroma in smokers and hypercholesterolaemic individuals.

Some evidence suggesting that an **increase in permeability** is important in atherogenesis is that atherosclerotic lesions contain large amounts of plasma-derived macromolecules, which would not normally be able to pass through the endothelial barrier.

The **aggregation of leucocytes** on the endothelial surface is well recognised as a response to local injury, as we have discussed under 'Cellular events' in Chapter 1. Now we need to know whether there is any evidence to link this with atheroma formation. Do areas of endothelial damage with platelet aggregation precede atheroma formation? The answer appears to be 'yes', as these changes are seen in both the aorta of rabbits subjected to cigarette smoke and in the arteries of the **white Carneau pigeon**. This unfortunate bird spontaneously suffers from atherosclerosis in the aorta and coronary arteries and, therefore, is a useful model to look for changes which might represent the early stages of an atheromatous lesion.

The next stage required in the 'response to injury theory' is that the aggregated platelets and monocytes release substances to promote smooth muscle proliferation and the

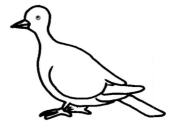

influx of more leucocytes.

Platelet-derived growth factor (PDGF) is believed to be important because smooth muscle proliferation is observed *in vivo* in zones where platelets adhere to damaged endothelium and *in vitro* PDGF can promote both proliferation and migration of smooth muscle cells. Interestingly, there are two animal models which provide supporting evidence. In one, the platelets lack α granules which contain PDGF and the animals do not develop atheroma. In the other, pigs lacking von Willebrand factor, which is necessary for platelet adherence and aggregation, are resistant both to thrombosis and to spontaneous atherosclerosis. Other growth factors, such as fibroblast growth factor, epidermal growth factor and transforming growth factor alpha (TGF-α), are probably involved as well as a reduction in the growth inhibitor (TGF-β) produced by macrophages and endothelial cells. The end result is that smooth muscle cells migrate from the media to the intima, they proliferate, they accumulate cholesterol and cholesterol esters to become one of the types of **foam** cells (the other is macrophage derived) and they also manufacture extracellular matrix.

The **influx of leucocytes** is apparent from simple observation, i.e. by counting the number of macrophages and lymphocytes in the atheromatous lesions and comparing this with the very small number present in non-atheromatous intima. Once lymphocytes and macrophages are involved, the whole complex army of cytokines can be called into action to promote chemotaxis, cell proliferation, altered permeability, etc. An important question is how does leucocytic infiltration and function in atherosclerotic plaques differ from that seen in ordinary inflammation?

Are specific immune mechanisms important in atherogenesis?

Very little is known about this but some recent evidence suggests that endothelial cells in rabbits that are hypercholesterolaemic express a new surface antigen which can act as a macrophage adhesion molecule and is nicknamed 'atheroELAM' (ELAM = endothelial leucocyte adhesion molecule). The T cells within the lesions could be just passing through in an inactive state, but this is unlikely because they express the IL-2 receptor, γ-interferon is present in the lesions and the adjacent smooth muscle cells are HLA class II antigen positive. These changes are evidence that there is specific activation of T cells. Specific activation means that specific antigens must be present in atheromatous lesions and the possible candidates are:

- oxidised lipoproteins
- heat shock proteins (e.g. HSP-70 produced by a variety of cells in response to stress)
- glycosylated lipoproteins in diabetes
- viruses (as suggested by the finding of the Marek virus in some chicken lesions and a herpes type virus in some human atherosclerotic plaques)

Oxidised lipoproteins (OLP) deserve further mention because they are a potential route for reducing atheroma formation through the use of antioxidants. It appears that they may be produced by reactive oxygen species altering the lipoprotein present in plaques. These reactive oxygen molecules are made by activated macrophages.OLP are thought to be able to cause:

- endothelial cell damage
- smooth muscle cell injury leading to central necrosis of the plaque
- foam cell formation as the OLP are taken up by the receptor for modified LDL
- recruitment and retention of macrophages

Even antibody-mediated damage in atheroma has some advocates, as certain experimental models of atheroma have antibodies directed against OLP or otherwise modified lipoproteins, and complement may be activated locally in hypercholesterolaemic rabbits resulting in deposition of the C5b–9 complex in the plaques.

Thus, there is a large literature supporting the 'response to injury' theory, although many questions remain unanswered.

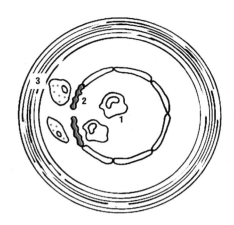

1. **Monocytes/macrophages**
   chemotaxis
   immobilisation
   foam cell formation
2. **Endothelium**
   damage
3. **Smooth muscle**
   damage
   foam cell formation

Fig 2.29 Effects of oxidised lipoproteins

What diet will prevent atheroma?

The popular press is fond of reporting the latest diet which will prevent atheroma and are then even more delighted to report the contradictions which follow; so what do we really know and what is speculation? We don't know a great deal about humans because the experiments take so long! Most of the evidence comes from comparing populations with distinctly different diets, for instance comparing the fish-eating Eskimos with meat-eating Danes or the butter lovers of Belgium with the olive oil fans of the Mediterranean. Let us digress for a second to consider how we should define a successful diet. Ideally, we would like to prevent the formation of atheromatous plaques but, as we cannot assess the size, number and distribution of plaques in millions of living people in different populations, most researchers opt to monitor the major life threatening complication of plaques, namely occlusive coronary heart disease (CHD). However by doing that they are really measuring the outcome of two different pathological mechanisms. The patient must not only suffer from atheroma in their coronary vessels but also undergo an occlusive event such as thrombosis; therefore there may be different dietary factors affecting the two processes, i.e. 'atherogenic' and 'thrombogenic' dietary factors. Obviously, it is likely that any atherogenic factors operate over decades and starting on a low-fat diet as you retire will cause little change to your plaques. However, the likelihood of thrombosis could be affected by an alteration of diet in later life.

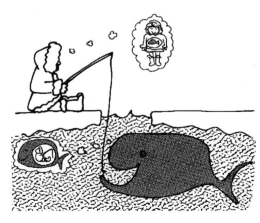

Fish-loving Eskimos

Saturated versus unsaturated fatty acids

In general terms, saturated fatty acids (SFA) are considered harmful while polyunsaturated fatty acids (PUFA) and monounsaturated fatty acids (MUFA) are good for you; hence the trend to quote the ratio of PUFA to SFA in foods. However, this is a gross oversimplification and while some SFA (e.g. lauric, myristic or palmitic fatty acids) do raise cholesterol levels, others (e.g. stearic acid and short chain SFA) do not. From our earlier discussion on the formation of atheroma, you will realise that SFAs are likely to be atherogenic if they cause hypercholesterolaemia. Another problem is that long chain SFA (but not PUFAs or MUFAs) promote thrombosis and can increase the likelihood of an acute occlusion.

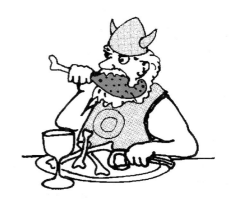

Meat-eating Danes

To recap on lipids: cholesterol and low density lipoproteins (LDL) appear harmful whereas high density lipoproteins (HDL) appear protective; therefore we need to know the effect of diet on these three components. The PUFAs include two important groups, the n-6 series derived from *linoleic acid* and commonly found in vegetable seed oils, and the n–3 series derived from *linolenic acid* and present in fish and fish oils. Diets rich in PUFAs of the n–6 group lower cholesterol, LDL *and* HDL. It is a pity that they reduce the cardioprotective HDL and this is of particular relevance if you are female because high LDL is not an important risk factor for atherogenesis in women. PUFAs of the n–3 group are much better because they reduce cholesterol and LDL but raise HDL concentration and also have an antithrombotic potential through a reduction in platelet aggregation mediated by PGI_3. MUFAs, such as olive oil, do not only reduce LDLs but also produce LDLs which are resistant to oxidation. The whole subject of lipoprotein oxidation begins to appear important in atherogenesis and may mean that diets rich in anti oxidants, such as vitamin C, will prove beneficial. It is even possible that this could be an explanation for the high levels of atherosclerosis in northern countries where fresh fruit and vegetables may be less common in the diet during the winter months.

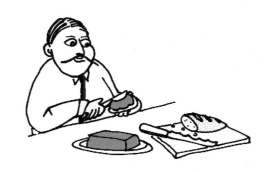

Butter-loving Belgians

What dietary advice should you give to your patients? 'Eat less fat' has received much publicity but there is very little correlation between CHD and total fat consumption. For example, there is a low incidence of CHD in Mediterranean countries where fat intake is high. 'Eat less red meat' ignores the facts that the UK has the second lowest meat consumption in the European community but the second highest incidence of CHD and that Greece has the highest red meat consumption but a low rate of CHD. It is probable that the best advice at the moment is to:

- replace butter and hard margarine with PUFA or oleic acid (a MUFA) alternatives
- use skimmed milk instead of full fat milk
- eat more fish
- eat lots of fresh fruit and vegetables

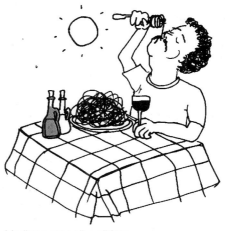

Mediterranean olive oil fans

What are the complications of atheroma?

The plaques in themselves do not cause any symptoms. They cause disease by reducing the size of the lumen of the blood vessel and hence causing ischaemia and infarction, by acting as a base for the formation of **thrombus** and **embolism** and by weakening the wall to cause local dilatation – an **aneurysm**. The luminal surface of the plaque may **ulcerate** and this commonly precipitates thrombus formation. **Haemorrhage** may also occur within plaques and the resulting haematoma may distend the plaque to cause ulceration. In almost all advanced atheromatous plaques, there is some degree of dystrophic **calcification** which, if extensive, will turn the artery into a stiff pipe.

The two commonest clinical manifestations of atherosclerosis are myocardial infarction and cerebral infarction. We will now discuss the clinical and pathological manifestations of myocardial infarction as an illustration of the role and significance of atherosclerosis in causing such overwhelming morbidity and mortality.

Myocardial infarction

Let us first briefly consider the clinical aspects. A typical scenario may be as follows. A 63 year old gentleman presented to the accident and emergency department complaining of chest pain. He had had central chest pain for 6–8 hours and the pain radiated down the left arm and into his neck. He was feeling nauseated and also complained of shortness of breath. He had a history of hypertension for the last five years and had been receiving treatment. He also smoked 25 cigarettes per day and was obese. He had a family history of hypertension and his father died at the age of 55 of a 'heart attack'. His brother was also hypertensive.

On examination he was found to have a pulse rate of 40 beats/min, blood pressure of 110/80 and he was in cardiac failure. An electrocardiogram (ECG) confirmed an inferior myocardial infarction and he was found to be in complete heart block. He received treatment for his pain, a temporary pacing wire was inserted and he was transferred to the intensive care unit for observation.

As house physicians and residents, you will encounter this sort of situation with alarming regularity. So what is the pathological sequence of events that leads to a myocardial infarction and what are the complications that may arise as a consequence?

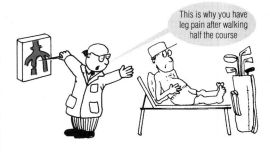

Luminal narrowing

- intermittent claudication

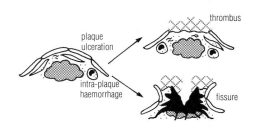

Thrombosis following plaque ulceration or fissuring complicated by:

- luminal narrowing
- luminal obstruction
- thromboembolism
- systemic infarction

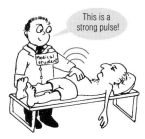

Aneurysm formation complicated by:

- thrombosis
- thromboembolism
- rupture

Fig. 2.30 The complications of atheroma

What mechanisms lead to myocardial infarction?

Myocardial infarction means that cardiac muscle cells die because of a lack of nutrients, most importantly oxygen. Generally, this results from poor blood flow through, or total occlusion of, one or more coronary arteries and the extent of the infarction will depend on the amount of collateral flow, the metabolic requirements of the cells and the duration of the insult. Atheroma of the coronary vessels accounts for the majority of cases but rarer causes include vascular spasm, emboli, arteritis and anaemia (see opposite).

Atheroma reduces the size of the arterial lumen and may cause clinical symptoms because it is suddenly complicated by thrombus to produce complete occlusion of a coronary artery or because the blood flow is insufficient for even a moderate increase in cardiac work, such as walking upstairs. Alternatively, the patient will complain of chest pain on exercise which is relieved on resting. This is called **angina** and occurs because the myocardial cells become ischaemic, but the damage is reversible. Obviously such a patient is precariously close to suffering an irreversible ischaemic cardiac episode, i.e. an infarction. How does an inactive atheromatous plaque suddenly occlude a vessel? It appears that the fibrous cap of the plaque splits so that blood can enter the soft necrotic centre. This can distort and enlarge the plaque but, most significantly, the plaque contents activate the thrombotic cascade. Platelets and fibrin will aggregate to block the lumen and the platelet constituents (thromboxane A_2, histamine and serotonin) may worsen the situation by promoting spasm in the vessel wall. It is not known why the plaque fissures but it may be influenced by macrophage activity in the soft atheromatous centre, by vasospasm in the wall, by bending and twisting of the vessel as the heart contracts or by altered distribution of stresses on the wall. It is often stated that coronary artery stenosis is not likely to produce clinical symptoms unless the cross-sectional area is reduced by 75%. This is true for long-standing fibrosed areas of atheroma, but the majority of plaques which fissure to produce occlusion are fairly small and have an abundance of soft lipid. Soft plaques are more likely to fissure than hard, fibrous plaques.

Vasospasm is an elusive mechanism for a pathologist to identify because there will be nothing to see at autopsy. However, it may be seen on angiography in some patients with angina or infarction and principally occurs in areas damaged by atheroma. It is potentially of great therapeutic importance because it may be influenced by drugs.

Occlusion of a single vessel, as described above, will produce a **regional infarct**, because it occurs in the region that is normally supplied by a particular coronary artery. The infarct may involve a variable thickness of the myocardial wall but when it involves the full thickness of the wall it is referred to as a **transmural infarction**; 90% of

List some rare causes of myocardial ischaemia/infarction

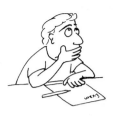

arteritis-
   SLE
   Polyarteritis
   Kawasaki's syndrome
vasospasm
↓↓ blood pressure
trauma to coronary arteries
emboli to coronary arteries

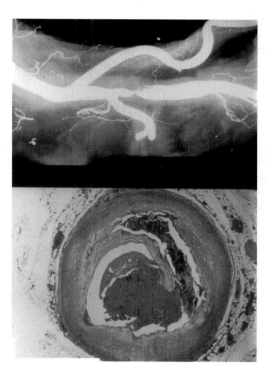

Fig 2.31 Angiogram showing an irregular area at the point of narrowing of a coronary vessel. This is due to thrombus formation where an atheromatous plaque has fissured as shown in the corresponding histological section.

transmural infarctions result from thrombosis complicating atheroma. In patients suffering an infarction, a third have severe atheroma affecting one vessel, a third have two vessels involved and a third have three vessels damaged. The left anterior descending coronary artery and left circumflex coronary artery are most likely to be damaged in their proximal 2 cm whereas the proximal and distal $^1/_3$ of the right coronary artery are worst affected. Myocardial infarction is much more common in the left ventricle and interventricular septum but approximately 25% of posterior infarctions will extend into the adjacent right ventricle or even into the atria. Occasionally, the infarcted region does not correlate with the thrombosed vessel and this is termed 'infarction at a distance'. It occurs because the patient has had previous coronary artery problems and has developed a collateral circulation so that, for example, long-standing poor flow through the left anterior descending coronary artery may make the anterior wall of the left ventricle dependent on collateral flow from the right coronary artery. Thus sudden occlusion of the right coronary artery may result in infarction of the region normally associated with the left anterior descending artery.

The other important pattern of myocardial damage is the **subendocardial infarction**. The pathogenesis of this type of infarction is different from the regional infarction as there is generally widespread atherosclerosis in all coronary vessels but no specific occlusion. The subendocardial region is the most vulnerable part of the myocardium for two reasons: firstly, any collateral supply that is developed tends to supply the subepicardial part of the myocardium and secondly, the subendocardium is under the greatest tension from the compressive forces of the myocardium and, hence, most likely to be ischaemic. Normally, blood will flow into the myocardium when the aortic root pressure exceeds the left ventricular cavity pressure as occurs during diastole. Generalised reduction in myocardial perfusion results from any combination of coronary stenosis, reduction in aortic root pressure, increase in left ventricular cavity pressure, myocardial thickening and shortening of diastole.

Subendocardial infarction is much less common than transmural infarction. It is confined to the inner half of the myocardium and may be **regional** or **circumferential**. A very thin layer of subendocardial muscle remains viable because it receives nutrients and oxygen from the ventricular luminal blood. It should be noted however that even a transmural, regional infarct probably begins in the subendocardial region and then spreads to the rest of the wall.

Is myocardial infarction preventable?

Hopefully you will realise from the preceding sections that any dietary or therapeutic factors which influence atherogenesis or thrombosis will alter the risk of myocardial infarction. If a patient has widespread severe atherosclerotic CHD, they may have their vessels bypassed by a graft from their leg veins or by synthetic vessels. If they have only a

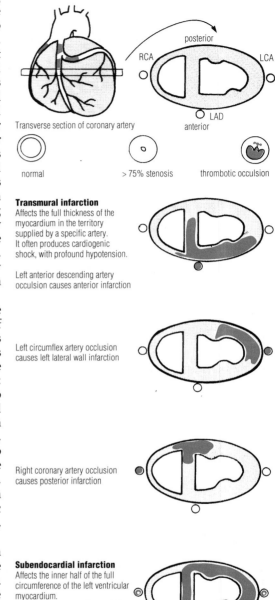

Transverse section of coronary artery

normal   > 75% stenosis   thrombotic occlusion

Transmural infarction
Affects the full thickness of the myocardium in the territory supplied by a specific artery. It often produces cardiogenic shock, with profound hypotension.

Left anterior descending artery occlusion causes anterior infarction

Left circumflex artery occlusion causes left lateral wall infarction

Right coronary artery occlusion causes posterior infarction

Subendocardial infarction
Affects the inner half of the full circumference of the left ventricular myocardium.
It results from severe, but partial, stenosis of several coronary vessels, and often follows an episode of hypotension

RCA = right coronary artery
LC = left circumflex artery
LAD = left anterior descending artery

Fig 2.32 Types of myocardial infarction and territories affected

localised lesion, they may have this treated by an intravenous balloon catheter. Low dose aspirin may be used to reduce any thrombotic tendency by acting on platelets. Once a coronary artery has become occluded, urgent action is required in the first 2 hours while ischaemic damage is in the reversible phase. An intravenous catheter may be used to attempt to dislodge the clot, lytic agents may help to dissolve it and the use of anti-thrombotic drugs will aim to prevent any extension of the thrombus.

What are the appearances of infarction?

Let us consider the clinical example described earlier in which the patient's ECG showed him to have had an inferior infarction. If he had died within a few hours, autopsy would have revealed a thrombus within the right coronary artery. This artery supplies the posterior wall of the left ventricle and the posterior third of the interventricular septum. Ischaemia of the septum would explain his complete heart block as this would damage the conduction pathway. No macroscopical abnormality would be seen, as the infarction would be only **6 hours** old, but the area of infarction could be highlighted using **histochemical techniques**. Normal heart muscle contains dehydrogenases which leak out of fibres that have been damaged by ischaemia. If a 1 cm slice of myocardium is dipped into a solution of the yellow dye nitroblue tetrazolium (NBTZ), the normal myocardium will appear blue due to the reduction of the dye by the dehydrogenase enzymes while the ischaemic myocardium will be pale and unstained. If the patient had died at **24 hours**, the infarcted area would either appear pale or be red-blue due to the trapped blood. Later the dead myocardium becomes pale yellow, softened and better defined with a rim of hyperaemic tissue at the periphery. Over the next few weeks, the necrotic muscle is replaced by fibrous scar tissue and this is usually complete by six weeks. The exact time course depends on the size of the infarct and any complications that may occur.

Under the light microscope the damaged area shows the changes depicted in Fig. 3.1. A more detailed account of reversible and irreversible ischaemic damage will be described in Chapter 3.

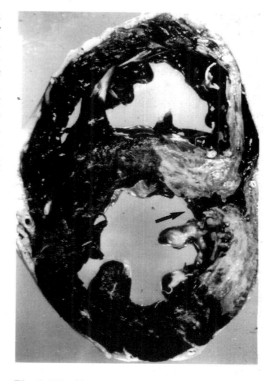

Fig 2.33 Heart slice through the right and left ventricle stained with NBTZ to demonstrate infarction in the area supplied by the left anterior descending artery. The left ventricular wall has ruptured (arrow) allowing blood into the pericardial space (slice viewed from below; right ventricle at top of photograph).

What complications may occur?

Our 63 year old gentleman was in cardiac failure and complete heart block, two of the commonest complications. First, we will consider the **arrhythmias.** This may be a type of heart block, ventricular tachycardia or bradycardia, ventricular fibrillation or asystole. Arrhythmias are responsible for many cases of sudden death following myocardial infarction and their prompt diagnosis is of crucial importance in the management of these patients. The arrhythmias occur either because of ischaemia or death of the specialised conducting tissue of the heart, or due to the interruption of the conduction of impulses within the damaged myocardium. A damaged atrioventricular node, for instance, may lead to complete heart block while damage to the conducting fibres within the ventricles will produce left or right bundle branch block. Damaged myocardial fibres may also be 'arrhythmogenic' and so initiate abnormal impulses which may terminate in ventricular fibrillation. It is interesting that many of the drugs used to treat arrhythmias, which act by altering the action potential, are also capable of inducing them.

The second complication mentioned was **cardiac failure**. His cardiac failure could be due to the complete heart block, so restoring normal sinus rhythm will be important in his treatment. Cardiac failure may also occur because of extensive death of muscle cells in the left ventricular wall or because they have been 'stunned' by a short period of ischaemia and are temporarily unable to contract, but may recover over a few days. If a **papillary muscle** is damaged then mitral incompetence will produce cardiac failure. Initially, the papillary muscle is likely to be intact but incapable of contraction. After 4–5 days, the infarction has softened and the muscle may rupture, allowing the valve leaflet to prolapse. Similar softening occurs in infarcted tissue in the left ventricular wall so that it may rupture. This occurs in transmural infarction (i.e. full thickness) but not in subendocardial infarction. Within 24–48 hours of transmural infarction, the damaged ventricular muscle stretches, i.e. it becomes thinner, and is liable to aneurysm formation or rupture. This is often referred to as '**infarct expansion**', but it should be appreciated that the amount of tissue damage is not increasing, it is merely a stretching of the damaged area. The **rupture** may take place in the septum, which creates a **ventricular septal defect** (VSD), or through the ventricular wall so that the blood leaks into the pericardial cavity, producing a **haemopericardium** which inhibits the normal action of the heart, so-called **cardiac tamponade**. Generally either of these complications is fatal.

The body's immune system responds to the infarction so that the pericardial surface overlying the infarcted area usually becomes inflamed (**pericarditis**) by the second or third day. In most cases, this is self-limiting, but the friction between the pericardial surfaces produces a **pericardial rub** which may be heard through a stethoscope. Similar changes occur on the endocardial surface of the infarct which, in combination with stasis, predispose it to **mural thrombosis**. Whenever there is thrombosis, there is a risk of **embolism**. In this case, these would be systemic emboli affecting organs such as the brain or kidneys.

Finally, the healed and fibrotic wall may balloon out to produce a **cardiac aneurysm**, which itself can be a site of thrombus because of stasis.

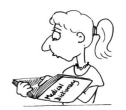

Tachycardia
increase in pulse rate

Bradycardia
abnormally slow heart rate

Arrhythmia
abnormal cardiac electrical rhythm

Asystole
absence of cardiac electrical activity

Fibrillation
unco-ordinated and ineffective muscle contraction

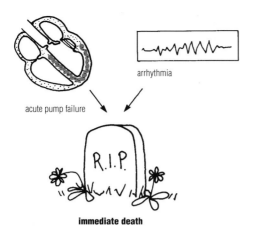

arrhythmia

acute pump failure

R.I.P.

immediate death

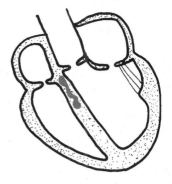

arrhythmia

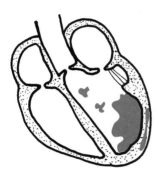

mural thrombus with thromboembolism

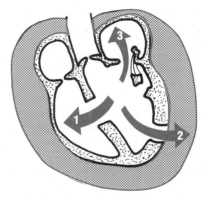

rupture of necrotic myocardium
1. Interventricular septum – septal defect
2. Left ventricular wall – cardiac tamponade
3. Papillary muscle – acute mitral regurgitation

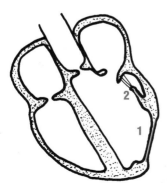

chronic pump failure
1.Scarred myocardium
2.Scarred papillary muscle with mitral valve regurgitation

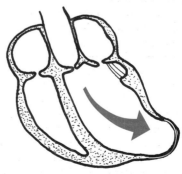

ventricular aneurysm formation

Fig 2.34 Complications of myocardial infarction

Aneurysms

Aneurysms only occasionally occur in the heart; they are commonest in large and medium-sized arteries, such as the aorta and cerebral arteries, where they produce a localised dilatation. Aneurysms may produce no symptoms or they may rupture with potentially devastating effects, cause problems through pressing on adjacent structures or they may become occluded as a complication of thrombosis.

Let us start with **berry aneurysms**. As the name suggests, these are more than just a dilatation, they look like a cherry stuck on the side of a vessel. These occur most commonly at the sites of bifurcation of the cerebral arteries and particularly at the junction between the carotid artery and the posterior communicating artery. Patients with berry aneurysms present with a sudden severe headache and some lose consciousness. Occasionally a patient will have ocular problems or facial pain because of pressure on the cranial nerves by an unruptured aneurysm. Frequently, these patients are young or middle-aged and are not normally hypertensive but are assumed to have raised their blood pressure by acute exertion. Up to 50% of patients will die without recovering consciousness and, in those who survive the first blow, there is a risk of re-bleeding. Permanent cerebral damage may occur if blood tracks into the brain parenchyma to produce an intracerebral haematoma or if ischaemia leads to cerebral infarction. Organised blood clot in the subarachnoid space may obstruct the normal flow of cerebrospinal fluid leading to raised intracranial pressure. Berry aneurysms are usually small, less than 1.5 cm in diameter and are globular in shape. Although referred to as congenital, they are not present at birth but develop because there is a defect in the media of the blood vessels at sites of bifurcation.

The other important type of aneurysm affecting cerebral vessels is the **microaneurysm**. These are present on small arteries within the cerebral hemispheres, are only a few millimetres in diameter, are generally multiple, occur in older, hypertensive individuals and are a common cause of intracerebral haemorrhage.

Congenital weakness of the vessel wall and hypertension are important aetiological factors in cerebral vessel aneurysms while most other vascular aneurysms are acquired, secondary to atherosclerosis, cystic medial necrosis or inflammatory damage.

Atherosclerotic aneurysms are commonest in the abdominal portion of the aorta and they may present with massive haemorrhage or as a pulsatile mass in the abdomen, which may compress structures such as the ureters. Often they become complicated by thrombosis with the risk of shedding emboli into lower limb vessels. These aneurysms occur in individuals with risk factors for atheroma and they develop due to thinning of the media exacerbated by hypertension. It is not known how atheroma, an intimal

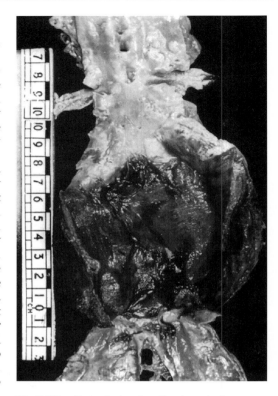

Fig 2.35 Abdominal aorta with a large fusiform aneurysm between the renal and iliac vessels. Thrombus is attached to the wall of the aneurysm.

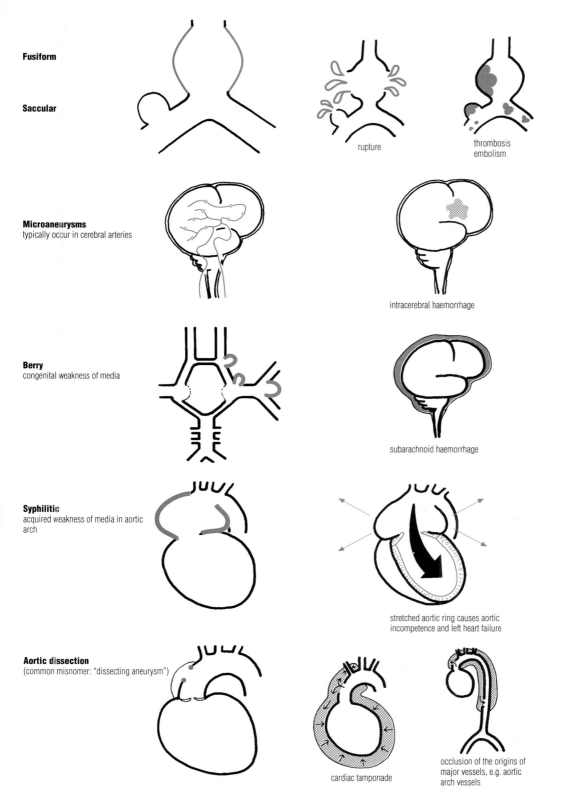

Fusiform

Saccular

rupture

thrombosis
embolism

Microaneurysms
typically occur in cerebral arteries

intracerebral haemorrhage

Berry
congenital weakness of media

subarachnoid haemorrhage

Syphilitic
acquired weakness of media in aortic arch

stretched aortic ring causes aortic incompetence and left heart failure

Aortic dissection
(common misnomer: "dissecting aneurysm")

cardiac tamponade

occlusion of the origins of major vessels, e.g. aortic arch vessels

Fig 2.36 Type of aneurysms and their complications

disease, produces medial damage. The aneurysms may be saccular or fusiform. Aneurysms greater than 6 cm in diameter are likely to rupture so it is recommended that these are replaced by prosthetic grafts as replacement after rupture carries a high mortality.

Cystic medial necrosis is a descriptive term for necrosis of the media associated with mucoid degeneration and the formation of mucoid cystic lakes. The cause of cystic medial necrosis is unknown but it is associated with hypertension and may involve production of abnormal collagen, elastin and proteoglycans of the media, as occurs in Marfan's syndrome. It is important as a possible aetiological factor in aortic dissection, in which blood tracks down through the media. Unfortunately, aortic dissection is often referred to as an aortic dissecting aneurysm despite the vessel not being dilated.

Aortic dissection usually occurs in the 40–60 year old group and affects men more commonly than women, although it does occur in pregnant women, possibly because of generalised hormonal actions which soften connective tissue. Patients complain of sudden severe pain in the centre of the chest, similar to that felt in myocardial infarction but this often radiates to the back and moves as the dissection progresses. The first event in aortic dissection is a tear in the intima so that blood enters the media and tracks down between the middle and outer thirds of the media. The tear often occurs in the ascending aorta and is thought to be due to shearing forces on the intima. It is possible that the intima may buckle into the aortic lumen in areas of medial weakness, where it is buffeted by the blood, particularly in areas of turbulence as are found in the ascending aorta. Any hypertension will exacerbate both the turbulence and the forces splitting the media. Once the blood begins to track along the media, it can travel in either direction; it may continue tracking or it can rupture back into the aorta or it can rupture out into the peritoneal cavity, pericardial sac or pleural cavity. Rupture outwards is catastrophic and common whereas rupture into the aorta is rare but has a good prognosis and will produce a **double-barrelled aorta**. Extension of the dissection will occlude the mouths of any tributaries which become involved and this commonly affects the coronary, renal, mesenteric, iliac or cerebral vessels.

Aneurysms secondary to inflammation will include those due to syphilis, arteritis and infection. Some of the clinical features of syphilis were covered in Chapter 1 (*page 47-49*). **Syphilitic aneurysms** tend to occur in the ascending aorta and arch of the aorta where they are ideally situated to cause mischief. Those that arise close to the aortic valve ring lead to dilatation of the ring and hence to **aortic incompetence**, the result of which is overload of the left ventricle and cardiac failure. Aneurysms may rupture into the trachea or oesophagus to produce haemoptysis (coughing up blood), haematemesis (vomiting blood) or death. Any cause of aortic expansion within the chest can produce difficulty in breathing or swallowing due to compression, persistent cough due to irritation of the recurrent laryngeal nerves, or problems of bone erosion. Fortunately, syphilis is now an uncommon disease in the western world and these complications are rare.

Aneurysms secondary to **vasculitis**, such as polyarteritis nodosa, tend to occur in the renal and mesenteric vessels where they lead to ischaemia. Patients, therefore, may present with renal failure or with intestinal infarction and peritonitis, all of which have a significant mortality. Aneurysms secondary to infection are called mycotic aneurysms.

Hypertension

Many of the diseases discussed in the second half of this chapter are related to hypertension. Atheroma, arteriolosclerosis, myocardial infarction and aneurysms are linked by their association with hypertension, so we cannot finish the chapter without discussing the aetiology and pathogenesis of hypertension.

Hypertension is extremely common, affecting around 25% of adults if a blood pressure of greater than 140/90mmHg is regarded as abnormal. Unfortunately, organ damage may be irreversible by the time a patient presents with symptoms, so, as it is important to screen people who are most susceptible, you need to know about risk factors. Hypertension is predominantly a condition of middle and later life but may be divided into 'benign' and 'malignant' forms. Fortunately, **'benign'** hypertension is much more common, is relatively stable and is treatable with long-term antihypertensive drugs. **'Malignant'** hypertension only affects 5% of hypertensive patients but it is more severe and is liable to affect men under 50 years of age. The major dangers of hypertension are coronary heart disease, cerebrovascular accidents, congestive heart failure and chronic renal failure. In 95% of cases, there is no obvious cause and this is termed primary or idiopathic hypertension. Most of the remainder are due to renal disease, with a small number due to endocrine abnormalities (secondary hypertension).

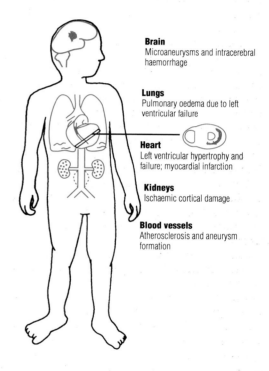

Brain
Microaneurysms and intracerebral haemorrhage

Lungs
Pulmonary oedema due to left ventricular failure

Heart
Left ventricular hypertrophy and failure; myocardial infarction

Kidneys
Ischaemic cortical damage

Blood vessels
Atherosclerosis and aneurysm formation

Fig 2.37 Complications of hypertension

What mechanisms may operate in hypertension?

We will have to be content with describing some of the theories concerning hypertension, as nobody knows the answers. First it is useful to review the factors influencing the control of blood pressure. In simple terms, the arterial pressure will depend on the **cardiac output** and the **total peripheral resistance**. The resistance is determined by the arteriolar lumen which may expand or contract depending on the state of the smooth muscle cells in the vessel wall.

This is called **local vascular tone** and is influenced by a variety of mediators (see list) which may act throughout the body or be produced and have their action locally, i.e. **autoregulation**. The cardiac output depends on the heart rate, its contractility and the blood volume.

It is suggested that **essential hypertension** could result from a primary defect in renal sodium excretion, possibly combined with abnormalities in sodium or calcium transport in other cells. The normal kidney will increase excretion of salt and water if the blood pressure rises, so that blood volume and hence blood pressure is reduced. It is not known what 'sets' the level at which this occurs but if it is 'set' too high, the blood pressure will be raised, although stable. Any defect in sodium or calcium transport which leads to a rise in calcium in vascular smooth muscle would increase vascular tone responses. Vascular tone would also be affected by alteration in any of the mediators already listed. The endothelial-derived ones are thought to be the most important. **Secondary hypertension** is most often related to renal disease and results from abnormalities in the renin–angiotensin system, abnormal salt and water balance and renal vasodepressor substances. Angiotensin II is increased in response to raised renin levels and will increase vascular resistance, by causing vascular smooth muscle contraction, and increase blood volume through aldosterone, which promotes distal tubular reabsorption of sodium. Negative feedback is provided through a lowering of renin levels secondary to the increase in angiotensin II, the raised pressure in the glomerular afferent arteriole and decreased proximal tubule sodium reabsorption which influences the macula densa. Increased renin secretion occurs in all of the renal causes of hypertension listed opposite, except for many cases of chronic renal failure. In chronic renal failure, there is sodium and water retention which is probably related to a reduced glomerular filtration rate influencing tubular sodium handling. Theoretically, renal disease might produce hypertension through a reduction in its secretion of vasodepressor substances such as prostaglandins or platelet activating factor. Recently a new group of powerful vasoconstricters, the **endothelins**, have been identified. Endothelin I is the most potent vasoconstrictor yet discovered. Its level is not raised in hypertensive individuals but it may have an important role in maintaining the blood pressure following a myocardial infarction and in endotoxic shock. It is also mitogenic for smooth muscle cells and so may have a role in the formation of atheroma.

The blood vessels in hypertension

We have already mentioned the morphological changes of hyperplastic arteriosclerosis (page 90) which occur in hypertension; now we should consider its relevance. Is this morphological change secondary to the hypertension or could it be the cause? Laplace's law defines the relationship

Which mediators may influence vascular tone?

constrictors-
angiotensin I
endothelin I
catecholamines
thromboxane
leukotrienes
dilators-
prostaglandins
kinins
PAF
endothelium-derived relaxing factor

Which renal diseases may cause hypertension?

acute glomerulonephritis
renal vasculitis
renal artery stenosis
renin-producing tumours
chronic renal disease

between tension in the wall (T), the pressure load (P), the radius of the lumen (R) and the wall thickness (W) as $T = (P \times R)/W$. If the wall tension is to remain constant as blood pressure rises, then the wall thickness must increase. This is exactly what we have described in hyperplastic arteriosclerosis; but the question still remains, is it cause or effect? An alternative way of approaching the problem is to consider what would happen if the *first* change is an increase in wall thickness leading to a decrease in lumen size. Poiseuille's formula shows that resistance to flow is proportional to the fourth power of the radius and so small changes in the radius will produce large changes in the resistance. The suggestion is that precapillary arterioles may constrict initially in response to a reversible vasoconstrictor but that they undergo remodelling with a permanent reduction in lumen size with chronic stimulation. This would, of course, lead to hypertension. It is only speculation, but it is interesting to note the overlap between substances that vasoconstrict and substances that promote growth. Vasoconstrictors, such as noradrenaline and angiotensin II, promote smooth muscle growth while growth factors, such as platelet-derived growth factor and epidermal growth factor, can cause vasoconstriction.

Does the wall thickness return to normal if the blood pressure is lowered? This is an important question because if vascular resistance was the result of morphological change, then reversal of these changes might produce a normotensive patient who did not require continuous anti-hypertensive therapy. At present, it is not possible to give a complete answer but, in humans, some antihypertensive drugs do produce some reduction in wall thickness and, in animals, the angiotensin converting enzyme (ACE) inhibitors are clearly effective while thiazide and hydralazine-like vasodilators have only a minor effect. Thus, simply lowering the blood pressure is not enough and, maybe, some antihypertensives are achieving the morphological changes through other actions on smooth muscle cells.

Clinicopathological summary

Clinical

A 65 year old man complains of transient loss of vision in his right eye. He had two episodes in the previous month, each lasting for approximately 7–10 minutes. Two months ago, he also had transient slurring of his speech.

Examination:
Blood pressure 180/110
Displaced apex beat and ejection systolic murmur

Carotid bruits present

No peripheral pulses palpable below the femorals

Chest X-ray confirmed cardiomegaly but with no evidence of pulmonary oedema
An ECG showed atrial fibrillation and features of an old anterior infarction
An echocardiogram demonstrated thrombus within the left atrium

Carotid doppler studies indicated moderate carotid artery stenosis
Urine analysis – no glucose detected

Blood tests – serial cardiac enzymes: normal
urea and creatinine: slightly raised

Management and progress:
It was decided that he should be treated with antihypertensive agents to reduce his blood pressure and anticoagulants to reduce the risk of further thrombosis/embolism. However, within 24 hours, he developed a right-sided weakness with hemiplegia and a right extensor plantar response. He died without regaining consciousness.

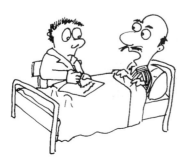

Pathology

Transient loss of vision or speech with full recovery is called a transient ischaemic attack. Generally it results from an embolus lodging in a small cerebral vessel and then being displaced or lysed. The commonest sites of origin are the heart or the carotid vessels.

He is hypertensive with an enlarged heart; i.e. left ventricular hypertrophy in response to increased workload.
The bruits indicate turbulent flow which is a result of stenosis and/or irregularities of the vessel wall due to atheroma.
Absent peripheral pulses indicate widespread arteriosclerotic disease.
The presence of pulmonary oedema would have indicated cardiac failure.
In atrial fibrillation, atria do not contract. The resultant stagnation of blood predisposes to thrombus formation.
Thrombus within the left atrium can be thrown into the systemic circulation. These can pass through the carotids to lodge in the cerebral vessels.
Dopplers detect turbulent flow. It is the electronic equivalent of the bruit.
A simple test for diabetes. Diabetics are at high risk of atheroma and may also suffer from sudden temporary loss of consciousness.
Test for myocardial infarction.
Mild renal impairment probably due to hypertension and atheroma.

The signs are of upper motor neurone damage involving the motor and sensory pathways with loss of consciousness. He has sustained a large left-sided cerebrovascular accident. The neural pathways cross, hence left-sided lesions give right-sided signs.

Postmortem findings:
Cardiovascular system – left ventricular hypertrophy. Atheroma in all three coronary arteries with an old anterior infarction. No evidence of recent infarct and no vegetations. A small amount of thrombus present in the left atrium. Extensive atheroma in aorta and carotids with narrowing of the mouth of the renal arteries.

Central nervous system – a large haematoma in the region of the left internal capsule. Extensive atheroma in the cerebral vessels.

Genitourinary tract – small scarred kidneys showing ischaemic damage.

Clinically the stroke could have been due to an embolus but, in his case, it was a result of rupture of a microaneurysm on the lenticulostriate branch of the middle cerebral, due to hypertention. These are called Charcot–Bouchard aneurysms.

This brings us to the end of this chapter on circulatory disorders. We started with the words of William Harvey, conveying his despair at trying to understand the physiology of the motions of the heart. Physiology and pathology are of fundamental importance in clinical medicine and the words of Sir William Osler, perhaps the greatest physician of recent times, provide an appropriate ending:

"A man cannot become a competent surgeon without the full knowledge of human anatomy and physiology, and the physician without physiology and chemistry flounders along in an aimless fashion, never able to gain any accurate conception of disease, practising a sort of popgun pharmacy, hitting now the malady and again the patient, he himself not knowing which."

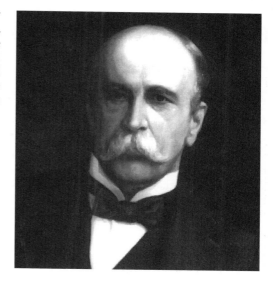

Fig 2.38   Sir William Osler (1849–1919) – Courtesy of the Wellcome Institute for the History of Medicine.

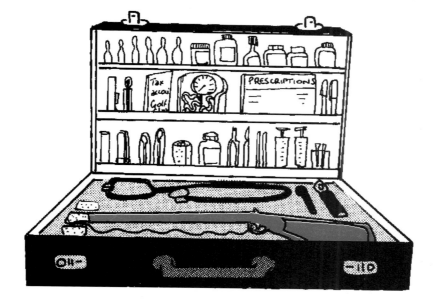

Further reading ————————————————————

G.B.M. Lindop, I.W. Percy-Robb & I.D. Walker. (1992). Disturbances of body fluids, haemostasis and the flow of Blood. Ch 3. *Muir's Textbook of Pathology*. Ed. R.N.M. MacSween & K. Whaley. 13th Edition. Edward Arnold. London.

R.S. Cotran, V. Kumar & S.L. Robbins. (1989). Fluid and hemodynamic derangements. Ch 3. *Robbins Pathologic Basis of Disease*. 4th Edition. W.B. Saunders Company. Philadelphia.

N. Woolf. (1992). Thrombosis. Embolism. Ischaemia and infarction. Ch 7.3, 7.4, 7.5. *Oxford Textbook of Pathology*. Ed. J. McGee, P.G. Isaacson & N.A. Wright. Oxford University Press. Oxford.

T.L.V. Ulbricht & D.A.T. Southgate. (1991). Coronary heart disease: seven dietary factors. *Lancet*. **338**: 985–992.

J.R. Vane, E.E. Anggard & R.M. Botting. (1990). Regulatory functions of the vascular endothelium. *New England Journal of Medicine*. **323**: 27–36.

Chapter 3

Cell and Tissue Damage

"It is a natural marvel. All of the life on earth dies, all of the time, in the same volume as the new life that dazzles us each morning, each spring. All we see of this is the odd stump, the fly struggling on the porch floor of the summer house in October, the fragment on the highway. I have lived all my life with an embarrassment of squirrels in my backyard, they are all over the place, all year long, and I have never seen, anywhere, a dead squirrel."

– Lewis Thomas

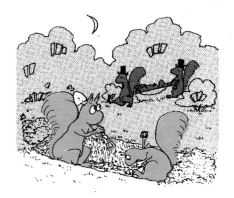

It would be terribly depressing if we saw dead things all around us all the time, but the fact that nature has a way of shielding us from such things also makes us view death as something abnormal and exceptional. In this chapter, we shall look at the pathology of cell and tissue damage and, while we will certainly examine situations in which cell damage and death occur due to an abnormal stress or injury, we will also see that cell death has an important role in embryogenesis, growth, differentiation and immune defence mechanisms.

We will use the model of ischaemic damage to introduce the subject and then consider other forms of lethal and non-lethal cell injury. The concept of **apoptosis** or programmed cell death will be discussed and it will be interesting to see how this type of cell death is mandatory for normal development and how it differs from **necrosis**, the cell death occurring as a result of injury. We will also consider two specific situations in which cells sustain damage – these are **amyloidosis** and **haemochromatosis**.

Cell damage

Let us begin this section by considering the clinical problem of myocardial ischaemia, a clinical scenario familiar from the previous chapter.

A middle-aged man complained of sudden onset of chest pain which radiated down his left arm. He was found to be in shock with a blood pressure of 90/50 mmHg and his ECG showed evidence of an anterior infarction. He had bilateral pulmonary oedema. The serum cardiac enzymes were elevated, including the creatine kinase MB isoenzyme. He developed ventricular fibrillation and, despite resuscitation attempts, died.

Let us use this example to consider the changes that take place in myocardial cells following an ischaemic insult. We know that the final outcome is dependent on a number of variables. These include the **severity** and **duration** of the ischaemia and the **volume of heart muscle** affected. It will also be influenced by any **collateral circulation** and the **metabolic demands** of the myocardial cells at the time of the insult. Hence, the extent of cell damage and death and whether the injury is reversible or irreversible depends on a number of factors and may be altered by medical intervention. The changes in the heart following ischaemia vary with time.

Macroscopical appearance

Although biochemical changes may take place very quickly, the gross appearance of the myocardium is generally entirely normal for the first 6–12 hours. As we have mentioned in the previous chapter, the NBTZ test can be used to highlight the area of infarction in this early period (page 103). After about 18 hours, the myocardium generally appears slightly pale but may look red-blue due to the entrapped red blood cells within the area of infarction. Each day that follows makes the area of infarction a little more defined, paler and softer. By the end of the first week, there is usually a rim of hyperaemia surrounding the pale yellow-brown area of infarction. This is due to the ingrowth of richly vascularised connective tissue that will be involved in the healing and repair process. As time goes by, the dead myocardial cell debris is removed and a pale firm fibrous scar laid down, a process which is complete by six weeks.

Microscopical appearance

As with the gross appearance, the light microscopical changes lag behind the biochemical changes. The earliest change (4–12 hours) is mild oedema and separation of the muscle fibres. The cells adjacent to the area of infarction may also show small droplets within the cytoplasm and this phenomenon is called **vacuolar degeneration**. By 24 hours, neutrophil polymorphs infiltrate the area of necrosis and the necrotic myocytes undergo cytoplasmic and nuclear changes typical of necrosis. The cytoplasm appears more pink (eosinophilic) and the nuclei become pyknotic. Later the nuclei are lost and the cross-striations disappear. By day 3, the infiltrate of neutrophils is heavy and, by the end of the week, the cellular debris from dead cells is being removed by macrophages. The fibrovascular connective tissue, which gives the hyperaemia seen macroscopically, is also evident. Examination at later stages shows the varying amounts of fibrous scar tissue seen on gross inspection.

Fig 3.1 summarises the main findings on gross and microscopical examination of the myocardium at different times following the ischaemic episode.

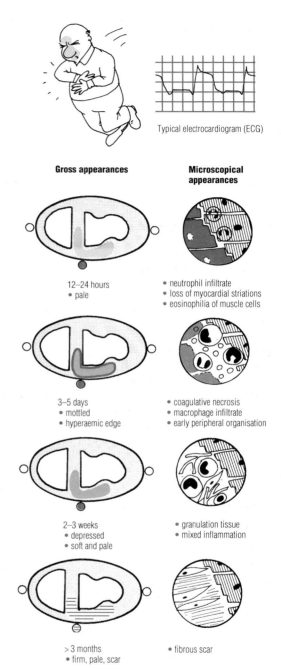

Typical electrocardiogram (ECG)

Gross appearances

Microscopical appearances

12–24 hours
• pale

• neutrophil infiltrate
• loss of myocardial striations
• eosinophilia of muscle cells

3–5 days
• mottled
• hyperaemic edge

• coagulative necrosis
• macrophage infiltrate
• early peripheral organisation

2–3 weeks
• depressed
• soft and pale

• granulation tissue
• mixed inflammation

>3 months
• firm, pale, scar

• fibrous scar

Note: Gross and microscopical changes take 8–12 hours to develop. Infarcts 2–8 hours old may be demonstrable by enzyme techniques.

Fig 3.1 Gross and microscopical appearances of myocardial infarction

Biochemical changes in the cells

There are two important questions to consider:

- What are the biochemical changes that occur in an injured cell?
- What distinguishes reversible from irreversible injury?

There are four sites within the cell that are of paramount importance in cell damage and death. These are the:

- mitochondria
- plasma membrane
- ionic channels in cell membranes
- cytoskeleton

The first effect of ischaemia is to reduce the production of ATP by the mitochondrial oxidative phosphorylation system. If the production of energy slows down or stops, then the cells cannot function; in the case of heart muscle, the cell cannot contract – as simple as that! Obviously, if the ischaemic cells cannot partake in aerobic metabolism, then they will switch over to anaerobic metabolism to derive energy from the stored glycogen. The enzyme creatine kinase, which is present in the myocardial cells, is also utilized to produce energy from the anaerobic metabolism of creatine phosphate. The net effect of these mechanisms is to deplete the cells of glycogen and to produce acidosis within the cells by the production of lactic acid and inorganic phosphates. This further inhibits the normal function of the myocardial cells. The acidosis within the cells is thought to be responsible for one of the observed histological hallmarks of cell damage – the clumping of the nuclear chromatin and **pyknosis** of the nuclei. Ischaemia also has profound effects on the plasma membranes and on the ionic channels situated within the membranes. You will recall that these are vital in maintaining the normal ionic gradients across the cell membranes, with sodium and calcium at low concentrations inside the cells and potassium lower in the extracellular space. These concentrations are maintained by pumps that are energy dependent; hence it is not difficult to see that the loss of the oxidative phosphorylation and any direct damage to the membranes will disrupt the function of these pumps. So what is the effect?

Firstly, the failure of the pumps will result in the leakage of sodium into the cells and potassium out of the cells. Sodium has a larger hydration shell than potassium so more water moves associated with sodium ions than exits with the potassium. Additional water enters because the acidosis and raised intracellular concentrations of high molecular weight phosphates will increase the osmotic pressure inside the cell. The result is acute swelling of the cell due to **cellular oedema**. The endoplasmic reticulum also swells, the ribosomes detach from the endoplasmic reticulum, the mitochondria become swollen and blebs begin to appear on the cell surface. This last phenomenon is intriguing as the

Reversible and irreversible cell damage

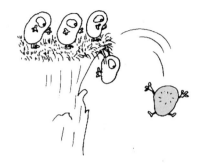

Reversible

cell swelling
mitochrondrial swelling
E.R. swelling
detachment of ribosomes
'myelin' figures
loss of microvilli
surface blebs
clumping of nuclear chromatin
lipid deposition

Irreversible

release of lysosomal enzymes
protein digestion
loss of basophilia
membrane disruption
leakage of cell enzymes and proteins
nuclear changes:
       pyknosis
       karyorrhexis
       karyolysis

('myelin' figures are derived from cell surface and organelle membranes that lose lipoprotein molecules and take up extra water)

changes in cell shape and surface blebbing implies alterations in the cytoskeleton of the cell. The changes in the microfilaments of the cytoskeleton are believed to be due to the increased concentration of calcium which also results from the failure of the membrane pumps. Calcium is a very important ion in cell death and we will see why in a minute.

You might find it difficult to believe, but all the changes described so far are reversible! If the oxygen supply is restored, the cells still have the capacity to return to the normal state and the ability of the myocardial cells to contract is restored. So what are the changes that finally tip the cell beyond the point of no return?

The morphological hallmarks are a severe disruption of the mitochondrial membranes with deposition of matrix lipoproteins, disruption of the plasma membranes and rupture of lysosomes with release of enzymes. **Calcium** is thought to play a central role in this final progression to irreversible cell death.

In the normal cell, the concentration of calcium is tightly controlled by the calcium pump in the cell membrane. Inside the cell, it binds to two important proteins, troponin and calmodulin. Troponin has a role in muscle contraction, and calcium binding to calmodulin is a switch to turn on phosphorylation of important enzyme systems inside the cell. Ischaemia disrupts oxidative phosphorylation, so affecting the energy dependent calcium pump, leading to a rapid influx of calcium and saturation of the calcium regulating proteins. The high levels of calcium are toxic to the cell leading to changes in the cytoskeleton, cell surface blebbing, and damage to the mitochondria, the lysosomal membranes and cell membranes. The calcium also binds to the phosphates within the cells leading to a precipitation of hydroxyapatite crystals which can be observed in the mitochondria. The release of enzymes from the ruptured lysosomes also contributes to the final destruction of the cellular components.

The biochemistry of cell damage and death is a complex process, with many systems interacting. In summary, ischaemia decreases the energy production by the oxidative phosphorylation system in mitochondria, which leads to loss of integrity of the plasma membrane, loss of function of the Na^+/K^+ and Ca^{++} pumps and severe injury to the mitochondria, nucleus, cytoskeleton and lysosomes. Experimental evidence suggests that calcium has a pivotal role in pushing the cell into irreversible cell damage and death.

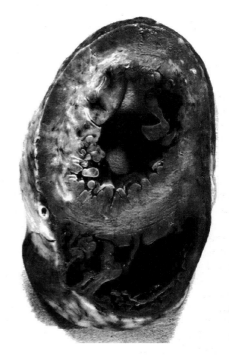

Fig 3.2 Section through the left and right ventricles with pale area in the left ventricular wall indicating infarction.

The clinical relevance of the cell changes

So much for science. Do these biochemical and micro-scopical changes help us to understand any of the clinical manifestations of our patient with chest pain and cardiac failure? We know that ischaemia leads to a decrease in mitochondrial function and, hence, a decrease in ATP formation so that the cells stop contracting. What is absolutely staggering is that an ischaemic episode lasting only 1 minute can produce this change!

The cellular damage may be reversible but the changes still profoundly affect the *function* of the organ. If the area of ischaemia is large, enough cells stop contracting to reduce the pumping power of the heart and cause **cardiac failure**. Any **arrhythmia** will exacerbate the cardiac failure. You will know that the rhythmic contraction of the heart is due to the passage of electrical impulses down the specialised conduction pathways and within the myocardium. Abnormal conduction can occur if there is damage to the sinoatrial or atrioventricular nodes, the conduction bundles or the myocardium. Conduction of electrical impulses requires an intact cell membrane and functioning ionic channels within the membrane, so ischaemia produces abnormal conduction.

The right coronary artery supplies the atrioventricular node in 85% of people; hence right coronary artery occlusion can produce complete heart block as well as inferior infarction. If the area of ischaemia involves the specialised bundles, the bundles may be selectively affected resulting in either a right bundle branch block or a left bundle branch block. Occlusion of the left anterior descending artery produces an anterior infarction which may be complicated by blockage of both conduction bundles. This is frequently fatal, not purely because of the conduction problem, but because it is associated with a large area of infarction. Finally, the myocardium itself may affect the passage of impulses. An infarcted area of myocardium may not only slow down or stop the passage of electrical current, but may also generate an arrythmia.

An **ECG** is a standard investigation for these patients and will detect disorders of cardiac rhythm, and the approximate position and size of the infarction. The 12 lead ECG essentially produces a three-dimensional electrical picture of the heart. When part of the myocardium is damaged by ischaemia, the normal path of the electrical wave is impeded and the impulse has to travel via an alternative route. Consequently, the ECG pattern is altered and the type of change on the tracing helps to identify the area and the approximate size of the infarction.

Our patient had elevated levels of **cardiac enzymes** in the blood. Many enzymes are common to a variety of cells but other enzymes are associated with the cell's specialist functions and will be restricted to only a few cell types. The cardiac muscle cell contains creatine kinase (CK), aspartate aminotransferase (AST) and lactate dehydrogenase (LDH). Ischaemic damage to the myocardial cells disrupts the cell

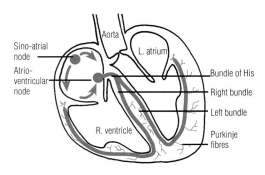

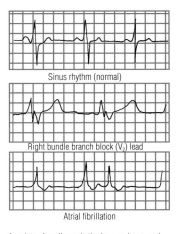

Sinus rhythm (normal)

Right bundle branch block (V_2) lead

Atrial fibrillation

A variety of cardiac arrhythmias may be caused by myocardial infarction affecting the conducting system. Two examples are shown here.

Fig 3.3 The conduction system of the heart

membranes, allowing leakage of these enzymes. If it is suspected that a patient has suffered a myocardial infarction, then serial measurements of these 'cardiac enzymes' can be helpful to confirm the diagnosis and give a rough indication of the size of the damage. Since CK is also found in skeletal muscle, it is customary to measure the CK-MB, which is an isoenzyme specific to cardiac muscle.

You can see how a knowledge of the cellular events helps us to understand the gross and histological appearances as well as the clinical measurements that are useful in diagnosis and management of the patient. Since mild reversible injury to cells is probably more common than irreversible injury we will examine the histological patterns of reversible sublethal injury before going on to look at types of necrosis.

Sublethal cell injury _____

There are two patterns that we need to consider – cloudy swelling and fatty change.

Cloudy swelling

This has already been mentioned when considering myocardial ischaemia. The insult affects membrane ion exchange mechanisms to alter the ionic gradients leading to increased intracellular sodium and water. This produces acute cellular oedema or 'cloudy swelling'. At the light microscopical level, this appears as expansion of the cell and a pale granular look to the cytoplasm. Vesicles may also appear due to the distension of the endoplasmic reticulum. This picture of cellular oedema is also referred to as **hydropic** or **vacuolar degeneration**. Remember that cellular oedema may be precipitated by a whole range of insults and that it is not specific to ischaemia. Chemical toxins, infections and radiation can all induce similar changes. Remember also that cellular oedema is reversible.

Fatty change

This refers to an excess of intracellular lipid which appears as vacuoles of varying size within the cytoplasm. Like cellular oedema, it is entirely reversible and a non-specific reaction to a variety of insults. Sometimes it is present adjacent to tissues that are more severely damaged or show frank evidence of necrosis. Fatty change can occur in any organ but is most frequent in the liver, which is not surprising since the liver is the major site of lipid metabolism. For this reason, we will use the liver as an example to discuss the pathogenesis of fatty change.

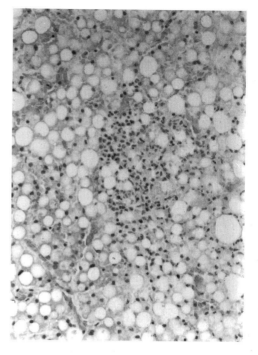

Fig 3.4 Photomicrograph of severe fatty change in a liver. The fat dissolves during the processing of the tissue to leave round holes of different sizes.

Fig. 3.5 illustrates the fate of fatty acids after uptake by the liver and the possible sites at which alteration may lead to an increased accumulation of lipid within the liver cells. Very simply, adipose tissue releases fat as free fatty acids which enter the hepatocytes where they are converted to triglycerides and, to a smaller extent, cholesterol. Triglycerides are complexed with apoproteins to form lipoproteins which are then secreted into the blood. Changes at any of the illustrated sites will lead to lipid accumulation within the hepatocytes. This is not just a hypothetical model derived from experimental systems but a common problem in people who abuse alcohol. **Alcohol** is a hepatotoxin that has wide ranging effects on fatty acid metabolism. It increases peripheral tissue release of fatty acids so that more is delivered to the liver and, within the liver, it is implicated in increasing fatty acid synthesis, in decreasing the utilisation of triglyceride, decreasing fatty acid oxidation and blocking lipoprotein excretion. Thus, it is common for the causative agent to interfere with a variety of biochemical pathways.

Other causes of fatty change include malnutrition, carbon tetrachloride and diabetes. **Malnutrition** particularly affects two steps. It increases the release of fatty acids from peripheral tissue and protein deficiency reduces the cell's ability to combine the triglyceride with apoprotein. **Carbon tetrachloride** also exerts its effect through reducing the availability of apoprotein. Disordered carbohydrate metabolism in uncontrolled **diabetes** leads to excessive peripheral release of fatty acids.

Gross examination of the organs affected by fatty change will show that they are enlarged, yellow and tend to be greasy to touch. Microscopically, the characteristic finding is of vacuoles within the cytoplasm. These may begin as small vacuoles but, if the fatty accumulation continues, the vacuoles will coalesce to form larger vacuoles or 'fatty cysts'.

To reiterate, this type of change is entirely reversible if the insult is withdrawn. A binge in the medical school bar on a Friday night may produce fatty change but this will disappear if one is able to abstain for a few days afterwards! Chronic abuse of alcohol may produce sufficient fatty change to interfere with the normal function of the hepatocytes and, in the long term, excessive alcohol consumption will lead to cell death, scarring and cirrhosis, which is *not* reversible.

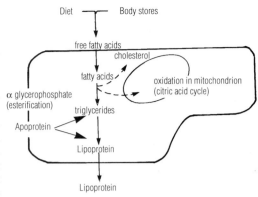

Actions of alcohol contributing to fatty change:

- ↑substrate for esterification
- ↓oxidation in mitochondrion
- ↑triglyceride production by ↑ amount of smooth endoplasmic reticulum
- ↓lipoprotein secretion
- ?↑dietary uptake
- ?↑breakdown of body fat
- ?↓apoprotein production

Fig 3.5 Alcohol and fatty change in the liver

What are the causes of fatty change in the liver?

alcohol
protein malnutrition
diabetes
acute fatty liver of pregnancy
congestive cardiac failure
ischaemia/anaemia
drugs — steroids
        methotrexate
        i.v. tetracycline
carbon tetrachloride
obesity

Necrosis

Necrosis is cell death due to injury.

In general terms, the microscopical changes include **eosinophilia** of the cytoplasm, shrinkage (**pyknosis)** and disintegration of the nuclei (**karyorrhexis**) and finally complete dissolution of the nuclei (**karyolysis**). However, there are different patterns of necrosis under different circumstances. The principal types are:

- coagulative
- colliquative or liquefactive
- caseous

Coagulative necrosis

If you consider the two pictures below, one is of a normal kidney with normal glomeruli and tubules. The adjacent picture is from a kidney that has suffered an ischaemic insult and is showing coagulative necrosis. Spot the difference?

The second picture is essentially the ghost outline of the first! The difference between the two is that the damaged kidney shows loss of nuclei from the cells and the cytoplasm stains a little darker. In a colour photograph, this would appear as eosinophilia (increased red-pink staining with eosin). This pattern of necrosis is the most common type and occurs in many solid organs like the heart and kidney. The necrosis following a myocardial infarction is therefore of the coagulative type. Strange isn't it? Why should the basic architecture and cellular outline be preserved if the cells are dead?

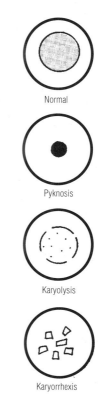

Normal

Pyknosis

Karyolysis

Karyorrhexis

Fig 3.6 Nuclear changes in cell death

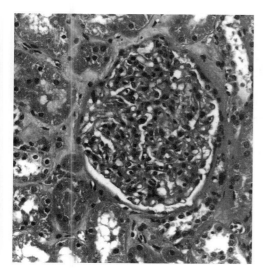
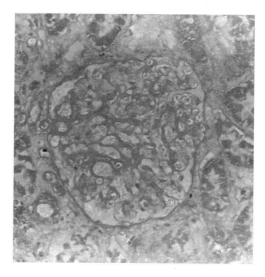

Perhaps the offending injury not only destroys the vital structural proteins within the membrane, cytoplasm and nucleus but also destroys the enzymes within the lysosomes that would otherwise degrade the cellular and extra cellular components. The tissue, of course, doesn't remain in that state for ever. If you remember the example of myocardial infarction, we stated that polymorphs move in within 24 hours of infarction. These inflammatory cells release enzymes that digest the cellular components and the resulting debris will be removed by phagocytic cells such as the macrophages. It should be clear from this that the appearance of an area of coagulative necrosis will change with time.

Colliquative or liquefactive necrosis

The hallmark of this type of necrosis is the release of powerful hydrolytic enzymes that degrade cellular components and extracellular material to produce a proteinaceous soup. Characteristically, it occurs in the brain where it produces a cystic cavity containing fluid and necrotic debris. Liquefaction may also be encountered in tissues when there is a superadded bacterial infection. Then, enzymes are released from both the bacteria and the inflammatory cells that have been recruited to fight the infection.

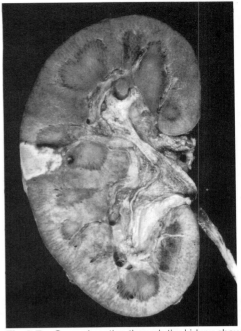

Fig 3.7 Coronal section through the kidney showing a pale triangular well-demarcated area of coagulative necrosis.

Caseous necrosis

Caseous necrosis typically occurs in tuberculosis and is so-called because of a resemblance to soft crumbly cheese! The necrotic area is not quite liquid but neither is the outline of the tissue retained as in coagulative necrosis. On microscopical sections stained with haematoxylin and eosin (H&E), the necrotic area appears homogeneously pink (eosinophilic) with a surrounding inflammatory response involving multinucleate giant cells, macrophages and lymphocytes (see granulomatous inflammation, page 40). It is believed that lipopolysaccharides in the capsules of the mycobacteria may be responsible for this peculiar reaction but the mechanism is unclear.

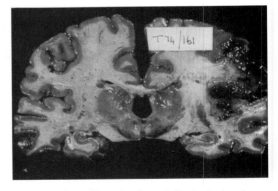

Fig 3.8 Coronal section through the brain showing softening and haemorrhage in the right parietal lobe in an area of liquefactive necrosis.

Other types of necrosis

Although these are the main types of necrosis, for completeness we should briefly mention four others. These are fat necrosis, gangrene, fibrinoid necrosis and autolysis.

Fat necrosis is peculiar to fatty tissue and is most commonly encountered in the breast following trauma and within the peritoneal fat due to pancreatitis. Within the breast, trauma may lead to the rupture of adipocytes and release of fatty acids. This will elicit an inflammatory response and the area will become firm due to scarring. Clinically, the lump may be mistaken for a carcinoma and excision and microscopical examination may be required to determine the diagnosis.

In pancreatitis, damage to the pancreatic acini results in the release of proteolytic and lipolytic enzymes which denature fat cells in the peritoneum and lead to an inflammatory reaction. Calcium is also deposited in the tissues in combination with fatty acids to form calcium soaps. This is a form of dystrophic calcification and we will consider calcification again in the section on tissue response to necrosis.

Gangrene does not represent a distinctive type of necrosis but is a term used in clinical practice to describe black, dead tissue. It is most commonly seen in the lower limb in patients with severe atherosclerosis, which often causes irreversible ischaemic damage to the most peripheral tissues in the body. If the pattern of necrosis is mainly of the coagulative type, it is referred to as **dry gangrene**, while the presence of infection with Gram negative bacteria converts it into a liquefactive type of necrosis, when it is called **wet gangrene**. It will be apparent from the preceding discussion that the type of necrosis encountered depends on a number of different factors, including the type of tissue involved and the nature of the offending agent.

Fibrinoid necrosis or fibrinoid change refers to the microscopical appearance seen when an area loses its normal structure and resembles fibrin (*see page 0000*). It does not have any distinctive gross appearance.

Autolytic change is completely different from the others as it refers to cell death occurring after the person has died. Obviously, the heart stops pumping and all the tissues become irreversibly ischaemic. Enzymes leaking from the cells digest adjacent structures but there is no inflammatory response because the inflammatory system is dead!

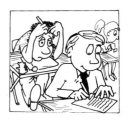

Compare and contrast coagulative and liquefactive necrosis

Coagulative	Liquefactive
Mechanism	
severe ischaemia destroying proteolytic enzymes	strong proteolytic enzyme action destroying tissue
Appearance	
initial preservation of cell outlines and tissue architecture	loss of cell outlines tissue becomes cystic or fluid
Occurrence	
kidney heart	brain bacterial infection

Causes and mechanisms of cell death

We have considered the biochemical and morphological changes that occur with cell injury and death, but what are the causes and what are the mechanisms?

There is a wide range of insults that can cause cell death, ranging from the obvious – such as trauma and burns – to more subtle causes arising as a result of specific metabolic abnormalities. The causes include:

- ischaemia
- physical agents, e.g. temperature, radiation, trauma
- chemical agents, e.g. corrosive agents, alcohol, carbon tetrachloride
- infections, e.g. bacterial, viral, parasitic
- nutritional disorders, e.g .obesity, malnutrition

- immunological disorders, e.g. autoimmune disease, hypersensitivity reactions
- genetic disorders, e.g. sickle cell disease

Let us consider the possible mechanisms involved in these varied causes of cell injury and death bearing in mind that it is not always possible to define the exact site of action of the initial insult. Since the cell membrane, oxidative phosphorylation and DNA are vital to the cell, it is very likely that these will be involved. You will also recall that the final outcome is dependent on the severity and duration of the insult and the metabolic demands of the tissues at the time of the insult.

Physical and chemical agents are well known for causing cell death. We are all aware of the devastating effects of dropping an atomic bomb and the mass destruction caused by chemical warfare. Radiation and chemicals produce cell death by the production of oxygen free radicals, the details of which have been illustrated in Chapter 1. Temperature is another important factor. Heat applied to the skin in low doses may induce a coagulative type of necrosis, but with intense heat the tissue may simply vaporise! Those interested in Arctic exploration will be aware of the gangrene induced by extreme cold which is due to a combination of thrombosis in small vessels and ice crystal formation in tissues (frostbite).

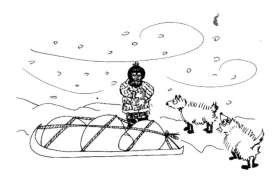

The role of infections in tissue death was discussed earlier. Briefly, microorganisms may injure tissues by producing toxins, by competing for essential nutrients, by a direct cytopathic effect as a result of cell invasion or by provoking attack by the immune system. In the course of fighting infection, there is usually some damage to the normal tissue through the release of degradative enzymes and chemical mediators of inflammation. Similar indirect mechanisms operate in the autoimmune diseases as well as in immunologically mediated injury as discussed under hypersensitivity reactions (page 34).

Sickle cell disease is caused by a genetic change in DNA which results in the production of an abnormal haemoglobin molecule. This molecule is susceptible to changes in oxygen concentration and hypoxia leads to a configurational change which results in red blood cells 'sickling'. These cells are unable to pass through the capillaries and so block the local circulation to produce local tissue ischaemia. The abnormal red cells are also prone to be removed from the circulation by the reticuloendothelial system. Sickle cell disease is therefore a good example of a genetic abnormality that results in cell injury and death. It is dealt with in more detail in Chapter 5.

So the tissue receives an insult in the form of infection, alcohol or ischaemia and the result is cell death and some type of necrosis. What then? What are the possible tissue responses and sequels to necrosis?

Tissue response to necrosis

Haemorrhage

Haemorrhage is not really a reaction to necrosis but is the consequence of endothelial cells being damaged. This may be due to the same agent as is causing the necrosis of the parenchymal cells or may be a secondary effect related to the inflammatory response. Severe endothelial cell damage may result in leakage of blood from the vessels and so areas of haemorrhage are common in necrotic tissues. The blood will eventually be removed by the phagocytic mechanisms involved in repairing the area of necrosis.

Tumours also often show macroscopically evident haemorrhage. This is thought to be due to the action of cytokines like tumour necrosis factor (TNF), which damage endothelial cells and induce thrombosis in small vessels, resulting in haemorrhage and necrosis in the tumours.

Repair and its complications

In the first chapter, we looked at the processes of inflammation and repair. Well, the healing and repair associated with necrosis follow identical pathways, which is not surprising because inflammation is one of the causes of necrosis. The inflammatory process is responsible for clearing cell debris from areas of necrosis and the final result is dependent on the site of injury and the extent of the damage. In the liver, for instance, minor degrees of injury may not be noticeable after the liver cells have regenerated. More severe damage with loss of the supporting tissue will produce scarring and fibrosis and may lead to cirrhosis.

Cirrhosis is an example of a problem caused by the healing and repair process. What happens is that the hepatocytes regenerate as parenchymal nodules without central veins or portal tracts. This ruins the normal blood flow through the liver and means that the liver vasculature cannot cope with the blood coming through the portal vein so the pressure rises to produce **portal hypertension**. The blood takes alternative routes through anastomoses which link the portal and systemic circulations, but this can produce more problems as the dilated anastomotic vessels, termed **varices**, are liable to rupture and cause life-threatening haemorrhage.

Almost every organ will have a set of complications related to the repair of necrosis. In the heart, a myocardial infarction may be followed by rupture or aneurysm formation. Lung fibrosis may impair both ventilation and gas transfer. Scarring of the skin may be disfiguring and induce contractures. All of these problems involve the formation of fibrous tissue and now we will turn to a complication which may affect the fibrosis itself, namely calcification.

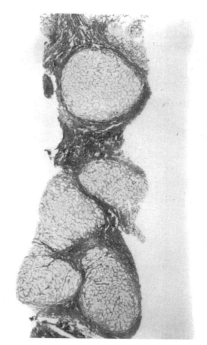

Fig 3.9 Photomicrograph of a liver biopsy stained to show fibrosis and regenerative nodules in cirrhosis (reticulin stain).

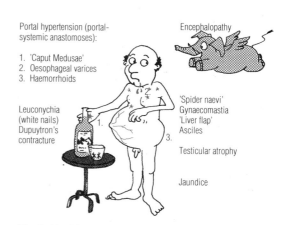

Portal hypertension (portal-systemic anastomoses):

1. 'Caput Medusae'
2. Oesophageal varices
3. Haemorrhoids

Leuconychia (white nails)
Dupuytron's contracture

Encephalopathy

'Spider naevi'
Gynaecomastia
'Liver flap'
Asciles

Testicular atrophy

Jaundice

Fig 3.10 Stigmata of liver failure

Calcification

Calcification in tissues is divided into two types:

- dystrophic calcification
- metastatic calcification

The table opposite illustrates the salient features of these two types of calcification. In this discussion, it is the first type that is important. **Dystrophic calcification** occurs in tissues that are dying or are non-viable following some type of injury, involution or alteration. The patient has a normal serum calcium level, which contrasts with the situation in **metastatic calcification**, where patients with high serum calcium levels calcify their previously normal tissues.

In this chapter, we have already mentioned the calcification that occurs in fat necrosis following an episode of pancreatitis and, in previous chapters, we have described the calcification that commonly complicates atheroma. Sometimes dystrophic calcification can be an aid for detecting lesions by X-ray examination, as occurs in breast screening programmes which use mammography. Dystrophic calcification can be intracellular and/or extracellular and may progress to bone formation (osseous metaplasia). The mechanism of dystrophic calcification involves two stages, **initiation** followed by **propagation**, which result in the formation of hydroxyapatite crystals. When the cell undergoes necrosis, large amounts of calcium enter the cell as the membrane ionic pumps fail. This calcium combines with the phosphates within the mitochondria to produce the hydroxyapatite crystals. The mechanism for extracellular calcification is similar, with crystals forming in membrane-bound vesicles derived from degenerating cells. After this initiation, the propagation of crystal formation depends on the local concentration of calcium and phosphate, whether there are inhibitors and the amount of collagen, since collagen enhances crystal production. Generally dystrophic calcification acts only as a sign of previous injury but at certain sites, such as the heart valves, it may affect function.

Metastatic calcification is due to an abnormality of calcium metabolism resulting in high levels of serum calcium. There are many causes of hypercalcaemia, which include primary and tertiary hyperparathyroidism, hyperthyroidism, sarcoidosis, metastatic cancer to bone and excess vitamin D ingestion. This form of calcification occurs in normal tissues and the favoured sites are soft tissues, blood vessels, lungs and kidneys. Extensive calcification in the kidney may impair renal function while soft tissue calcification may be nothing more than a minor nuisance. The mechanism of metastatic calcification is thought to be similar to the dystrophic variety, with the formation of hydroxyapatite crystals commencing in mitochondria.

Having considered necrosis and its complications, we will now move on to apoptosis, the paradox of cell death.

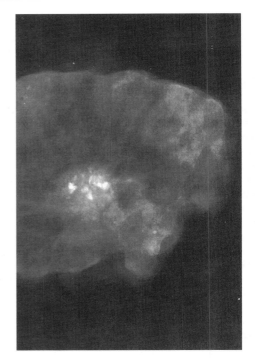

Fig 3.11 X-ray of breast tissue (mammogram) showing a circumscribed abnormality which is radio-opaque because of dystrophic calcification

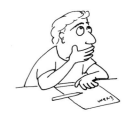

Compare and contrast dystrophic and metastatic calcification

	Dystrophic	Metastatic
Serum calcium	Normal	Raised
Tissues affected	Dead or damaged	Previously normal
Examples	Scars Atheroma Damaged heart valves Tuberculous lymph nodes Neoplasms Dead parasites	Renal failure Bone metastases Sarcoidosis Myeloma Primary and tertiary hyperparathyroidism

Apoptosis

The word apoptosis is derived from Greek and was originally used to describe the falling of individual leaves from a tree. In pathology, it is a specific type of cell death that involves single cells or small groups of cells in a tissue where the other cells are functioning normally. A similar pattern of cell death is also encountered in plants and invertebrates and is called programmed cell deletion. The term **programmed cell death** may be more appropriate than apoptosis as it emphasises that programmed cell death appears to be under physiological and, possibly, genetic control, whereas cell necrosis is due to injury. Genetic control of death! That is quite a statement to make for it implies that our own genes, selected by the pressures for survival, are also involved in causing cell death! Can death be a necessary part of life? The philosophers and gardeners amongst you will have no difficulty with this concept; after all, a good rose garden requires a certain amount of pruning.

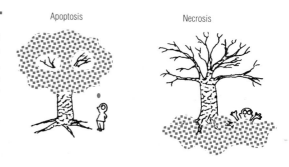

Apoptosis   Necrosis

Can cell death be useful?

The importance of controlled cell death is evident from the earliest stages of the embryo through to the involutional changes of the menopause.

Fetal development

Let us consider the production of a limb with its five digits. To achieve this, tissue growth has to occur by cell division but it is also necessary to produce interdigital cell death. It is either that or ending up as a duck! This type of cell death is genetically controlled. Similarly there are the stages of metamorphosis which take place to turn a tadpole into a frog. Metamorphosis requires not only mitotic activity and tissue growth but a large amount of controlled cell death. When a tadpole turns into a frog, the most obvious change is that limbs are formed and the tail is resorbed. During the process of resorption, there is an increase in thyroxine which appears to lead to the activation of collagenases and, hence, destruction of the tail. Here we have an example of how programmed cell death may depend on the production of a hormone with activation of protein enzyme systems to assist the process.

Hormonal effect on cell death is also important in the maturation of the human reproductive system. The reproductive system has an early indifferent phase when it is neither male nor female. The Wolffian duct will differentiate into the epidydimis and vas deferens in the male, while the Mullerian duct forms the uterus and Fallopian tubes in the female. We know from experimental observations that administration of oestrogens at a critical time will feminise the male while administration of testosterone will masculinise the female. In order for that to happen, there has to be regression of the primitive Woolfian or Mullerian structures and this occurs via controlled cell death.

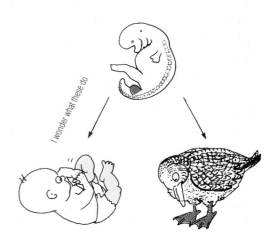

I wonder what these do

Fig 3.12 Apoptosis at the embryonic stage

Infancy

The thymus is large in the fetus and infant but atrophies before adulthood. This involution occurs via cell death which is thought to be steroid-sensitive. The steroid hormones are produced in the adrenal gland so that, in this case, one organ is responsible for the involution of another via its secreted product. This observation is useful in perinatal autopsies for deciding whether the death of a newborn baby is a sudden event or whether it follows several days of problems *in utero*. If the baby has been stressed *in utero*, adrenal steroids will cause premature involution of the thymus so that it is less than half of its normal size. If the baby has been normal *in utero* but has suffered a problem during delivery (e.g. birth asphyxia), then the thymus will be of normal size. There is some recent evidence that this steroid sensitivity is under the control of a single gene and the same gene may be involved in apoptosis caused by cytotoxic T lymphocytes (see later).

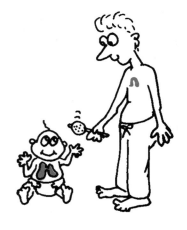

Adulthood

The endometrium is a hormone-dependent tissue that undergoes cyclical changes during the reproductive period as well as involutional changes after the menopause. The oestrogens secreted by the ovary in the early part of the menstrual cycle induce endometrial proliferation and, if pregnancy does not occur, there is programmed cell destruction that results in **menstrual shedding**. If pregnancy occurs, then there is hyperplasia of the breast in preparation for lactation, which will be followed by **physiological atrophy** involving apoptosis after weaning. This atrophy is not only due to cell loss but also results from a reduction in cell size and loss of extracellular material. Following the menopause, the withdrawal of the hormonal influence results in **involution of the uterus and ovaries**.

The immune system

Our examples so far have been of hormones affecting a particular tissue. Now we will discuss apoptosis initiated by immune cells, which differs in that individual target cells die after a **local** stimulus from an immune cell. For example, in a liver infected by hepatitis B virus, a liver biopsy will reveal many individual apoptotic cells; this is due to the immune cells attacking hepatocytes bearing the antigens of hepatitis B. It appears that cytotoxic T cells and natural killer cells are capable of directing a target cell to commence apoptosis, i.e. to commit suicide. This action is not confined to viral infection but is also likely to be involved in some autoimmune diseases and some tumour cell death.

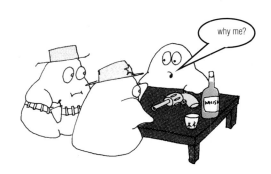

Apoptosis initiated by NK and T$_C$ cells

Cell events in apoptosis

Apoptosis is an energy-dependent process which requires the maintenance of the membrane pumping systems and the synthesis of cellular proteins. Apoptosis has two phases: **priming** and **triggering**. The initial or priming events in apoptosis involve the transcription of DNA into mRNA and the production of specific proteins which eventually dictate the path to destruction. One important protein that is transcribed by this method is an endonuclease which has the capacity to destroy the DNA which produced it in the first place. With the priming complete, the cell needs a triggering factor to drive the cell towards its death. This relies on a calcium-dependent system similar to that involved in the final stages of necrosis.

The original term for apoptosis was 'shrinkage necrosis' and apoptotic cells tend to shrink while necrotic cells initially swell. Apoptotic cells lose their contact with neighbouring cells early on. After 1–2 hours the nuclear chromatin condenses on the nuclear membrane and then the membrane 'packages' these small aggregates of nuclear material to give membrane-bound nuclear fragments. The cytoplasm shrinks and the cell's organelles also become parcelled into membrane-bound vesicles These are called **apoptotic bodies** and they contain morphologically intact mitochondria, lysosomes, ribosomes, etc. Finally, these apoptotic bodies are phagocytosed by neighbouring cells or by macrophages. Experimental evidence suggests that an apoptotic cell acquires molecules on its surface which allow neighbouring cells and macrophages to identify it as having committed suicide and hence leads to clearing of the fragments.

A crucial feature of apoptosis is that the cell's contents are not allowed to leak into the extracellular space, where enzymes may digest adjacent structures, or proteins may stimulate an immune response. Instead, the cell packages itself into small membrane-bound vesicles, which contain functioning mitochondria and other cell organelles. These survive long enough to be phagocytosed by macrophages which can degrade the components in secondary lysosomes. This mechanism is essential for allowing cell death without secondary inflammation and scarring.

Apoptosis versus necrosis

Cell death is certainly useful, as we have seen, both in normal development and under abnormal conditions such as with infection or malignancy. But what are the fundamental differences between apoptosis and necrosis? The figure on the following page compares the steps involved in necrosis and apoptosis.

Necrosis

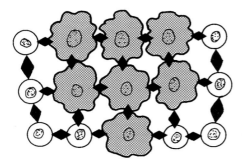

- groups of cells affected
- cells swell but initally retain inter-cellular bonds
- ↓ ATP causes membrane pump failure; influx of Na+ and Ca++ causes cell swelling and blebbing of membranes.
- cell-cell junctions break down.

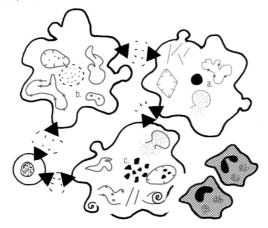

- lysis of endoplasmic reticulum
- cell membrane defects → 'myelin figures'
- rupture of lysosomes
- mitchondrial swelling
- nuclear changes:
  - a. pyknosis – condensation of chromatin
  - b. karyolysis – digestion by DNAase
  - c. karyorrhexis – fragmentation

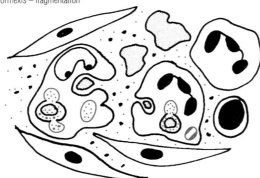

- disintegrating cells stimulate an inflammatory response
- neutrophils and macrophages digest cell debris and degrade it in 2° lysosomes

Apoptosis

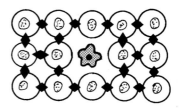

- single cell selected
- cell shrinks and loses inter-cellular bonds
- energy-driven
- endonuclease digests nuclear DNA

- nuclear chromatin condenses on nuclear membrane

- nuclear fragments and cell organelles are packed into membrane-bound vesicles

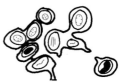

- cell shrinks further
- cytoplasm blebs to form apoptotic bodies
- new surface markers are expressed to encourage phagocytosis

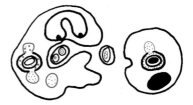

- the fragments are degraded in 2° lysosomes.
- there is no inflammatory response.

Fig 3.13 Necrosis and Apoptosis

Therapeutic cell death and its mechanisms _____

The study of cell death and apoptosis has raised important therapeutic issues, none more so that in the field of oncology. It is now generally accepted that tumour growth is a result of a fine and precarious balance between cell proliferation and cell loss. Tumours that grow fast do so not only by proliferating fast but also by keeping cell death to a minimum. The mainstay of cancer treatment has been surgery, radiation and chemotherapy. The mode of action of the latter two is to change the rate of cell proliferation and this has proved successful with many types of cancer. The first reported cure with radiotherapy was in 1899 on a basal cell carcinoma of the skin. Therapeutic radiation damages the cells, both malignant and normal, by generating ions in the tissue, the commonest of which are the oxygen free radicals derived from water. These are the same as those involved in bacterial killing in inflammation (page 14). Indirect biochemical damage includes peroxidation of molecules (especially lipids), interference with oxidative phosphorylation, changes in membrane permeability and inhibition of some enzymes. All of these would produce the necrosis type of cell death. In addition, radiation damages DNA (as we shall discuss in the next chapter on oncogenesis) producing breaks in the strands. These are normally repaired promptly but, on occasions, there may be errors in the repair leading to cell death.

There are numerous chemotherapeutic agents with a variety of modes of action. **Alkylating agents** (e.g. cyclophosphamide, melphalan) form covalent links with certain molecules, the most important of which is the guanine base in DNA. This lead to breaks in the DNA and faulty transcription. **Anti metabolites** (e.g. cytarabine, methotrexate) resemble naturally occurring substances but are subtly different so that they block an enzyme pathway or damage the macromolecular structure in which they are incorporated. Many are analogues of purine or pyrimidine bases and affect nucleic acid synthesis while methotrexate interferes with folic acid metabolism so blocking DNA and RNA synthesis. **Antibiotics** useful in chemotherapy (e.g. adriamycin, daunorubicin) often produce a local distortion of the DNA helix which interferes with the function of DNA and RNA polymerases. The **vinca alkaloids** (e.g. vinblastin) act in a completely different manner and bind to tubulin in the microtubules of the mitotic spindle to block division. The hallmark of both radiotherapy and chemotherapy is that the cell's metabolism becomes irreversibly damaged and the proliferating cell is most likely to perish, i.e. necrosis.

What about apoptosis? Does that have any therapeutic potential? We are still at an early stage but there is considerable interest in the various cytokines that might be able to promote apoptotic tumour cell death. Cytokines are produced by lymphocytes and macrophages following stimulation and, besides modifying the immune response, they may act directly to cause death of tumour cells.

Tumour necrosis factor (TNF, cachectin) is produced by activated macrophages and its action on tumour cells takes place by various distinct mechanisms. It has a role in inflammation which alters endothelial cells, promoting thrombosis and so causing ischaemic cell necrosis in the tumour. Although the death of cells in a tumour is rather complex with ischaemia playing a major role, there is evidence that at least some of the cells die due to attack by lymphocytes. In experimental models, TNF also causes an increase in apoptotic cell death, which appears to be a direct effect as there is an early rise in the synthesis of RNA in the affected cell. Various interleukins appear to produce tumour cell death secondary to stimulation of cytotoxic T cells and natural killer cells which then act on the tumour cells to initiate apoptosis.

Interferons, on the other hand, appear to exert their effects by acting in synergy with the above factors. They have been shown to enhance the cytotoxicity of T lymphocytes and natural killer cells and they also increase the phagocytic activities of macrophages for tumour cells. They are known to reduce the rate of tumour cell multiplication (in combination with TNF).

The study of mediators and mechanisms of cell death has raised a tremendous euphoria in clinical oncology. With the advent of genetic engineering, it is possible to produce quantities of cytokines necessary for cancer treatment. The initial euphoria has been dampened a little as some cytokine treatment is rather toxic, but advances will continue to be made in both the biology and the clinical regimens.

As Lewis Thomas says, cell death is indeed a natural marvel! It seems to be such an integral part of life yet until recently we have paid little attention to it. The study of cell death is assuming an increasingly important role in the understanding of such diverse processes as embryogenesis, infections and neoplasia.

We will now go on to consider the two specific types of tissue damage caused by amyloidosis and haemochromatosis.

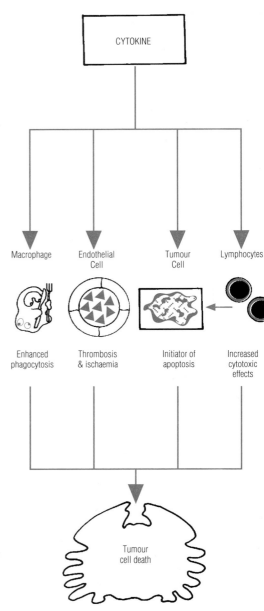

Fig 3.14 Postulated actions of cytokines on tumours

Amyloid _____

First a clinical history!

A 60 year old lady complained of tiredness, weakness, loss of weight, pain in her ribs and shortness of breath which had been getting worse for six months. Her exercise tolerance had decreased to 200 yards and she had noticed that her urine was frothy. On examination, she was thin, appeared anaemic and had a raised jugular venous pressure and peripheral oedema. She was tachycardic with a pulse rate of 110 beats/min and her blood pressure was 110/90 mmHg. Auscultation revealed evidence of pulmonary oedema. Dipstick testing of the urine sample showed the presence of protein.

Investigations showed that she was anaemic with a haemoglobin of 9 g/l, serum albumin was low at 20 g/l and calcium was raised at 3.5 mmol/l. Her urea was raised at 25 mmol/l and her creatinine was 180 μmol/l indicating impaired renal function. Urine analysis confirmed protein-uria and protein casts. Chest X-ray showed cardiomegaly with pulmonary oedema and, in addition, revealed lytic lesions in the ribs. This prompted a further skeletal survey which showed lytic lesions in the skull and pelvic bones and serum electrophoresis demonstrated the presence of a paraprotein band and reduction of other immunoglobulins. Bence Jones protein was found in the urine.

A diagnosis of myeloma appeared likely and it was felt that her cardiac and renal failure might be the result of amyloid deposition, so a renal biopsy was performed which confirmed the presence of amyloid.

We will follow our familiar pattern and consider the pathophysiology behind the signs and symptoms, the appearances on biopsy material that help us to make the diagnosis of amyloid and then the whole concept of amyloidosis.

How do we explain the signs and symptoms?

Myeloma is a disorder of plasma cells in which there is overproduction of part of one immunoglobulin. In essence, it is cancer of plasma cells. Amyloidosis is one of the complications of myeloma, as amyloid protein can be formed from the light chains of immunoglobulin molecules. The amyloid protein is deposited at various sites in the body, including the heart and kidneys and can interfere with normal function. In the heart, amyloid is deposited within the extracellular space of the myocardium and so infiltrates around the myocardial fibres. Here it restricts movement of the myocardial cells leading to poor ventricular contraction. This results in decreased cardiac output with cardiac failure and a compensatory increase in heart rate (**tachycardia**). Failure of the left ventricle will increase the hydrostatic pressure in the pulmonary veins to produce **pulmonary oedema** while failure of the right ventricle results in a **raised jugular venous pressure** and **peripheral oedema**. In addition, amyloid infiltration may affect the conduction system leading to arrythmias and hence exacerbation of the cardiac failure, which is also being worsened by the patient's anaemia.

This lady had evidence of **renal failure** with a raised plasma urea and creatinine concentration and protein in the urine which makes the urine frothy. Amyloid damages the kidney by being deposited within the glomerular tufts where it both reduces the amount of fluid filtered and

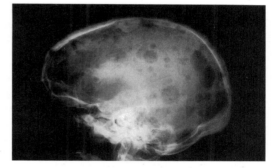

Fig 3.15 Skull X-ray with multiple 'punched out holes' in a patient with a myeloma

makes the filter more leaky so that protein can pass into the urine. The protein and immunoglobulin light chains in the tubular fluid can precipitate to cause obstruction and, hence, cause direct damage to the tubules which further compromises renal function. Amyloid is also found in the blood vessel walls and around tubular basement membranes. We will consider the microscopical appearances later in the chapter.

The other symptoms and signs in this patient are related to the malignant plasma cells which proliferate in the bone marrow. These may depress haemopoesis leading to **anaemia** and produce **bone pain** and **hypercalcaemia** as the tumour expands and erodes the bone to produce the lytic lesions seen on X-rays.

Now that we understand the reasons for the signs and symptoms, let us consider the microscopical features that may help us to make a diagnosis of amyloid. In this patient a renal biopsy was carried out to assess the degree of damage and to confirm the presence of amyloid. Where a renal biopsy is not indicated, a simpler way of looking for amyloid is to use a rectal biopsy or to obtain peritoneal fat by fine needle aspiration, which is easier and less traumatic.Figs 3.16 & 3.17 are of renal biopsies from a normal kidney and from a patient with myeloma.

Let us consider the glomeruli first. The glomerular tuft has an increase in matrix material (amyloid) in the mesangium (1) which is denser in some areas leading to obliteration of the capillary lumina (2). Compare this with the normal kidney where the mesangial cells are evenly distributed and the lumina of the vessels are widely patent. The blood vessel (3) in the case of amyloidosis shows thickening of the wall due to the deposition of hyaline material which can be demonstrated to be amyloid. The narrowing of these arterioles leads to ischaemia of the tubules and you can see that, compared with the normal kidney, there is evidence of tubular loss (atrophy). Some of the tubules also contain protein casts (4) within their lumina due to the leakage of albumin and immunoglobulin light chains. In one of the tubules, there is a laminated concretion (5); this is a deposit of calcium within the tubules. In the discussion of calcification earlier, we mentioned that metastatic calcification occurs when there is an abnormality of calcium metabolism. Myeloma is one of the causes of hypercalcaemia and metastatic calcification is a recognised finding which may also contribute to the renal failure. There is an inflammatory infiltrate within the interstitium of the myeloma kidney and this is secondary to the tubular damage caused by ischaemia. It is not uncommon for these patients to develop ascending infections related to the tubular blockage caused by the protein casts, and severe interstitial inflammation with polymorphs in the tubular lumina is an indication of pyelonephritis.

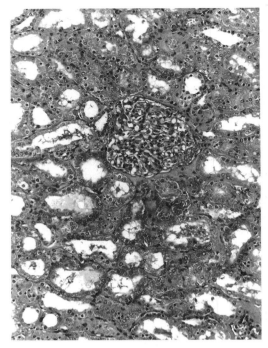

Fig 3.16 Normal kidney

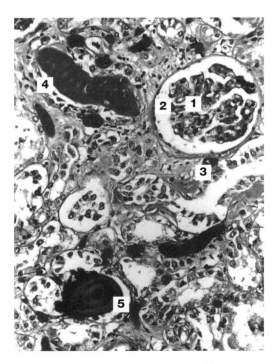

Fig 3.17 Kidney from a patient with myeloma

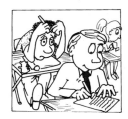

Well, now we know about the clinical aspects of amyloid, we need to ask:

- What is amyloid?
- Under what circumstances is it formed?
- Which organs are affected?
- How are they damaged?
- How can we be sure that the amorphous pink material in a biopsy is amyloid?

We have known about amyloid for a very long time and, as early as 1842, Rokitansky had reported the presence of a 'waxy, eosinophilic' material in tissues. It was Rudolf Virchow, however, who coined and popularised the term 'amyloid' because of the reaction of the material with iodine and sulphuric acid, an indication that the material is 'starch-like'. Organs affected by amyloid are generally enlarged and firmer than normal. An imaginative pathologist has likened an amyloid spleen to a cricket ball. The amyloid is not toxic but causes damage by producing **atrophy of parenchymal cells** through pressure or ischaemia, or by interfering with function by impairing the heart's contractions or the kidney's glomerular permeability, as already described. The list summarises the functional effects of amyloid.

Amyloid is an extracellular deposit of proteinaceous material. This deposition may be **localised** or **systemic**. The important point is that, despite the fact that amyloid appears identical on light microscopy in different disorders, the chemical composition differs! Therefore amyloidosis is not a single entity, but a group of disorders whose amyloid has a different composition but common physical properties because of the three-dimensional folding pattern of the protein.

What are the functional effects of amyloid?

Heart
    restrictive cardiomyopathy
    heart failure
    arrhythmias
Kidney
    proteinuria
    renal failure
Gut
    malabsorption
    altered motility
    perforation
Liver/spleen
    pressure atrophy
    often no clinical effect
Haemorrhage due to amyloid in vessels &/or Factor X deficiency

The nature of amyloid

Amyloid's rather uninteresting and bland appearance on routine microscopy belies quite a complex structure. Electron microscopy reveals that it is a fibrillary protein with fibrils arranged in non-branching rods which are orientated longitudinally. The length of the fibres is indefinite but the diameter is between 7.5 and 10 nm. Each of the fibrils is composed of two or more filamentous subunits of 2.5 – 3.5 nm in diameter. The feature that gives amyloid its common properties is its 'cross-beta' pleated configuration which can be visualised using X-ray diffraction crystallography. For some unknown reason, this prevents the material from being digested and removed by phagocytic cells. The chemical properties of amyloid protein are more variable but fall into distinct groups as indicated in Table 3.1.

There are two protein components in amyloid: the variable component and a glycoprotein common to all amyloid except cerebral amyloid, which is called **amyloid P component**. This may be derived from serum amyloid P component, which is an identical acute phase reactant

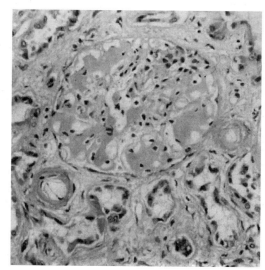

Fig 3.18 A glomerulus showing severe involvement with amyloid.

molecule found in the plasma. Component P does not contribute to the fibrils but combines as five globular subunits to form a pentagonal doughnut shape with an internal diameter of 4 nm and external diameter of 9 nm.

Before we proceed to discuss the different types of amyloid, it is important to appreciate that only amyloid related to immune disorders (AL) and amyloid related to chronic reactive conditions (AA) are reasonably common and cause significant disease. Familial amyloid is rare; endocrine-related and dermal amyloid are of little clinical importance. Senile amyloid is common but of uncertain significance. It may turn out to be very important because of the presence of amyloid in the brain in many dementias.

Systemic amyloidosis

Table 3.1 is a recent classification of amyloidosis. Looking at the table, you can see that the amyloid types are designated using two letters. The first, A, refers to amyloid. The second letter – L, A, F, H, Sc, E, D – refers to the biochemical classification. We will now consider these individual groups in a little more detail.

AL or immune-associated amyloid
Although the reactive type (AA) of amyloid is most common worldwide, the AL form is the commonest in most developed countries. It is the type of amyloid which is associated with plasma cell dyscrasias, such as multiple myeloma, Waldenstrom's macroglobulinaemia and monoclonal gammopathies. Approximately 6–15% of the patients with myeloma develop amyloid and most will die within a year of the diagnosis; 50% die from cardiac failure, since the heart is the most important organ affected by AL-type amyloid. It is important to appreciate that AL amyloid affects a somewhat different group of tissues to AA amyloid, which is reflected in the patient's presentation and problems (see opposite).

AL amyloid is so designated because it is derived from the *light* chains of immunoglobulin molecules, which is why it occurs in disorders of the immunoglobulin-producing cells, i.e. plasma cells. Only part of the light chain is involved in amyloid production and this part is derived from the variable region of the molecule. Interestingly, although more myelomas produce kappa light chains than lambda light chains, it is more common to find amyloid in patients with lambda light chain myeloma. It is thought that this is because the light chains must undergo proteolysis before fibril formation and only some light chains have suitable regions for proteolysis. Similarly, AA amyloid precursors are believed to require cleavage and some patient's serum AA protein is not suitable for proteolysis, so not all patients with predisposing conditions will actually develop amyloid.

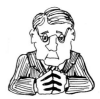

Which organs are commonly involved in AL and AA amyloid?

AL–immune associated	AA–reactive
1. Restrictive cardiomyopathy	Kidney
2. Kidney	Spleen
3. Peripheral neuropathy	Liver
4. Skin	
5. Polyarthropathy ("padded shoulder"sign)	
6. Macroglossia (enlarged tongue)	
7. Isolated factor X deficiency	
8. Idiopathic carpal tunnel syndrome	

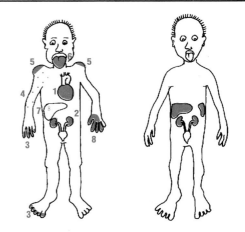

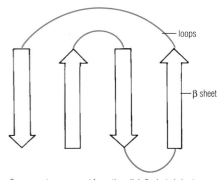

Commonest arrangement for antiparallel β-pleated sheet

Table 3.1 Classification of amyloidosis

Clinical disorder	Amyloid fibril	Related serum protein
Systemic amyloidosis		
Immunocyte dyscrasias with amyloidosis – Monoclonal gammopathy alone – Myeloma – Waldenström's macroglobulinaemia	AL	Ig light chains
Reactive systemic amyloidosis	AA	SAA

Heredofamilial systemic amyloidosis
– Neuropathic form
  (type 1)
– Non-neuropathic form
  (familial Mediterranean fever)
	AF
	
	AA
		Transthyretin
		
		SAA

Haemodialysis-associated amyloidosis	AH	β_2-Microglobulin
Senile amyloid	ASc ASc I	Transthyretin Atrial naturetic peptide
Localised amyloidosis		

Cerebral amyloid
– Alzheimer's disease
– Down's syndrome
– Hereditary cerebral angiopathy
  – Dutch
  – Iceland
	A4 β-Protein
	
	Crystatin C
		–
		
		–

Endocrine-related amyloid – Medullary carcinoma of thyroid – Endocrine tumours of pancreas	AE	Calcitonin Islet peptides
Plasmacytoma – light chains	AL	Ig light chains
Cutaneous amyloid	AD	?Keratin
Dystrophic amyloid	?	?

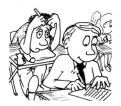

Amyloid is composed of antiparallel β pleated sheets. What is a β sheet?

The amino acid sequence of a protein is called its primary structure. Different regions of the sequence form local regular secondary structures, such as alpha helices and beta strands joined by loop regions. β strands can combine to form β sheets. Proteins have a C terminal with a free COOH group and an N terminal with an NH_2 group. If all the β strands lie in the same direction, it is called a parallel sheet; if their directions alternate, it is an antiparallel sheet. Molecules like immunoglobulin light chains and β2 microglobulin have abundant β strands.

AA or reactive amyloid

This type of amyloid is called secondary or reactive amyloid because it is associated with chronic infective or inflammatory disorders, such as rheumatoid arthritis, tuberculosis, chronic inflammatory bowel disease and osteomyelitis. Approximately 10% of patients with rheumatoid arthritis will develop amyloid, generally after 10–15 years of active rheumatoid disease. The kidney is most commonly affected (70%) and half of the patients will die from the effects of amyloid within five years.

Amyloid A protein is not derived from immunoglobulins but is a 76 amino acid protein with a molecular weight of 8500. It is produced by cleavage of a circulating 12000 molecular weight protein, termed SAA (serum amyloid A associated) protein, which is produced by the liver and is one of the acute phase proteins.

The AA type of amyloid is also associated with familial Mediterranean fever (FMF) and some neoplasms, such as renal cell carcinoma and Hodgkin's disease. FMF is an autosomal recessive disorder in which there is inflammation affecting pleura, peritoneum, skin and synovium. FMF is the 'odd man out' of the familial forms of amyloid because its protein component is derived from SAA, probably related to recurrent bouts of inflammation.

AF or familial amyloid

This is a group of inherited disorders in which the amyloid is deposited principally in nerves (familial amyloid polyneuropathy). It occurs in small clusters throughout the world and has an autosomal dominant pattern of inheritance. The genetic abnormality appears to affect the production of transthyretin (previously called prealbumin), whose normal role is the *trans*port of *thy*roxine and *retin*ol – hence the name. The abnormal transthyretin molecules can aggregate to form amyloid fibrils. In contrast to AL and AA amyloid, where the relevant light chain or precursor (SAA) serum level is elevated, the serum transthyretin levels are normal but it is the structural abnormality of the molecule which is important.

AH or haemodialysis-associated amyloid

A distinct form of amyloid has been identified in patients receiving *haemodialysis* for chronic renal failure which particularly affects the joints and tendons and may cause carpal tunnel syndrome. In patients with renal failure, there is an accumulation of β_2-microglobulin because this molecule is not filtered during haemodialysis. β_2-microglobulin is a normal serum protein and a component of MHC class I molecules. Here is an example of amyloid which is not due to overproduction of the precursor or an abnormality in the precursor but is simply a failure of normal excretion of a normal molecule.

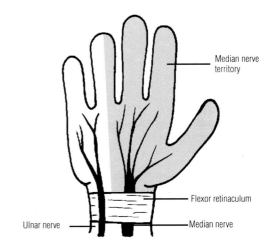

Median nerve territory

Flexor retinaculum

Ulnar nerve

Median nerve

Fig 3.19 Carpal tunnel syndrome

Intermittent compression of the median nerve in the carpal tunnel produces tingling of the fingers supplied by the median nerve.

ASc or senile amyloid

How many people have senile amyloid? Well, it depends on how hard you look. Autopsy studies report that 25% of people over 65 years old and 100% of people over 80 years have some deposits. Often the deposits are localised, most commonly in the heart, but 25% of people have widespread deposits, especially affecting the heart, lung, pancreas and spleen. A more important question is: how many people *suffer* from senile amyloid? The answer is very few as the amyloid deposition is generally asymptomatic except for occasional cases of senile cardiac amyloid. The amyloid protein of generalised senile amyloidosis is formed from an abnormal transthyretin molecule suggesting a genetic predisposition. It is called ASc. Senile cardiac amyloid, however, is derived from atrial naturetic peptide and is referred to as ASc I. Cerebral amyloid is sometimes included under senile amyloid but it is biochemically different and can also occur in young people, so we will discuss it separately.

Localised amyloidosis

Cerebral amyloid

Our knowledge and theories concerning cerebral amyloid are changing quite rapidly. Cerebral amyloid differs from other forms of amyloid in that it does not contain component P and it can occur in intracellular (neuro-fibrillary tangles) as well as extracellular locations. The functional significance of cerebral amyloid is not known but it occurs in Alzheimer's dementia, Down's syndrome, transmissible encephalopathies, some hereditary cerebral angiopathies and some elderly normal individuals. The amyloid may be deposited in:

- vessel walls
- neuritic plaques
- neurofibrillary tangles

A4β protein has been isolated from these lesions and the gene coding for it is on chromosome 21. It is also interesting that this type of amyloid is believed to be synthesised locally rather than being derived from a serum precursor like the other types of amyloid.

AE or endocrine-related amyloid

Certain endocrine tumours, such as medullary carcinoma of the thyroid and islet cell tumours of the pancreas, contain amyloid derived from the hormone or prohormone produced at that site. Thus, in medullary thyroid carcinoma, the amyloid is derived from calcitonin and precalcitonin and, in islet cell tumours, insulin and proinsulin are often implicated. The amyloid does not appear to have any clinical significance.

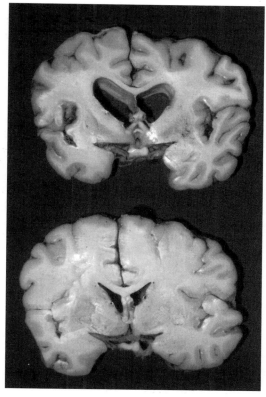

Fig 3.20 Coronal sections of normal brain (bottom) and an atrophic brain (top) showing dilatation of the ventricles and widening of the cerebral sulci as occur in Alzheimer's disease.

AD or dermal amyloid

Primary cutaneous amyloid deposits have been noted and it is thought that the amyloid is derived from keratin. The skin may also be involved in immune-associated systemic amyloid (AL) when the deposits involve degraded immunoglobulin light chains.

Dystrophic amyloidosis

This category did not feature in our table on classification because this entity is not yet easy to categorise. Originally it was used to describe localised amyloid in damaged cardiac valves which were not associated with systemic disease or old age. Similar deposits were noted in a quarter to a half of all osteoarthritic joints and it has also been found in damaged or abnormal tissue, such as endometriotic cyst walls, fibrotic epidermal cysts, hernial sacs and skin ulcers. The biochemical nature of the amyloid has not been identified.

Pathogenesis

The pathogenesis of amyloid formation is far from clear but the mechanism illustrated below is the currently held view. It is generally believed that there is production of 'amyloidogenic' fragments through catabolism of precursor molecules. These precursors may result from:

- elevated production of normal proteins, e.g. light chains, SAA
- reduced excretion of normal protein, e.g. β2-microglobulin
- abnormal form of protein, e.g. transthyretin

Staining characteristics of amyloid

At autopsy, amyloid can be demonstrated in fresh organ slices by applying 1% acetic acid followed by iodine. If amyloid is present, the tissue will stain a deep brown colour, which will turn blue-violet when 10% sulphuric acid is added. In formalin-fixed, paraffin-embedded microscopical sections, amyloid may be demonstrated using Congo red, crystal violet, methyl violet or thioflavine T. Congo red is most commonly used and it stains amyloid a pink-red colour. Collagen and elastic fibres may also stain pink but these may be distinguished by viewing the section under polarised light when only amyloid will give an apple green colour. All of the forms of amyloid will stain by these techniques and it is sometimes useful to distinguish the various types. If AA or AH amyloid is treated with potassium permanganate before Congo red staining, it fails to stain whereas the other forms of amyloid are resistant to potassium permanganate. Alternatively, specific antisera to the different forms of amyloid may be used on tissue sections by the immunoperoxidase technique.

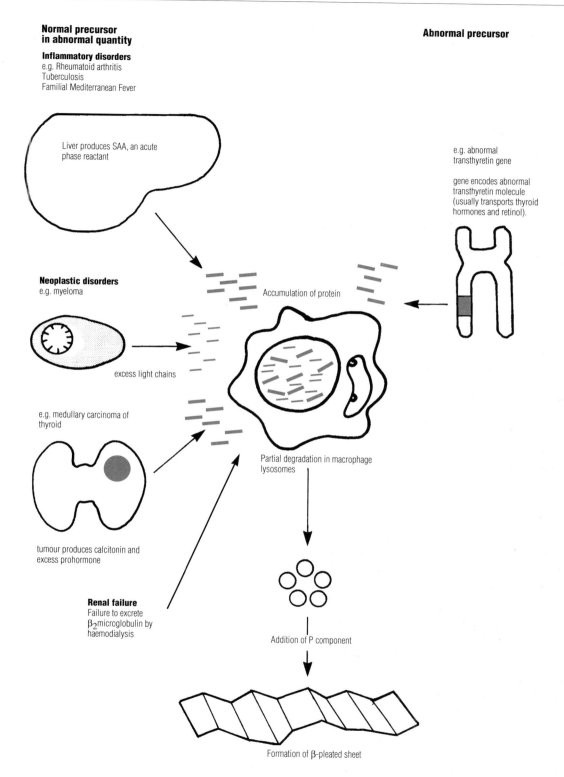

Normal precursor in abnormal quantity

Inflammatory disorders
e.g. Rheumatoid arthritis
Tuberculosis
Familial Mediterranean Fever

Abnormal precursor

Liver produces SAA, an acute phase reactant

e.g. abnormal transthyretin gene

gene encodes abnormal transthyretin molecule (usually transports thyroid hormones and retinol).

Neoplastic disorders
e.g. myeloma

Accumulation of protein

excess light chains

e.g. medullary carcinoma of thyroid

Partial degradation in macrophage lysosomes

tumour produces calcitonin and excess prohormone

Renal failure
Failure to excrete $\beta_2$microglobulin by haemodialysis

Addition of P component

Formation of β-pleated sheet

Fig 3.21 Mechanisms operating in amyloid production

Now we know how to prove that the amorphous pink material is amyloid, but what if it isn't? Amyloid is not the only amorphous pink material and two common causes of a similar microscopical (but not clinical) picture are hyaline and fibrinoid change.

Hyaline change does not refer to a specific entity but is a descriptive term for a variety of intracellular and extracellular materials (Table 3.2). These have nothing in common except for their microscopical appearance. **Fibrinoid change** refers to a similar pink homogeneous material which has the histochemical staining characteristics of fibrin and may be due to deposition of fibrin in tissues. Fibrinoid necrosis classically occurs in blood vessel walls as a result of immune complex disease or malignant hypertension and also occurs in the subcutaneous nodules of rheumatoid arthritis, so called rheumatoid nodules.

Haemochromatosis

Haemochromatosis is the other form of tissue damage that we should like to discuss in more detail because it allows us to look at various aspects of iron metabolism and the diseases associated with accumulation of excess iron. First, let us begin with a clinical history.

A 40 year old gentleman complained of tiredness, weight loss and increased frequency of micturition. The symptoms had been present for nine months but had been worse for the last three months. He gave no other relevant history. The doctor noticed that the patient appeared sun tanned although he had not been on a recent holiday. Examination showed a mild degree of pulmonary oedema, an enlarged liver and small testes. Dip stick examination of the urine revealed glycosuria but no proteinuria or blood. The patient had a raised fasting blood sugar, abnormal liver function tests with raised alanine transaminase, γ-glutamyl transferase and alkaline phosphatase. Serum ferritin and iron levels were also raised and a chest X-ray showed a normal-sized heart with a mild degree of pulmonary oedema. Liver biopsy showed increased parenchymal iron but no evidence of cirrhosis or malignancy. The doctor concluded that his patient had 'bronzed diabetes' or haemochromatosis.

Let us consider this gentleman's symptoms and see if they could all be due to haemochromatosis. The fundamental problem in haemochromatosis is an increase in the total body iron and we will discuss the possible causes and mechanisms of the increased iron later. For the present, how can we explain the symptoms on the basis of the increased iron?

Excess iron in the body is deposited in the macrophages of the reticuloendothelial system (lymph nodes, bone marrow, spleen and Kupffer cells of the liver) and in the parenchymal cells of various organs, most commonly the pancreas, liver and heart. Deposition of iron in the **pancreas** leads to

Table 3.2 Hyaline change

	Material
Intracellular site	
Proximal renal tubule in proteinuria	Protein
Russell bodies in plasma cells	Immunoglobulins
Viral inclusions in many cells	Viral proteins
Mallory's alcoholic hyaline in hepatocytes	Intermediate filaments
Extracellular site	
Hyaline arteriosclerosis and glomerular hyalinisation	Basement membrane material and plasma proteins
Hyaline membranes in lung	Surfactant and degenerate pneumocytes

destruction of islet cells resulting in deficient insulin secretion and, hence, **diabetes**. The symptoms of tiredness, weight loss and increased frequency of micturition are all explained by the presence of diabetes. This also accounts for the glycosuria and raised blood sugar. Mild iron deposition in the **skin** leads to a massive increase in melanin production and, thus, the tanned skin. Note that most of the colour is due to melanin and not iron. The combination of the above two is the reason for the old name of 'bronzed diabetes'. Deposition of iron in the **liver** may have serious consequences and, in this gentleman, had produced an enlarged liver and abnormal liver function. Iron within parenchymal cells is toxic and leads to hepatocyte cell death with resultant scarring and fibrosis. If left untreated, the liver will eventually become cirrhotic and predispose the patient to **carcinoma of the liver (hepatocellular carcinoma)**. His heart failure is explained by deposition of iron in myocardial cells, necrosis of the myocytes and, ultimately, fibrosis. His small testes are most likely to be due to some toxic effect of iron on the hypothalamic–pituitary axis resulting in secondary atrophy of the testes since iron is not found in large amounts within the testes.

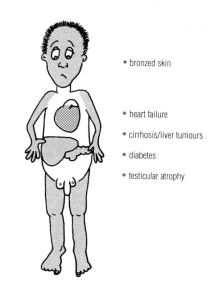

- bronzed skin
- heart failure
- cirrhosis/liver tumours
- diabetes
- testicular atrophy

Fig 3.22 Haemochromatosis

What causes haemochromatosis and what is the pathogenesis?

Primary haemochromatosis is a disorder of iron metabolism that is inherited in an autosomal recessive fashion and has an association with HLA-A3, -B7 and -B14. Males are affected more than females, in a ratio of 7:1. It is called primary haemochromatosis to distinguish it from haemochromatosis secondary to haemolytic anaemias, liver disease or high iron ingestion. The other form of systemic iron overload is much less severe and is termed **haemosiderosis**. It results from similar causes to secondary haemochromatosis but the excess iron is insufficient to swamp the reticuloendothelial cells of the bone marrow, lymph nodes, spleen and liver, so the iron remains in macrophages and does not cause toxic damage to parenchymal cells. These disorders result from an imbalance between the amount of iron ingested and the amount excreted, so it is a convenient moment to remind ourselves of how iron is absorbed, transported and excreted in normal circumstances.

Iron is an important element with well-known roles in haemoglobin, myoglobin, cytochromes and various enzyme systems in the cells. Approximately 80% of the body's iron is in one of these functional forms while the remaining 20% is stored as ferritin or haemosiderin. There is no control over the excretion of iron and so the total iron in the body is regulated by its absorption. Some iron is lost through exfoliation of cells at epithelial surfaces and small amounts of blood are lost in the gastrointestinal tract. Menstruation is an important route of iron loss in premenopausal females

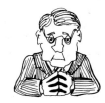

What are the causes of haemochromatosis?

Primary – Hereditary

Secondary
↑ iron ingestion
    iron tablets
    some wine and beer
    frequent transfusions

↑ breakdown of red blood cells
    thalassaemia major
    sideroblastic anaemia

Liver disease
    alcoholic cirrhosis

and may account for the higher incidence of haemo-chromatosis in men.

Food contains iron in two forms. The more important one is **haem** iron from animal haemoglobin and myoglobin. First, this is released from its apoproteins by the action of gastric acids and taken into the epithelial cell where enzyme degradation releases the iron. This iron can be stored temporarily in the cell as the protein–iron complex **ferritin**, or immediately despatched into the plasma for transfer to other sites bound to the glycoprotein **transferrin**. Approximately 25% of haem-iron in food is absorbed whereas only 1–2% of non-haem iron is absorbed. **Non-haem iron** absorption requires a different mechanism and probably involves secreting transferrin into the gut where it binds to iron and then joins to a specific receptor on the epithelial surface. The iron–transferrin–receptor complex would undergo endocytosis so that the iron enters the epithelial cell's cytoplasm. Most iron is absorbed in the duodenum, although some enters through the stomach, ileum and colon.

The normal total adult body iron is between 2 and 6 grams but this is increased to 50–60 grams in haemochromatosis. The hypothesis is that the basic defect in haemochromatosis resides at the level of iron absorption in the gastrointestinal tract. The exact defect is not known but it may be an alteration in the transport proteins or membrane receptors of the mucosal cells that allows excess iron to enter. Alternatively, there may be a lack of the immediate postabsorption excretion of iron or an impairment in the normal role of macrophages in controlling mucosal absorption.

Once the iron has been absorbed in excess in primary haemochromatosis, it accumulates in parenchymal cells of various organs. What happens to the cells that have accumulated a lot of iron and does it inevitably lead to cell death? The answers are 'don't know' and 'no'. It is possible that iron is involved in the production of free radicals which may damage the cell's membranes and organelles. Iron also tends to accumulate in the lysosomes and any damage to the lysosomal membrane will release degradative enzymes which could damage the cellular components and lead to cell death. However, we also know that cells containing excess iron do not inevitably die and their iron content can sometimes be reduced with iron-chelating drugs such as desferrioxamine.

The appearance of the involved organs

The affected organs will have a dark-brown colour to their cut surface and they can be stained for iron using Prussian Blue. The texture of the organs may be altered because of the fibrosis which makes them firmer and may cause shrinkage. Microscopical examination will show large amounts of golden-yellow pigment within the cells and often some atrophy or loss of normal cells with varying degrees of fibrosis. The liver classically shows micronodular cirrhosis.

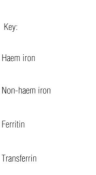

Key:

Haem iron

Non-haem iron

Ferritin

Transferrin

Senescent cell

Haemosiderin

Fig 3.23 Iron metabolism

Body iron is derived predominantly from the breakdown of haemoglobin, myoglobin and cytochrome pigments by macrophages in the spleen, liver & bone marrow.

Dietary iron replaces iron lost through daily cell loss, menstruation, haemorrhage etc. Children & adult males must eat 5-10mg iron/day, whereas pregnant or menstruating females require 7-20mg/day. Haem iron can enter the enterocytes directly whereas non-haem iron must be bound by mucosal transferrin.

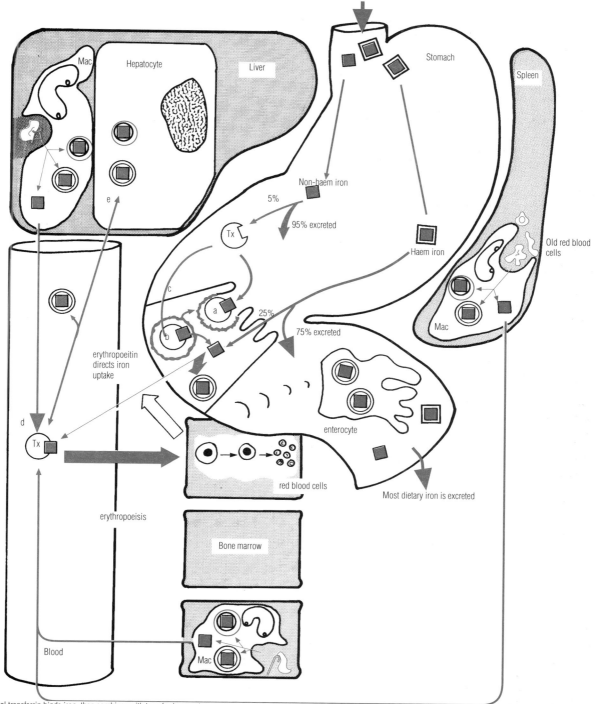

a. mucosal transferrin binds iron, then combines with transferrin receptor
b. Iron-transferrin-receptor complex is endocytosed
c. transferrin and receptor recycled; most iron is stored in enterocyte as ferritin, a small amount enters the bloodstream.

d. 95% of plasma iron is carried by transferrin, which transports it to the bone marrow for use in erythropoiesis, or to the liver for storage.
e. Surplus iron is stored as soluble ferritin or insoluble haemosiderin, mainly in the liver, but also in the macrophages of the liver, spleen and bone marrow.

Distinguishing pigments by light microscopy

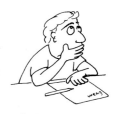

Iron is not the only pigment that appears brown or golden-yellow on light microscopy; the others are melanin, lipofuscin and bile. Identifying the type of pigment present may be essential for reaching a diagnosis. For example, excess brown pigment in the liver may be iron suggesting haemochromatosis, bile suggesting obstructive liver disease, or lipofuscin which is probably of no significance.

Distinguishing these pigments at light microscopy depends on their appearance, their distribution and their histochemical staining pattern.

List the histochemical stains that are commonly used for distinguishing brown pigments

Prussian Blue	iron
Masson-Fontana	melanin
Sudan Black	lipofuscin
Fouchet	bile

Iron

Iron stored as haemoglobin is brown or golden-yellow, tends to be granular, and is found in the cells of the reticuloendothelial system as well as the parenchymal cells. The technique most commonly used for demonstrating iron is **Prussian blue** stain which makes iron blue.

Melanin

Melanin can vary in colour from light brown to black. It is found in normal skin and retina but can also be seen in benign naevi and in malignant melanoma. Whilst malignant melanomas often contain melanin, they may also contain iron, due to haemorrhage within the tumour and the two pigments may appear very similar on H&E sections. Thus distinguishing melanin from iron in a tumour may establish the diagnosis of melanoma. This can be achieved by the **Masson–Fontana** technique, with which melanin stains black.

Jaundice: Yellow discoloration of skin and sclera due to excess serum bilirubin.
Causes of jaundice:
i.   Pre-hepatic: e.g. ↑ red cell breakdown, as in haemolytic anaemia (↑ unconjugated bilirubin)
ii. Intra-hepatic: e.g. viral hepatitis (often a mixed type of hyperbilirubinaemia)
iii. Post-hepatic: e.g. bile duct obstruction by gallstone or pancreatic carcinoma (↑ conjugated bilirubin)

Lipofuscin

Lipofuscin is composed of pigments derived from oxidation of lipids and lipoproteins and is found mainly in lysosomes but can also be seen in mitochondria. They have been referred to as 'aging' or 'wear and tear' pigments because their amount increases with the patient's age. It is thought that they represent the residue of degradation, i.e. what is left after everything else has been processed for excretion or recycling. The most common sites of deposition are the liver and heart.

The **Sudan black** technique turns lipofuscin black.

Key:

Albumin	(Alb)		
Unconjugated bilirubin	■	Conjugated bilirubin (mono- & di-glucuronides)	
Biliverdin	□		
Macrophage		Usual route	→
Senescent cells		Unusual route	- - →

Fig 3.24 Bilirubin metabolism and jaundice

Bile

Bile pigments result from the breakdown of red cells (*see* Fig 3.24). Following the removal of haemoglobin and iron, bilirubin is transported to the liver where it is conjugated with glucuronic acid and excreted into the hepatic duct. These pigments can be seen in the bile canaliculi as well as in the hepatocytes and appear either as brown or green-yellow pigment. There are a number of methods that can be used to demonstrate this pigment. The **Fouchet** technique stains bile pigments blue-green.

a. Macrophages in the liver, spleen and bone marrow break down haemoglobin and myoglobin to release bilirubin. Bilirubin is water insoluble and is transported in the blood bound to albumin.

b. The liver enzyme, UD Glucuronyltransferase, catalyses the formation of mono- and di-glucuronides (conjugated bilirubin).

c. Most of the glucuronides enter the gut via the bile, but some enter the bloodstream. They are soluble and are loosely bound to albumin. If blood levels are raised, e.g. by blockage to bile outflow, they are excreted via the kidney, producing dark brown urine, and also in sweat.

d. Normally the majority of glucuronides are broken down by gut bacteria to form faecal pigments, such as biliverdin. Most of these are excreted via the gut, but some are reabsorbed and excreted in the urine, producing a yellow/green tint.

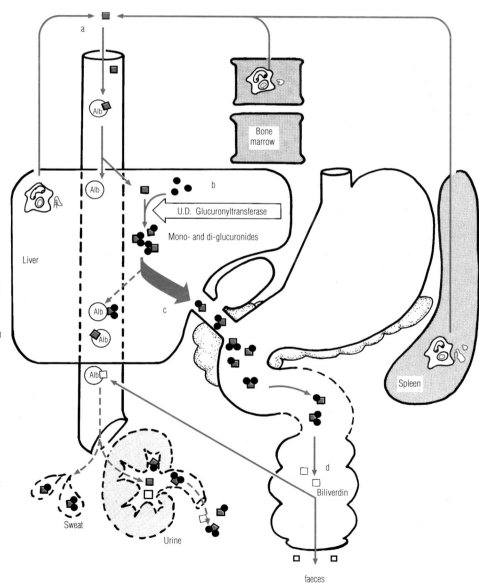

Bilirubin

a

Bone marrow

Alb

Alb

Liver

U.D. Glucuronyltransferase

Mono- and di-glucuronides

Alb

Alb

c

Spleen

Alb

Sweat

Urine

d

Biliverdin

faeces

Clinicopathological summary

Clinical

A 60 year old man, with long-standing history of alcohol abuse presented with a three-week history of general malaise, weight loss, loss of appetite and a productive cough.

Examination:
He was noted to be short of breath with an increased respiratory rate and was jaundiced. He had a fever and tachycardia of 110 beats/min. He also had supraclavicular lymphadenopathy and a mildly enlarged and tender liver. Auscultation of his chest revealed coarse crackles over both lung fields.

Investigations:
The liver function tests were abnormal with a raised bilirubin of 45 µmol/l and a raised gamma-GT of 90 IU/l. His chest X-ray showed bilateral consolidation with a small right pleural effusion. A lymph node and liver biopsies were carried out.

The lymph node showed numerous caseating granulomata with calcification. The Ziehl–Neelson stain showed abundant acid-fast mycobacteria. The liver biopsy showed an acute alcoholic hepatitis with marked **fatty change** and liver fibrosis, but without cirrhosis.

Management and progress:
He was started on antituberculous therapy and rehabilitation was instituted to help him with his alcohol abuse.

While in the hospital, he complained of abdominal pain and nausea. He also had one bout of diarrhoea. He therefore underwent a gastroscopy and a sigmoidoscopy. The gastroscopy revealed a patchy gastritis which was confirmed on histological examination of the gastric biopsy. Sigmoidoscopy was unremarkable; however, histological examination revealed the presence of **amyloid** within the mucosa.

He was started on antacids for his gastritis, continued with his antituberculous treatment and was sent for rehabilitation. He failed to complete his rehabilitation and after two months was lost to follow-up from the medical out-patient clinic. All attempts to trace him were unsuccessful.

Pathology

He had a long history of alcohol abuse and this predisposes to many illnesses. Alcoholics tend to be malnourished as they derive their calories mainly from the alcohol and are therefore deficient in many vitamins, especially the B group. They damage the liver by episodes of hepatitis which heals with scarring, producing fibrosis and eventually cirrhosis. They are also predisposed to infections because of depression of the immune system caused by the alcohol and, in this man, clinical examination revealed signs of a chest infection. Tuberculosis is a particular problem in alcoholics.

The liver function tests were in keeping with alcoholic damage with raised bilirubin and liver cell enzymes. The chest X-ray confirmed a pneumonic process involving both lungs.

Caseous necrosis *with granuloma formation is a classical picture of tuberculosis and special stains revealed the mycobacteria. Immune suppression due to the alcohol abuse is responsible for the reactivation or secondary infection.*

*In areas of necrosis, calcification is common and this type is called **dystrophic calcification**. The serum calcium levels are normal, as opposed to metastatic calcification in which the serum calcium levels are raised.*

*His liver biopsy showed the classical **fatty change** common in alcohol abuse with some hepatitis, i.e. inflammation of the hepatocytes with liver cell necrosis. The result is healing by scarring with resultant fibrosis. He was lucky in not yet having reached the cirrhotic phase, which is irreversible. Fatty change is reversible.*

Alcoholics are predisposed to gastritis, i.e. inflammation of the gastric mucosa. They may also have gastric ulcers. Other complications include oesophageal varices that occur with portal hypertension in cirrhosis, and this is a serious complication demanding urgent treatment.

*Patients with long-standing chronic inflammatory diseases such as rheumatoid arthritis and tuberculosis are prone to a reactive **amyloidosis**, type amyloid AA. Rectal biopsies are convenient ways of diagnosing amyloid. The amyloid may have been the cause of the diarrhoea, but in such a patient infective causes should always be ruled out.*

Lack of compliance is a common problem with alcoholics.

This brings us to the end of this chapter on cell and tissue damage. A basic understanding of cell death and how tissues react to injury is vital not only for understanding clinical signs and symptoms but also in allowing us to formulate theories on embryogenesis and normal development. Paradoxically, this study of death is fundamental to our knowledge of life, and as Lewis Thomas says:

"We will have to give up the notion that death is catastrophe, or detestable, or avoidable, or even strange. We will need to learn more about the cycling of life in the rest of the system, and about our connection to the process. Everything that comes alive seems to be in trade for something that dies, cell for cell."

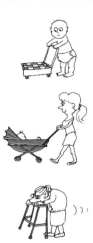

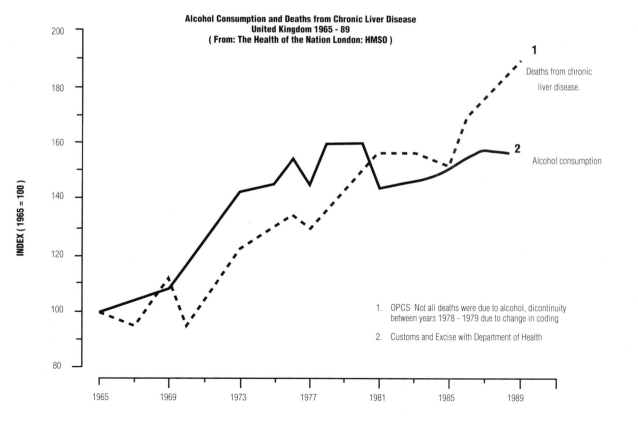

Alcohol Consumption and Deaths from Chronic Liver Disease
United Kingdom 1965 - 89
(From: The Health of the Nation London: HMSO)

1 Deaths from chronic liver disease.

2 Alcohol consumption

1. OPCS Not all deaths were due to alcohol, dicontinuity between years 1978 - 1979 due to change in coding

2. Customs and Excise with Department of Health

INDEX (1965 = 100)

Further reading

J.M. Lackie & I.A.R. More. (1992). Cells and tissues in health and disease. Ch 1. *Muir's Textbook of Pathology*. Ed. R.N.M. MacSween & K. Whaley. 13th Edition. Edward Arnold. London.

R.S. Cotran, V. Kumar & S.L. Robbins. (1989). Cellular injury and adaptation. Ch 1. Robbins *Pathologic Basis of Disease*. 4th Edition. W.B. Saunders Company. Philadelphia.

I.D. Bowen & S.M. Bowen. (1990). *Programmed Cell Death in Tumours and Tissues*. Chapman and Hall. London.

B. Alberts, D. Bray, J. Lewis, M. Raff, K. Roberts & J.D. Watson. (1989). Molecular Biology of the Cell. 2nd Edition. Garland Publishing,. New York & London.

A.H. Wyllie & E. Duvall. (1992). Cell death. Ch 3.1. *Oxford Textbook of Pathology*. Ed. J. McGee, P.G. Isaacson & N.A. Wright. Oxford University Press. Oxford.

S. Young. (1992). *Life and death in the condemned cell*. New Scientist. 133: 34–37.

Chapter 4

Cell Growth and its Disorders ___

Does early death come
As a punishment?
Or
Does it come too late,
For those who are tortured
By incurable pain?
Is death really cruel?
Or
Is it merciful?

– Gitanjali 1961–1977

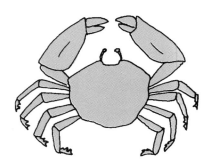

Gitanjali, as beautiful as the poem by Rabindranath Tagore, died at the age of 16 with cancer. To many people, cancer is regarded as a disease that appears suddenly, takes a tight grip, progresses relentlessly and causes a slow and painful death.

In 1731, Lorenz Heister, a German surgeon wrote: "The name *Scirrhus* is given to a painless tumour that occurs in all parts of the body, but especially in the glands, and is due to stagnation and drying of the blood in the hardened part. … When a scirrus is not reabsorbed, cannot be arrested, or is not removed by time, it either spontaneously or from maltreatment becomes malignant, that is, painful and inflamed, and then we begin to call it *cancer* or *carcinoma*; at the same time the veins swell up and distend like the feet of a crab (but this does not happen in all cases), whence the disease gets its name; it is in fact, one of the worst, most horrible, and most painful of diseases."

Is this pessimism really justified? About 20% of people will die of cancer, which is less than the number dying from cardiovascular disease, but heart disease does not usually generate such intense dread.

In this chapter, we shall look at the symptoms which occur in cancer, how it is diagnosed and which features are important for prognosis and treatment. Then we will turn to the aetiology and pathogenesis of tumours, how they spread and what treatments are available. Finally we shall consider the benign disorders of cell growth and the premalignant changes which are clues of early cancer and are important in screening programmes.

First a few words on the history of cancer. Johannes Müller, a German microscopist, established that tumours were made of cells (1883). This laid the foundation for his pupil, Rudolf Virchow, whose book on cellular pathology dealt extensively with tumours, which he divided into 'homologous' and 'heterologous'. The homologous group resulted from proliferation of cells already present and were generally benign, while the heterologous group showed a change in the character of the cell and were generally malignant. However, Virchow failed to recognise the mechanism of metastasis which was described by Billroth (1856) and Von Recklinhausen (1883). Many investigators looked for causes of cancer. One of the most famous was Percival Pott who, in 1775, identified that scrotal cancer in chimney sweeps was related to chronic contact with soot.

Occupational exposure to industrial tar and paraffin was recognised by Von Volkmann in 1875 as causing cancers and many such associations have since been described. Techniques in molecular cell biology have advanced considerably and we are now in a position to attempt to answer some of the fundamental questions relating to the control of normal cells and the mechanisms involved in the production of cancer cells.

Malignant neoplasms

We will begin by considering a clinical problem and will take the example of a 50 year old lady who presented to her family doctor with a lump in her left breast. She had noticed a recent enlargement in its size but the mass was not painful. She had no other medical problems but she had a positive family history, her mother having died of breast cancer five years previously.

Her family doctor could feel a 2 cm diameter mass below the nipple in her left breast. This was hard, poorly defined and fixed to the surrounding tissues. The nipple and areola on that side had an eczematous appearance but the right breast and nipple were normal. He did not find any enlarged lymph nodes in either axilla or supraclavicular fossa and no abnormalities in the rest of the body. The family practitioner suspected that this was a malignant tumour and so referred her to hospital for further investigation. Let us digress for a moment to discuss why the doctor decided that this mass was malignant.

Clinical features of malignant tumours

It should be stressed that it was not a single criterion that allowed him to draw a reasonable conclusion, but a combination of factors. In this case, the lump was **ill-defined, hard and involved adjacent tissues** and skin. A characteristic feature of malignant tumours is that they infiltrate surrounding structures, whereas benign tumours grow with a smooth pushing edge (Fig. 4.4). Thus the malignant lumps lack a well-defined edge and, because they are attached by infiltrating tongues of tissue, it is often impossible to move them relative to the surrounding tissues. Many malignant tumours induce a proliferation of benign fibroblasts which produce collagenous connective tissue. This reaction is termed **desmoplasia** and gives the tumour its hard texture.

The lesion's **size** was greater than most benign lesions, although this is a variable feature. More importantly, there was a recent **rapid increase in size**, which often indicates malignant growth. In this example, there was one other important clue for the doctor which is a peculiarity of some breast cancers. The 'eczema' that was noted over the nipple is referred to as **Paget's disease of the nipple** and is due to

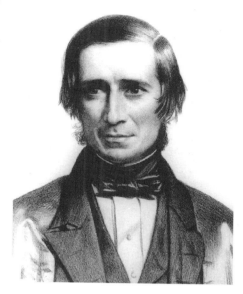

Fig 4.1 Sir James Paget (1814–1899). Courtesy of the Wellcome Institute for the History of Medicine.

James Paget was born in Yarmouth, Norfolk. He was apprenticed to a surgeon at the local hospital at the age of 16 and enrolled as a medical student at St. Bartholomew's Hospital, London at the age of 20 years. In 1837, a year after obtaining his M.R.C.S., he was appointed Curator of the Museum at the hospital.

Paget was an excellent clinical observer, and an eloquent lecturer. He is best remembered for his descriptions of Paget's disease of bone (osteitis deformans) and Paget's disease of the nipple.

He was elected F.R.S. (1851) and Surgeon Extraordinary to Queen Victoria (1858). He was created a Baronet in 1871.

carcinoma cells growing along the breast ducts towards the nipple and then into the epidermis of the skin. Two other factors, had they been present, would have influenced the doctor; these are **pain** and **metastasis**. Many tumours, both benign and malignant, are painless, but the presence of unremitting pain is suggestive of malignancy. The presence of metastatic disease is the definitive evidence that a tumour is malignant so it is important to understand possible routes of spread, in order that the most likely sites for metastasis can be examined especially carefully. In this lady's case, there was no pain or metastatic tumour spread, so the doctor suspected that it was a localised malignant growth and the patient was referred to hospital.

Here a series of tests were performed to make a more precise diagnosis and to assess the extent of her disease; this included mammography, a chest X-ray and bone scan to look for tumour spread and haematological and biochemical blood tests to look for anaemia and changes in liver function.

The surgeon must make a definite diagnosis by obtaining some tissue from the breast lump. He has various options, he could:

- anaesthetise the patient and remove the whole lump
- anaesthetise the patient and remove a part of it
- insert a needle attached to a syringe to suck out some cells for examination (fine needle aspiration (FNA) cytology)
- he could insert a special biopsy needle which would ream out a core of tumour about 3 mm wide and 10–15 mm long

In this particular case the surgeon opted for FNA cytology, which showed malignant cells and the surgeon went on to excise the lump and sample the axillary lymph nodes. In the fullness of time, the surgeon received the pathologist's report on these tissues and used that information to guide his management of the patient. The report is reproduced opposite and we shall discuss its relevance for patient management and some points it raises about the biology of tumours.

First, there is the gross appearance which records points similar to the criteria used by the family practitioner for distinguishing malignant from benign lumps. This includes the size, the infiltrating margin and the consistency of the tumour. Most importantly, there is an assessment of whether the tumour appears completely excised, since incomplete excision will result in rapid recurrence and increased opportunity for spread. The report of the microscopical appearances records the pathologist's conclusion, i.e. that it is a primary malignant tumour of breast tissue. Let us consider how this conclusion has been reached.

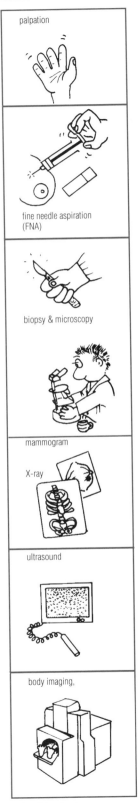

palpation

fine needle aspiration (FNA)

biopsy & microscopy

mammogram

X-ray

ultrasound

body imaging,

Fig 4.2 Tools of the trade

Gross appearance

A simple mastectomy specimen consisting of skin, including nipple, which measures 170 mm × 90 mm and covers fatty tissue with maximum dimension of 80 mm (Total weight = 280 g). In the tissue beneath the nipple, there is a pale, firm, gritty mass measuring 25 mm × 20 mm × 20 mm which has an irregular, poorly defined margin. The closest excision margin (medial) is 15 mm from the mass. There is an area of erythema around the nipple. The axillary dissection measures 80 mm x 50 mm × 50 mm and 13 lymph nodes have been identified.

Microscopical appearance

Sections show an insitu and invasive ductal carcinoma exhibiting a moderate amount of tubule formation, mild nuclear pleomorphism and occasional mitotic figures (grade 1), with maximum dimension of 22 mm. There is no evidence of lymphatic or vascular permeation and resection margins are tumour free. The sections of the nipple confirm the presence of Paget's disease. None of the 13 axillary lymph nodes contain tumour.

Conclusion

Breast: in situ and invasive ductal carcinoma.

Reported by Dr. S.P. Ecimen.

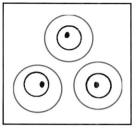

Benign
- Cell size & shape regular
- Nuclear membrane smooth & even
- Nuclear chromatin evenly distributed
- Nucleoli usually round, single & inconspicuous
- Nuclear:cytoplasmic ratio low, e.g. 1:4

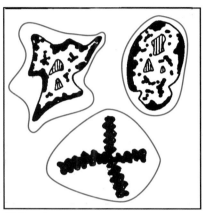

Malignant
- Cells pleomorphic, i.e. highly variable in size and shape
- Nuclear membrane irregular in shape and thickness; often angulated
- Nuclear chromatin pattern uneven
- Nucleoli variable in size and shape, frequently multiple & conspicuous
- N:C ratio high, e.g. 1:1

Fig 4.3 Cytological features of malignancy

What are the microscopical features that distinguish malignant tumours?

Malignant tissues differ from benign tissues in that they have an abnormal architectural arrangement and an atypical appearance to the individual cells. The **disordered growth pattern** can only be appreciated by comparing it with the normal appearance of that tissue. For example, the normally regular glands of the stomach mucosa contrast with the complex glandular pattern and extension of the glands through the basement membrane in a gastric adenocarcinoma. A crucial factor, which is often essential for diagnosing carcinoma, is that cells should invade through the basement membrane, which marks the boundary between epithelial and sub-epithelial tissues (although in some sites it is possible to identify an in situ, i.e. non-invasive, carcinoma).

An atypical appearance of individual cells (cytological **atypia**) is a rather more subtle change and may involve both nucleus and cytoplasm. The nucleus is often many times the size of a normal nucleus, has an altered distribution of chromatin and is a darker colour in stained sections, so called **hyperchromatism**. These alterations reflect the increased amount and abnormalities of nuclear chromatin, which is common in tumours as they are frequently **aneuploid**. Most normal cells have a small single nucleolus.

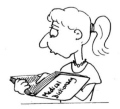

Aneuploid: an abnormal number of chromosomes that is not an exact multiple of the haploid (23) number.

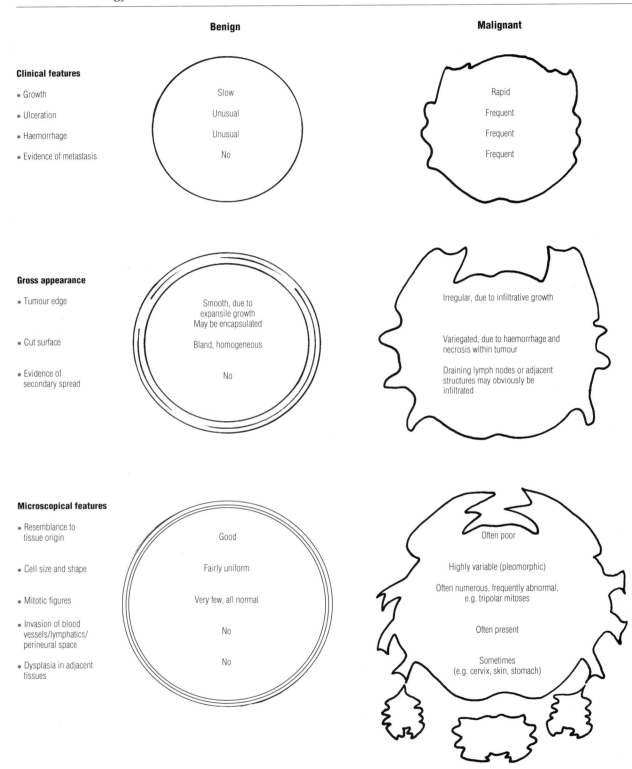

Benign

Malignant

Clinical features

- Growth
- Ulceration
- Haemorrhage
- Evidence of metastasis

Slow

Unusual

Unusual

No

Rapid

Frequent

Frequent

Frequent

Gross appearance

- Tumour edge

- Cut surface

- Evidence of
  secondary spread

Smooth, due to
expansile growth
May be encapsulated

Bland, homogeneous

No

Irregular, due to infiltrative growth

Variegated, due to haemorrhage and
necrosis within tumour

Draining lymph nodes or adjacent
structures may obviously be
infiltrated

Microscopical features

- Resemblance to
  tissue origin

- Cell size and shape

- Mitotic figures

- Invasion of blood
  vessels/lymphatics/
  perineural space

- Dysplasia in adjacent
  tissues

Good

Fairly uniform

Very few, all normal

No

No

Often poor

Highly variable (pleomorphic)

Often numerous, frequently abnormal,
e.g. tripolar mitoses

Often present

Sometimes
(e.g. cervix, skin, stomach)

Fig 4.4 Features of benign and malignant tumours

In malignant cells, there may be many nucleoli of varying sizes or, alternatively, a large single nucleolus. The position of the nucleus is often abnormal, i.e. it exhibits a **loss of polarity**. Thus, the nucleus of a normal colonic cell is situated at the cell's base with mucus in the cytoplasm nearer the surface whereas the nucleus is more central in a malignant cell. The general appearance of the cells is altered as there is an **increase in nuclear-cytoplasmic ratio**, either because the amount of cytoplasm is less or the nucleus is larger or a combination of the two.

The cytoplasmic changes vary depending on the tissue but generally involve a **loss of specialised features**, e.g. absence or reduction in mucin content in a colonic adenocarcinoma. The malignant cells do not only differ from normal cells but also from each other and this variation is referred to as **pleomorphism**. Ultimately, however, all of these features are only guidelines and the real test is whether the tumour behaves in a malignant fashion. Of course we cannot leave patients untreated just to see how the tumour behaves. Pathologists have learnt much about the behaviour of tumours from autopsy studies and, fortunately, tumours of similar appearance usually show similar behaviour in different patients.

What factors influence prognosis?

Here we are concerned with factors which influence prognosis and can be assessed routinely by histo-pathologists. As we shall see later, there are specialist techniques which can be used for certain tumours, but here the discussion will be limited to the information in a routine report.

The important points are:

- the type of tumour
- the grade of tumour
- the stage of the disease

First it is essential to decide whether the tumour has arisen locally or whether it is a metastasis. Two points help make this distinction and these are whether there are precancerous changes or in situ carcinoma present and whether the lesion resembles tumours known to occur at that site.

In situ carcinoma is an alteration in architecture and cytological appearance which is similar to that seen in malignant tumours but does not show any invasion. **Precancerous lesions** are harder to define but are changes which have been shown in large studies to be associated with the development of cancer and are believed to represent an early, but possibly reversible, stage of malignancy.

In most organs, there is one type of malignant tumour which is far more common than any other and this generally corresponds with the type of tissue which is proliferating in

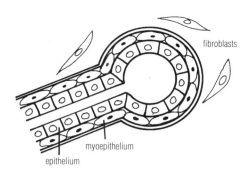

Normal breast lobule lined by two cell layers.

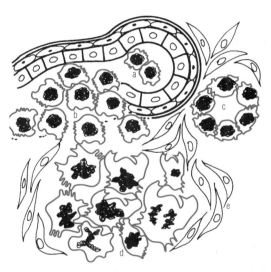

a. In-situ carcinoma: malignant epithelial cells distend the lobule.

b. Early invasion.

c. Well differentiated adenocarcinoma: tubular (duct-like) architecture and fairly uniform cells with few mitoses.

d. Poorly differentiated adenocarcinoma: the tumour lacks any architectural pattern and is composed of cells varying in size and shape, and many mitoses are present.

e. "Desmoplastic" stromal response to infiltrating tumour cells.

Fig 4.5 In-situ and invasive adenocarcinoma of breast

that normal organ. For example, the breast and colon have active glandular epithelium so the commonest malignant tumour at both sites is an adenocarcinoma composed of malignant glandular epithelium. The bladder is lined by transitional epithelium which gives rise to transitional cell carcinoma and the oesophagus has squamous epithelium and squamous carcinomas. Remembering the normal histology can be a great help in predicting the commonest tumours for a particular site.

To return to our patient; she has an adenocarcinoma of ductal type which has in situ and invasive components. Therefore, this is a primary tumour of the breast. If it was entirely in situ then it would have an extremely good prognosis because the lack of local invasion would mean that the tumour had no ability to extend into lymphatic or blood vessels and no possibility of metastasis. In our patient however, there was local invasion, but tumour was not seen in lymphatic or blood vessels. The most important prognostic feature is the type of tumour but after that the prognosis is influenced by the grade and stage. (In most organs there is just one type of adenocarcinoma but the breast has two histologically and clinically distinct forms of adenocarcinoma termed ductal and lobular. This need not concern us here. The grade of a tumour depends on its histological appearance while the stage of a tumour depends on its size and extent of spread. The **histological grade** is a crude measure of how much the tumour resembles normal tissue combined with an estimate of its mitotic activity. There is a well-defined scoring system for breast tumours (see Table 4.1), based on tubule formation, nuclear pleomorphism and the mitotic count. This divides them into three grades, with grade 1 tumours having a better prognosis than grade 3 tumours. Many sites have no formal grading system and so the pathologist will merely record whether the tumour is well-differentiated, moderately differentiated or poorly differentiated, by assessing similar features but in a less mathematical way.

The **stage of a tumour** depends on both pathological and clinical information, including CT scans, ultrasound scans, bone marrow examination, etc. A TNM staging system is often used for breast carcinoma where T is for primary tumour, N is for regional node involvement and M for metastatic disease (see Fig. 4.7). This provides an easy shorthand for indicating the disease stage, which is helpful for deciding treatment and comparing the outcome of patients treated with new therapeutic regimens. Obviously, assessment of a new treatment regimen must take account of the stage of a patient's disease to avoid spurious results.

The pathology report on our patient states that none of the lymph nodes contained tumour and the clinical investigation did not show metastases. Therefore, she would be categorised as T2, N0, M0 which translates as stage II disease. This short coded message tells the doctor that she is in a relatively good prognostic group.

Table 4.1 Grading of breast cancer

This is based on assessment of 3 criteria: tubule formation, nuclear pleomorphism and mitotic count. Scores are given as follows:

Tubule formation:
Good tubule formation (>75%)	1
Moderate (10–75%)	2
Poor (<10%)	3

Nuclear pleomorphism:
Mild	1
Moderate	2
Severe	3

Mitotic Count: Mitoses are counted per 10 high power fields. (Varies with type of lens).
0–5	1
6–10	2
>11	3

Grade		
1	= Score	3–5
2	= Score	6–7
3	= Score	8–9

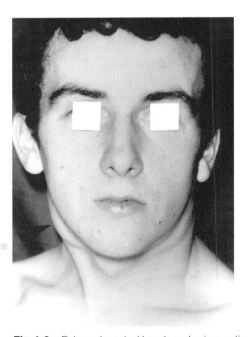

Fig 4.6   Enlarged cervical lymph nodes in a patient with Hodgkin's disease.

TNM system, e.g. Ca breast

T = tumour size:
T0: impalpable
T1: 0-2 cm
T2: 2-5 cm
T3: >5 cm ± fixation to underlying muscle
T4: any size, with fixation to chest wall or skin

N = Lymph node status:
N1: regional nodes involved
N2, 3: more distant nodal groups

M = Metastases
M0: No detectable spread
M1: Metastases present (specify sites)

Dukes' staging of colorectal carcinoma

Comment: 5 year survival figures:
Dukes' A: 85%
Dukes' B: 45%
Dukes' C: 15%

mucosa,
m. mucosae
submucosa

m. propria

lymph nodes

Dukes' A: Tumour confined within bowel wall; no spread through main muscle layer

Dukes' B: Spread through m. propria into serosal fat, without lymph node involvement

C_1

C_2

Dukes' C: Tumour spread to lymph nodes.
C_1: Pericolic nodes involved
C_2: Involvement of higher mesenteric nodes

Cotswolds revision of Ann Arbor staging system for Hodgkin's Disease

Comment: The presence of "B" symptoms, e.g. fever, drenching sweats, weight loss, adversely affects the prognosis, and is included in the stage, e.g. Stage II A (no B symptoms), or Stage II B.

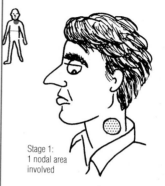

Stage 1:
1 nodal area involved

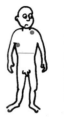

Stage II: ≥ 2 nodal areas on same side of diaphragm involved (no. of involved sites recorded)

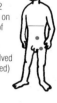

Stage III: Nodal areas on each side of diaphragm:
III_1 upper abdo,
III_2 lower abdo

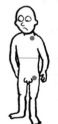

Stage IV:
Visceral involvement

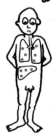

The spleen is part of the reticuloendothelial system. Splenic involvement does not carry the same staging implications as, for instance, bone marrow or liver

Fig 4.7 Staging of tumours

When the doctor talks to his patient about these results, she may well ask him a variety of questions about her prognosis but before we attempt to answer those questions, we should digress to discuss the classification of tumours.

Classification of tumours

You will recall that a knowledge of the normal structures at a particular site can be of great help in predicting the commonest tumours. This is because the tumour resembles part of the parent tissue and the classification is based on the assumed histogenesis, i.e. because a transitional cell carcinoma has some similarities with transitional epithelium, it is assumed to arise from it.

The broad classification divides tumours into those arising from epithelia (carcinomas), from connective tissue (sarcomas), from lymphoid tissue (lymphomas) and 'the rest', which includes specialised tissues such as the brain. Included in Fig. 4.8 are the benign counterparts arising from the same tissues.

At this point there needs to be a word of caution because, although this classification originated from ideas on histogenesis, it is now apparent that cells of one tissue type may 'differentiate' to resemble cells of another type. For example, bronchial glandular epithelium may become squamous. This can occur in cells under normal control, where it is termed metaplasia (see later), but its malignant counterpart destroys the histogenetic approach to classification, because we have a tumour that appears squamous on microscopy but which originally arose from glandular epithelium. Fortunately, we only have to claim that we will classify tumours according to their type of differentiation and we eliminate the problem! Thus a tumour resembling squamous cells is a squamous cell carcinoma regardless of the true origin. Sometimes a tumour cell is very poorly differentiated so that, even to the trained histopathologist's eye, it does not resemble a particular type of normal cell. In this situation, special stains to demonstrate cytoplasmic or surface molecules can be helpful. Thus the presence of intracellular mucins would suggest an adenocarcinoma, and immunohistochemical stains for different intermediate filaments or lymphoid antigens would help to distinguish between a wide variety of tumours. Some of these substances are also released into the blood, which is useful both for diagnosis and for following the patient's response to treatment.

Now we must turn to the patient's questions. What causes cancer? How will it behave? What treatments are available? Will there be a lot of pain?

If we are not to be stumped by the the patient, we have to understand a little more about cancer biology.

What causes cancer?

Cancer occurs because of changes that take place at the cellular level. However, we still do not completely understand what happens to a cell in order to produce a tumour. A little more clear are the factors that predispose to cancer and it is by identifying these that we may deduce

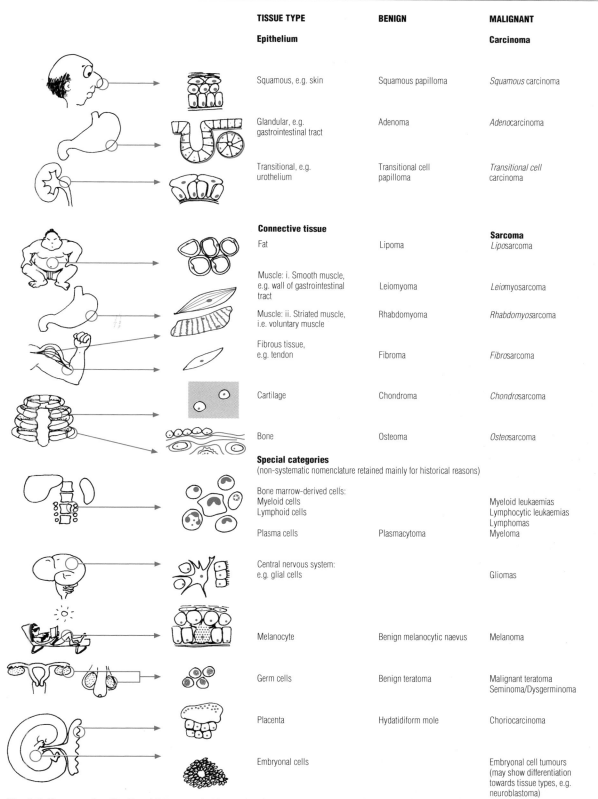

TISSUE TYPE	BENIGN	MALIGNANT
Epithelium		**Carcinoma**
Squamous, e.g. skin	Squamous papilloma	*Squamous* carcinoma
Glandular, e.g. gastrointestinal tract	Adenoma	*Adeno*carcinoma
Transitional, e.g. urothelium	Transitional cell papilloma	*Transitional cell* carcinoma
Connective tissue		**Sarcoma**
Fat	Lipoma	*Lipo*sarcoma
Muscle: i. Smooth muscle, e.g. wall of gastrointestinal tract	Leiomyoma	*Leio*myosarcoma
Muscle: ii. Striated muscle, i.e. voluntary muscle	Rhabdomyoma	*Rhabdomyos*arcoma
Fibrous tissue, e.g. tendon	Fibroma	*Fibro*sarcoma
Cartilage	Chondroma	*Chondro*sarcoma
Bone	Osteoma	*Osteo*sarcoma

Special categories
(non-systematic nomenclature retained mainly for historical reasons)

Bone marrow-derived cells: Myeloid cells		Myeloid leukaemias
Lymphoid cells		Lymphocytic leukaemias Lymphomas
Plasma cells	Plasmacytoma	Myeloma
Central nervous system: e.g. glial cells		Gliomas
Melanocyte	Benign melanocytic naevus	Melanoma
Germ cells	Benign teratoma	Malignant teratoma Seminoma/Dysgerminoma
Placenta	Hydatidiform mole	Choriocarcinoma
Embryonal cells		Embryonal cell tumours (may show differentiation towards tissue types, e.g. neuroblastoma)

Fig 4.8 Tumour classification: histogenesis (tissue type)

clues about the causes of cancer. There is a whole host of predisposing factors which can be discussed under the broad headings: 'genetic' and 'environmental'; however, there is often considerable overlap.

Age

The advent of antibiotics, improved sanitation and good nutrition has extended people's expected lifespan so that they achieve an age in which there is a high incidence of malignant tumours, particularly those of colon, lung, prostate and bronchus. However, tumours are not confined to the elderly and certain tumours, such as leukaemias, predominate in the young. It is postulated that carcinogens may have a cumulative effect over time which may explain an increased incidence with age or that age-related metabolic or hormonal changes are important. In some childhood tumours (e.g. retinoblastoma) heredity plays a major part, as the first 'hit' for carcinogenesis is inherited through chromosomal changes. However, as regards most tumours we are left with the situation that we know that age is an important factor but we don't know why!

Genetic factors

In our case of breast carcinoma, the doctor discovered that the patient's mother had died of breast carcinoma. This is of relevance in several tumours where the risk of the cancer in close family members is increased. How much the risk is increased in individual cases and with different tumours is not easy to specify but, in general, it is about two to three times normal. Obviously, tumour development is not inevitable and many other factors such as environmental and dietary influences may modify the risk.

In some tumours, the genetic susceptibility is better understood than most and in two autosomal dominant conditions, familial polyposis coli and retinoblastoma, it involves loss of a **tumour suppressor gene** or **antioncogene** (page 174). Familial polyposis coli (familial adenomatous polyposis) is a disorder in which individuals develop hundreds of polyps in the gastrointestinal tract. These appear benign by light microscopy but should be regarded as premalignant because practically all of these patients will develop a colonic carcinoma if the colon is not removed. Retinoblastoma is a malignant tumour of the eye which is commonest in children; 40% of cases of retinoblastoma are hereditary and the sporadic cases involve the same changes to the genome but require two 'hits', one for each chromosome (page 175).

Geographical and racial factors

Geographical factors merge with environmental factors, as a geographical factor is only an environmental factor which affects the population of a particular area. This may be a sunny climate, radioactive rock formations or a carcinogen in the water supply.

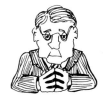

What are the major aetiological factors involved in tumour formation?

Age
Genetic factors
Geographical and Racial factors
Environmental agents
Carcinogenic agents
    Chemicals
    Radiation
    Viruses

Let us discuss the increased incidence of stomach cancer in Japan compared with North America. The tumour is seven times more common in Japanese people living in Japan than in Americans living in the United States. Is this a racial difference or an effect of some climatic, geological or dietary factor which operates in Japan? To answer this we need to know the incidence in Japanese people who move to America and raise families. They will keep their racial (genetic) factors and may import their dietary factors but not their geographical factors. We find that the incidence drops in these immigrants and is halved in their first generation offspring but is still higher than in white Americans; so we haven't achieved a definite answer to our question. Some reports suggest that the incidence drops further in future generations until it equals the American rate. This would appear to rule out a racial factor and may implicate a cultural dietary change.

A much easier example is the incidence of melanomas in white-skinned Australians. Here there is a *racial predisposition*, because they do not have sufficient skin pigmentation to protect them from ultraviolet light, and the *geographical facto*r of a sunny climate. If the Australian emigrates at birth to a cold grey country, then his risk of melanoma drops dramatically.

Environmental agents

Numerous environmental agents have been implicated in the causation of cancer. Everybody knows that there is a strong association between tobacco smoking and lung cancer (and yet people still smoke!). This problem may not only affect the smoker but also the 'innocent bystander' who inhales exhaled tobacco smoke (passive smoking).

Asbestos exposure increases the risk of developing lung carcinoma and malignant mesothelioma of the pleura and peritoneum. Exposure to β-naphthylamine, which may occur in the rubber and dye industries, increases the risk of transitional cell tumours of the bladder. Exposure to vinyl chloride in the plastics industry enhances the development of liver cell carcinoma.

One of the first examples of an environmental cancer was described in 1775 by Percival Pott, surgeon to St. Bartholomew's Hospital. He had observed that chimmney sweeps had a very high incidence of scrotal cancer, and correctly deduced that this was due to chronic contact with soot. In fact, Percival Pott achieved a double – he described an environmental carcinogen and an occupational cancer in one go! He is also remembered for his description of spinal tuberculosis, referred to as Pott's disease.

Carcinogenic agents

So far we have discussed carcinogenesis under the broad headings of age, genetics, race, geography and environment. The next step is to consider what type of agent is operating (the aetiological agent) and to look at ideas on how the agent converts a normal cell to a malignant cell (pathogenesis).

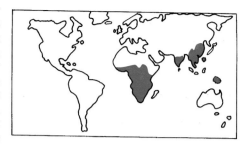

Hepatocellular carcinoma
Sub-Saharan black Africa
Far-East

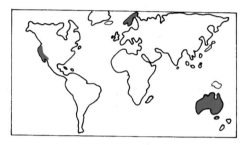

Malignant melanoma
Australia
Scandinavia
N. America: Californian whites, highest risk

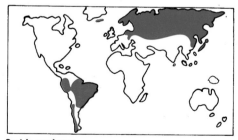

Gastric carcinoma
Japan, China
Brazil, Colombia, Chile
Iceland, Finland
USSR, Poland, Hungary

Fig 4.9 Geographical variation in tumour incidence

It is worth remembering that, as in the case we were discussing of the lady with breast cancer, by the time the patient presents with a tumour, a large number of cellular events and many thousands of cell divisions have already taken place. Consequently, we are looking at a growth that has been in existence for quite some time. In order to understand the cellular mechanisms involved in cancer formation, we must discuss the multistep theory.

The '**multistep theory of neoplasia**' states that cancers do not arise from a single event but that multiple steps are involved. It also implies that many of the so-called aetiological agents do not actually induce cancer, but cause an alteration in a cell that predisposes it to further changes which eventually lead to cancer. The next question must be: what are these multiple steps and are any of them reversible?

There are three major groups of agents involved in carcinogenesis that we need to consider in order to address this question. These are:

- chemical carcinogens
- radiation
- viruses

Chemical carcinogen
Fig. 4.10 illustrates classical experiments of chemical carcinogenesis using mouse skin, which provide the basis for the multistep theory and lead to the descriptions of **initiation** and **promotion**.

Let us consider Fig. 4.10. If you apply a polycyclic hydrocarbon (initiator) to the shaved skin of the mouse and don't do any more, then no tumours will result. However, if you later apply another chemical, croton oil (promoter), to the same skin, tumours will grow. The important points are that the initiator must be applied before the promoter and that the promoter must be applied repeatedly and at regular intervals. There may be a long time interval between initiation and promotion which suggests that initiation provokes an irreversible change in the DNA which is fixed by cell division. In contrast, the promoter acts in a dose-related, reversible fashion and appears to modify the expression of altered genes.

Some chemicals (**complete carcinogens**) can act as both initiator and promoter whereas others (**incomplete carcinogens**) only fulfil one action. Sometimes a carcinogen needs to be converted from an inactive **procarcinogen** to an active **ultimate carcinogen**. These are called **indirect carcinogens** while others, which can act without modification, are called **direct carcinogens**. It is interesting that the enzymes involved in the activation of indirectly acting chemicals, the cytochrome P-450 dependent mono-oxygenase system, can be induced by a variety of drugs including phenobarbitone. Hence the carcinogenic effect of chemicals can be modified by altering the enzymes involved in the activation process. Since many other factors can also modify these enzyme systems, it is not difficult to see why

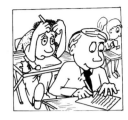

Discuss the different types of chemical carcinogens

Direct-acting carcinogens

Busulphan
Cyclophosphamide
Chlorambucil
Melphalan
β-Propiolactone
Dimethyl sulphate

Indirect-acting carcinogens

2-Acetoaminofluorene
Benzene
Benzidene
2-Naphthylamine (β-naphthylamine)

Naturally occurring carcinogens

Aflatoxin B1
Betel nut
Cycasin
Griseofulvin

Others

Fungicides
Insecticides
Nickel
Nitrosamines

age, nutrition, hormonal status and so on are important variables in the aetiology of cancer.

The table opposite lists some of the major chemical carcinogens associated with cancer. We have already mentioned some of these in previous sections. Sir Percival Pott recognised the importance of soot in causing carcinoma of the scrotum, and we now know that soot contains a mixture of polycyclic hydrocarbons which are carcinogenic in animals. Similar polycyclic hydrocarbons are present in tobacco smoke and assumed to be involved in the production of bronchial tumours.

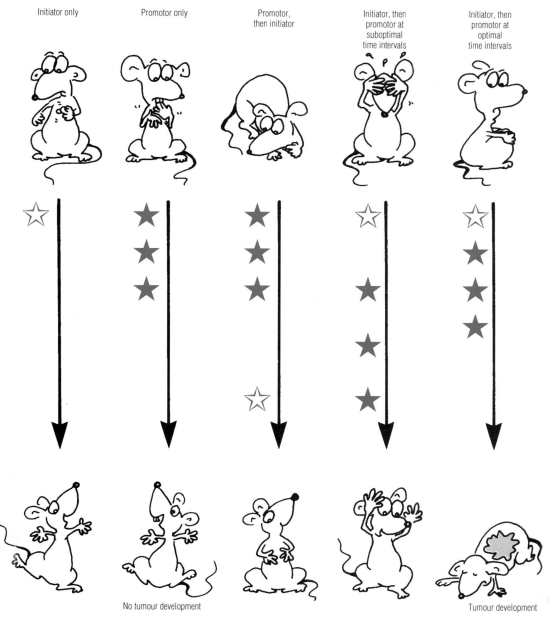

Fig 4.10 Chemical carcinogenesis: the effects of tumour promotors and initiators

Radiation

Ionising radiation includes **electromagnetic rays**, such as ultra-violet light, X-rays and gamma rays, and **particulate radiation**, such as alpha particles, beta particles, neutrons and protons. All of these are carcinogenic. As ionising radiation passes through tissue, it interacts with atoms in its path to destabilise them. This disturbance in the electron shell of atoms may lead to chemical changes.

The precise mechanisms are still obscure. Radiation causes chromosomal breakage, translocations and mutations. Various protein molecules are also damaged and there are two principal theories to account for the observations. The **direct theory** states that ionising radiation directly ionises important molecules within the cell while the **indirect theory** states that ionisation first affects water within the cell, which leads to the production of oxygen free radicals which cause the damage. Whichever mechanism operates, the end result is that DNA is altered, analogous to the initiator effect in chemical carcinogenesis.

The carcinogenic effect of radiation is related to this ability to produce mutations and it is known that this depends on the type and strength of the radiation and the duration of exposure. Some tissues, such as bone marrow and thyroid, are particularly sensitive to the effects of radiation and children are more susceptible than adults.

Ultraviolet light is particularly important clinically, as sun exposure causes vast numbers of melanomas, squamous cell carcinomas and basal cell carcinomas of the skin. Fortunately, squamous cell carcinomas and basal cell carcinomas generally can be cured by complete local excision, but melanomas metastasise early and kill. Many of the pioneers who studied radioactive materials and X-rays developed skin cancers, and miners of radioactive elements have a high incidence of lung cancers. The radiation from the atomic bombs dropped on Hiroshima and Nagasaki resulted in increased incidence of leukaemia, especially acute and chronic myeloid leukaemia, breast, lung and colonic cancers.

Viruses

A large number of viruses have been implicated in the causation of cancer and these are listed on the next page. We will discuss:

- Epstein–Barr virus
- human papilloma virus
- hepatitis B virus
- human T cell leukaemia virus 1 (HTLV-1)

Epstein–Barr virus (EBV) is a member of the herpes family. It is implicated in two types of cancers, **Burkitt's lymphoma** and **nasopharyngeal carcinoma**. There is a very strong association between EBV and the African variety of Burkitt's lymphoma, since over 98% of the cases show EBV genome in the tumour cells and all the patients have a raised level of antibodies to EBV membrane antigens. Fortunately,

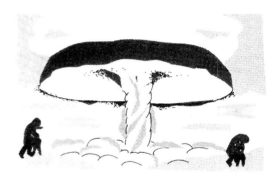

Immediate effects
Death from blast/burn injuries
Acute radiation syndromes:
- bone marrow depression
- gastrointestinal tract effects
- cerebral effects

Delayed malignancies depend on age at time of exposure:

Childhood exposure
- Leukaemias*
- Thyroid cancer
- Breast cancer

Adult exposure
- Leukaemias*
- Lung/breast/salivary gland cancer
- All other cancers increased to some extent

*All leukaemias except chronic lymphocytic leukaemia are increased

Fig 4.11 Radiation effects e.g. bombing of Hiroshima/Nagasaki

EBV does not inevitably cause cancer, as EBV is a common infection in developed countries, where it causes a flu-like illness called infectious mononucleosis or glandular fever. That production of Burkitt's lymphoma can occur without EBV is demonstrated by how few non-African Burkitt lymphomas (15–20%) have the EBV genome. Therefore, EBV must be just one factor involved in the transformation of B lymphocytes to a B–cell malignancy.

It is interesting that the African regions where Burkitt's lymphoma is common are also regions where malaria is endemic. It would appear that malaria causes a degree of immunoincompetence that allows the EBV-infected B cells to proliferate and hence gives them an increased risk of mutation. Burkitt's lymphoma exhibits a specific mutation resulting in translocation 8;14 regardless of whether EBV is involved. This translocation moves the c-*myc* gene from its position on chromosome 8 to be adjacent to the immunoglobulin heavy chain gene on chromosome 14. c-*myc* codes for proteins which control cell proliferation and the effect of this translocation is to increase its transcription, possibly because that zone of chromosome 14 is an area of frequent transcriptional activity.

Human papilloma virus (HPV) is a papova virus which has long been known to be associated with **skin papillomas** (warts). Its role in causing cancer was recognised during the study of a very rare disease, epidermodysplasia verruciformis, in which patients have defective cell-mediated immunity and numerous skin papillomas. These papillomas may transform into squamous cell carcinomas which frequently contain the genome of HPV 5, 8 or 14. HPV is not a single virus but a group of around 50 genetically distinct viruses. Interestingly, some types appear to produce benign tumours while others predispose to malignancy. Thus HPV 16 and 18 are implicated in squamous cell carcinoma of the uterine cervix while HPV 6 and 11 are common in benign cervical lesions. It is not known how HPV alters the cells.

HPV can be transmitted by sexual intercourse and it is noted that there is a high incidence of carcinoma of the cervix in those who begin sexual activity at an early age and in those who are promiscuous. The question is: why doesn't our immune system eradicate the virus? Many people have skin warts on their hands and feet (verrucae) as children but appear to develop immunity so that the warts are less common in later life.

Now that we know the viral types involved in some cancers, it opens the door for developing vaccines. Unfortunately, immunising people to prevent cervical cancer is not yet available but immunisation for the prevention of hepatitis B and its associated hepatocellular carcinoma is already in progress.

Hepatitis B virus (HBV) is associated with the production of a chronic hepatitis, cirrhosis and **carcinoma of the liver**. In sub-Saharan Africa and south-east Asia, where infection with HBV is endemic, the infection is transmitted vertically from mother to child during pregnancy. These children,

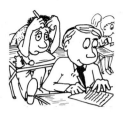

Which viruses are implicated in human cancers?

Virus	Associated tumour
Oncovirus	
HTLV-1	Adult T cell leukaemia/ lymphoma
Hepadnavirus	
Hepatitis B	Liver cancer
Papovirus	
Papilloma types:	
6, 11, 2, 4	Genital, laryngeal and skin warts
16, 18	Cervical cancer
10, 16	Laryngeal cancer
5	Skin cancer
Herpes virus	
Epstein–Barr (EBV)	Burkitt's lymphoma Immunoblastic lymphoma Nasopharyngeal carcinoma
Herpes simplex types 1 and 2	?Cervical cancer
Cytomegalovirus	?Kaposi's sarcoma ?Cervical cancer

therefore, have chronic HBV infection and a high incidence of hepatocellular carcinoma.

The importance of HBV in hepatocellular carcinoma is apparent from this sort of epidemiological work and also from molecular biological investigation looking for integrated HBV DNA sequences. These have been identified in the hepatocytes of some patients with chronic HBV infection and some hepatocellular carcinoma cells. It appears that integration of the viral genome precedes malignant transformation by several years but, to date, no known oncogenic sequences have been identified. The HBV genome does contain a **transactivating gene**, termed X, which codes for a product that alters the level of transcription of other genes, including the genes in the hepatocytes.

Liver cell carcinomas are also associated with alcoholic liver disease, androgenic steroids and aflatoxins. Aflatoxins are toxic metabolites of a fungus, *Aspergillus flavus*, which can contaminate food in the tropics. Aflatoxin B is thought to contribute to the high incidence of liver cancer in parts of south-east Asia and Africa. Possibly these agents act by causing damage which leads to regenerative activity and, hence, the production of proliferative nodules that are susceptible to further cellular alterations by HBV.

Human T cell leukaemia virus 1 (HTLV-1) is important because it is the only example (so far!) of a retrovirus causing a human cancer. It is implicated in adult T cell **leukaemia/lymphoma** (ATLL) which is a rare tumour of the lymphoid system. HTLV-1 infection is commonest in southern Japan, South America and parts of Africa and precedes the development of malignancy by decades. It has a transactivating gene, *tat*, that increases IL-2 receptor expression in infected T cells, which promotes their growth. The study of **retroviruses** has advanced our knowledge of the role of genes in tumour biology by allowing the identification of specific transforming genes. (This is discussed in greater detail in Chapter 5.) However, to date, they have not been shown to be important in common human tumours.

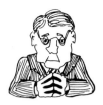

What are oncogenes and anti-oncogenes?

Oncogenes are genes that can transform cells into cancer cells. They may be derived from exogenous sources (e.g. a virus: v-onc) or they may be endogenous, formed by mutation of proto-oncogenes (p-onc) to cellular oncogenes (c-onc). Oncogenes work by stimulating cell growth.

Anti-oncogenes, better called tumour suppressor genes, have an inhibitory effect on cell growth, hence their **loss** leads to excessive cell proliferation.

In summary, regardless of aetiology, cancer appears to develop through a series of steps commencing with **initiation**. This is followed by **promotion** which results in the production of a focal proliferative lesion which can undergo further changes that allow the cells to become **autonomous**. These cells are almost identical genetically and are called a **clone**. The autonomous cells are independent of normal control mechanisms for growth and spread and, hence, are cancerous. This theory helps to explain the apparent long 'lag' phase that occurs in many tumours.

It also fits with the observations of tumour development in diseases such as familial polyposis coli in which the affected individuals develop numerous colonic polyps and have a high incidence of colonic cancer. Colons removed in these cases not only show polyps and sometimes carcinoma but also focal changes in the architecture and microscopical appearances of the epithelial cells, which are similar to those of malignancy but do not show evidence of invasion. These alterations are believed to indicate a **precancerous** stage. This 'human model' demonstrates multiple steps in the evolution of cancer from normal epithelium through abnormal epithelial cells and polyps to carcinoma.

This is referred to as the **'multistep theory of neoplasia'**. The theory suggests that tumours do not arise from a single event that takes place at the cellular level but, in order to produce disordered cell growth, a number of events (e.g. mutations) have to occur. The spectrum of lesions from benign neoplasia through precancer to frank malignancy is then explained on the basis that, at the benign end, only a few events have taken place and further changes are required to lead to cancer.

We have talked about viruses, radiation and chemicals causing changes in genes that lead to malignant transformation of the cells. Often the exact changes are unknown but, in some cases, the genetic abnormality has been defined and this leads us to a discussion of oncogenes.

Oncogenes

Oncogenes are genes that can transform normal cells into cancer cells; but where do they come from? There are both exogenous and endogenous sources. The **exogenous** sources include viral oncogenes (v-*onc*) which may be introduced into cells by tumour viruses. **Endogenous** genes are called cellular oncogenes (c-*onc*) and these are genes that are normally present in the cell but have been altered to produce the oncogene. The normal gene from which the oncogene is derived is called the proto-oncogene (p-*onc*).

So far so good! Let us now add a level of complexity. The viral or exogenous oncogenes can be divided into two types: those that show similarity to normal cellular genes and those that are completely different. This is important because viral oncogenes that resemble cellular genes are actually derived from the cell's genes. This is quite amazing when you think about it! A virus infects a cell and incorporates some of the cellular genes into its own genome. These genes, finding themselves in a new piece of DNA or RNA, become altered in their properties and are then viral oncogenes. When the virus infects another cell, it can introduce the viral oncogene (a process called **transduction**), which leads to altered growth of the infected cell. **Retroviruses**, which consist of RNA that becomes incorporated into the host DNA through the action of reverse transcriptase, can readily 'pick up' some host DNA and so can carry viral oncogenes derived from cellular oncogenes. Oncogenic DNA viruses generally possess gene sequences that are uniquely viral and have no homology with cellular oncogenes.

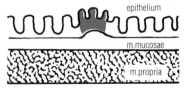

Mutation, e.g. to chromosome 5, produces a hyperproliferative epithelial focus.

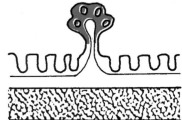

Further DNA alterations, e.g. ↓methylation, leads to the formation of a type I adenoma

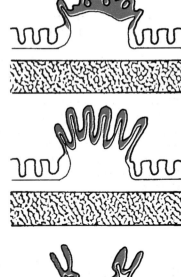

Further mutation, e.g. to ras gene, produces a type II adenoma

Further mutation, e.g. allele loss from chromosome 18, produces a type III adenoma

Another mutation, e.g. allele loss from chromosome 17, leads to the development of invasive cancer.

Other mutations may confer the ability to metastasise

Fig 4.12 Multistep theory of carcinogenesis: e.g. colonic polyp-carcinoma sequence

How can oncogenes promote cell growth?

Normal cell growth is believed to be influenced by growth factors binding to receptors on the surface of the cell. This produces a stimulus through a 'transducer' molecule which influences the cell's nucleus to produce instructions for proliferation. Therefore, cell growth could be stimulated by:

- increased growth factor production
- increase in growth factor receptors on the cell's surface
- abnormal growth factor receptors
- abnormal transducers which will act as if growth factor has bound to its receptor
- nuclear acting molecules

Oncogenes have been identified which act through each of these mechanisms.

Growth factors

Growth factors are polypeptides that act locally to stimulate proliferation and, sometimes, differentiation. If tumour cells produce substances that act as growth factors, then they will be continually self-stimulating (**autocrine stimulation**). The oncogene, c-*sis*, codes for a protein with homology to the known growth factor, platelet-derived growth factor. The oncogene *int*-2 produces a protein similar to fibroblast growth factor.

Growth factor receptors

When the normal cell surface receptors are activated by growth factors, there is an increase in their **tyrosine kinase** activity. Some proto-oncogenes code for receptors, and their related oncogenes produce receptors with altered kinase activity. For example, c-*erb-B1* codes for an epidermal growth factor receptor with increased kinase activity. Some tyrosine kinases are not attached to a receptor but are anchored to the plasma membrane and participate in signalling. The c-*src* oncogene alters the activity of one of these **non-receptor tyrosine kinases**.

Intracellular messengers

In the normal cell, intracellular messages involve G- and N-proteins that control adenylate cyclase activity. The *ras* family of oncogenes probably act by interfering with this pathway through their actions on GTP.

Nuclear acting molecules

Nuclear associated proteins are involved in the regulation of the normal cell cycle. Their precise localisation and function are unknown but oncogenes, such as *myc*, are thought to act in this way.

↑ Growth factor
c-sis

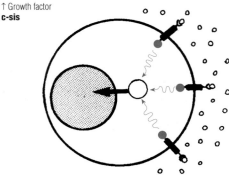

Permanent activation of receptor
v-erb B

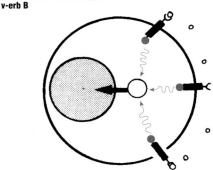

↑ Growth factor receptor
c-neu

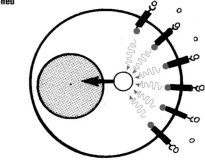

Abnormal signal transduction
c-K-ras

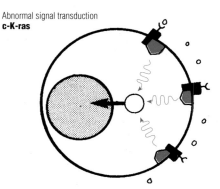

Fig 4.13 Examples of possible mechanisms of cell activation by oncogenes

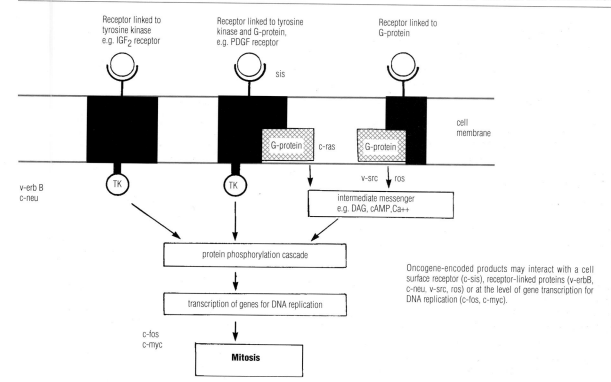

Fig 4.14 Oncogenes and cellular signalling and transduction mechanisms

Oncogene-encoded products may interact with a cell surface receptor (c-sis), receptor-linked proteins (v-erbB, c-neu, v-src, ros) or at the level of gene transcription for DNA replication (c-fos, c-myc).

How are proto-oncogenes activated?

Proto-oncogenes can undergo change within the cell to produce an oncogene, either by spontaneous mutation or secondary to the effects of chemical carcinogens, radiation or viral infections.

The actual change in the DNA may involve:

- translocation
- point mutation
- amplification

We have already mentioned **translocation** when discussing Burkitt's lymphoma. Here c-*myc* moves from chromosome 8 to the immunoglobulin heavy chain region on chromosome 14. **Point mutation**, by substitution at codon 12, activates *ras* which is present in 30–40% of colonic tumours and 50% of lung adenocarcinomas. **Amplification** of the proto-oncogene, so that there are multiple copies, is another method of tumour production. Several hundred copies of the N-*myc* gene can be found in neuroblastomas and the tumours showing greatest amplification of genes behave most aggressively. This type of amplification of genes, and hence their protein products, also occurs in breast cancer where *c-neu* is implicated. The subject of how these genes move and the effects of the move on the molecular biology of the cell will be covered in greater detail in Chapter 5.

Anti-oncogenes or tumour suppressor genes

We have been considering how the abnormal activation of genes that promote cell growth can lead to abnormal growth. We have already mentioned that the cell is under both positive and negative regulatory stimuli. In other words, there are genes that code for proteins that normally inhibit cell growth.

The fact that these genes may be involved in the production of cancer is a relatively new idea. The prototype is the **retinoblastoma gene**. Retinoblastoma, a tumour of childhood, occurs in two forms: 40% are familial while the rest occur in a sporadic fashion. It is also known that the familial tumour is often bilateral while the sporadic tumours tends to to be unilateral. In order to account for this interesting observation, it was proposed that the tumour must arise by a 'two hit' mechanism. What this means is that, for retinoblastoma to occur, both the alleles on the chromosome must be inactivated. It is then postulated that in the familial cases, the child inherits one inactivated gene from the parents. Consequently, it only requires one more spontaneous mutation in order to produce the tumour. In sporadic cases, both genes are normal at birth and two mutations are needed to produce the tumour. This explains beautifully why the familial cases tend to be bilateral while the sporadic cases are unilateral. After all, the chances of one mutation occurring in a retinoblast are much higher than two mutations occurring in the same cell.

The retinoblastoma gene has been traced to the *RB-1* gene within chromosome 13q14 that produces a nuclear protein that may have suppressive effects on DNA synthesis. The exact role of this protein and how mutations in the genes lead to cancer is not known at present. What is interesting is that patients with retinoblastoma are also at increased risk of developing osteosarcoma and soft tissue tumours.

In **familial polyposis coli**, affected people inherit a defective copy of the *APC* gene situated on chromosome 5 in the q21–22 region. Any deletion of the area on the paired chromosome will increase the development of tumours. Another possible oncosuppressor is *NF-1* on chromosome 17q which is associated with the inheritance of **neurofibro-matosis**, a condition in which patients develop numerous skin manifestations and nerve sheath tumours, some of which turn malignant. Chromosomal deletions are also found in a variety of sporadic tumours and it is assumed that the deleted area may have coded for a suppressor protein. For example, part of the short arm of chromosome 17 is lost in many small cell lung cancers, colorectal and breast cancers. This codes for a suppressor protein termed p53. The p53 story is a little more complex than that for the other tumour suppressor proteins as it can develop alterations which appear to have a direct oncogenic action.

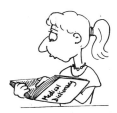

Allele: alternate form of a gene found at the same locus in homologous chromosomes

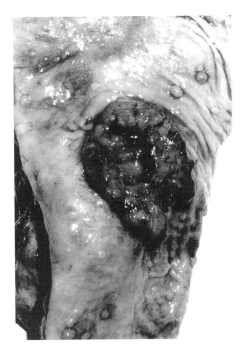

Fig 4.15 Large bowel with an adenocarcinoma in a patient with multiple adenomatous polyps.

In addition, normal p53 may be inactivated by binding to protein E6 which is produced by HPV-16, the virus implicated in human cervical cancer. HPV also produces a protein E7 which can inactivate the retinoblastoma gene product. Thus it appears that some viruses may exert their effects through stimulating cell growth by increasing growth factor actions whilst others may cause cell proliferation by inactivating inhibitory controls.

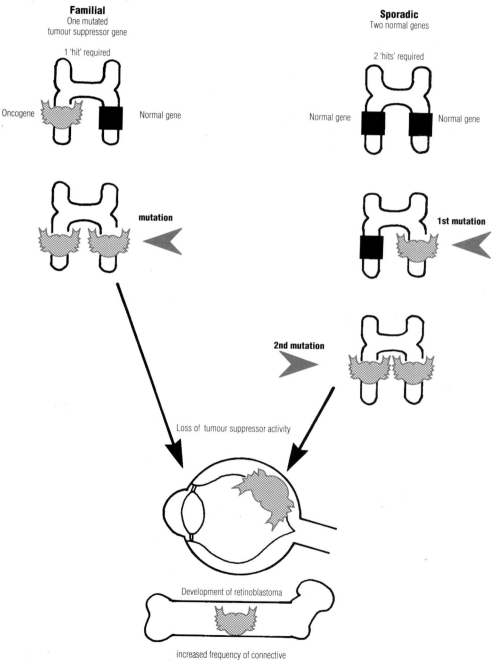

Fig 4.16 Development of retinoblastoma and other malignancies

Investigation of these genes is likely to provide us with greater insight into neoplasia. That brings us to the end of our discussion on the cellular events involved in producing the cancer cell. Of course, we have a long way to go before we have a full understanding, but our knowledge is advancing at an exciting pace, and a whole new language of tumour terminology is emerging. For the scientist, the battle is the biology; for the clinicians and students trying to understand and apply the new knowledge, it is often the terminology!

The next question we need to address and one that will be in the forefront of the patient's mind is, how will it behave?

How will it behave?

The behaviour of a tumour can be considered under a number of headings covering how fast it will grow, whether it is likely to metastasise, which sites are affected and what symptoms and complications the patient is likely to suffer.

The growth of tumours

It is often assumed that tumours grow faster than normal tissues because they expand to compress the surrounding structures. However, this does not necessarily mean that the cells are dividing more often or quicker, but that there is an **imbalance between production and loss**. The time taken for tumour cell division varies between 20 and 60 hours, with leukaemias having shorter cell cycles than solid tumours but, in general, tumour cells take *longer* than their normal counterparts. Cells can be in a resting phase or in growth phase. Some normal tissues have a high turnover of cells, such as the intestine, where around 16% of the cells will be in the growth fraction. In contrast, most tumours have only 2–8% of their cells actively dividing. This is important therapeutically because the cells in the growth phase are most readily damaged by chemotherapy and so tumours with a large growth fraction (e.g. leukaemias, lymphomas and lung anaplastic small cell carcinoma) will respond better than tumours with few cells proliferating (e.g. colon and breast).

Can we predict how fast a tumour is growing? To some extent, yes. The number of mitotic figures present per unit area in a light microscopical section is a crude measure of how active the proliferation is within a tumour. A tumour with a large number of cells in mitosis is likely to behave aggressively and this is why a mitotic count is one of the criteria for grading tumours (see page 160). However, the number of cells seen to be in mitosis is not only influenced by the growth fraction and the cell cycle time but also by whether they get ''stuck', i.e. the tumour cell can enter mitosis but, possibly because of an irregularity in chromosome number or in the internal organisation of the mitotic spindle, may fail to complete the mitosis. Thus it appears to be proliferating indefinitely but it is really 'stuck'.

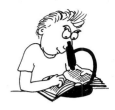

Name some of the methods for assessing cellular proliferation.

Mitotic count
Measuring DNA content
   Thymidine labelling
   Flow cytometry
Immunohistochemical methods
   Ki67 staining
   Proliferating cell nuclear
   antigen (PCNA)
Nucleolar organiser regions
   AgNORs

Tumour growth will also be influenced by factors like the blood supply and, possibly, the host's immune response (pages 182 and 184), so-called 'proliferation markers' may give additional information.

It would be wrong to assume that every cell in a tumour behaves the same. The cells of a particular tumour are almost identical genetically and are said to be a **clone**, i.e. they are all derived from one original cell. However, there is genetic instability which results in **subclones** forming that have certain survival advantages; for example, they may have enhanced invasive or metastatic capabilities. This is referred to as **tumour heterogeneity** and it is important to consider when planning treatments because it means that some tumour cells may respond differently to particular chemotherapeutic agents. This is rather analogous to bacterial resistance to antibiotics. Just as a combination of antibiotics is most effective against an unknown organism, so a mixture of drugs should be used against a tumour and, if a tumour recurs after chemotherapy, a different drug should be used.

How do tumours spread?

Just over a hundred years ago, Stephen Paget (no, not the man who described Paget's disease – that was Sir James Paget) collected postmortem records of 735 patients who had died of breast cancer and he found that the majority of the metastases were in the liver and brain. He concluded therefore that certain tumours were predisposed to metastasise to certain tissues. He wrote, "When a plant goes to seed, its seeds are carried in all directions; but they can only live and grow if they fall on congenial soil". Not surprisingly, it came to be known as the 'seed and soil' theory. James Ewing, 40 years later, suggested that tumours went to particular organs not because of the seed and soil effect, but depending on the routes of lymphatic and venous drainage of the primary organ.

We know now that they are both partially correct. Tumours of the colon do indeed go to the liver which is in line through the portal circulation, but then so do many other tumours much farther away, such as melanomas arising in the eye. We also know that organs such as the heart and skeletal muscle, despite being exposed to large volumes of blood, rarely have metastases. In broad terms, tumour spread through lymphatics will produce metastases in the anatomically related lymph nodes whilst spread through the blood is influenced more by 'seed and soil' considerations although anatomy is still of some importance.

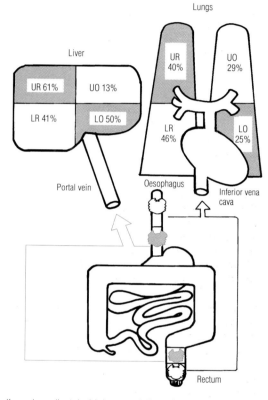

If spread were directed solely by venous drainage, the tumours in the upper oesophagus (UO) and lower rectum (LR), which drain via the inferior cava should metastasise to the lungs, whereas lower oesophageal (LO) and upper rectal (UR) tumours, which drain via the portal vein, should metastasise to the liver. This study highlights a surprising variation in metastatic patterns of these tumours, illustrating that "seed and soil" are not the only factors determining metastasis.

Figures are percentages of metastases from each tumour group involving each site, determined at post mortem.

Fig 4.17 Seed and soil theory of tumour metastasis

The main **routes of spread** are via:

- lymphatics
- veins
- transcoelomic cavities
- cerebrospinal fluid
- arteries

Lymphatic spread is common in carcinomas and the nodes which are involved first are the nodes which drain the tumour site. Thus a knowledge of the lymphatic anatomy is useful for predicting where the tumour will spread and is the basis for many of the staging protocols (page 161). However, lymph nodes near tumours can enlarge as part of an immune reaction that particularly results in expansion of the macrophage compartment (sinus histiocytosis). This means that the doctor must try to distinguish between soft, mobile nodes, which are likely to be reactive, and the hard, fixed nodes which contain metastatic tumour.

Venous spread will take tumours of the gastrointestinal tract to the **liver** and tumours from a variety of sites to the **lungs**. It is also the favoured route of spread for **sarcomas**. Some tumours may even grow along a vein, causing its obstruction, e.g. renal cell carcinoma in the renal vein. **Arteries** are not often penetrated by tumours but, in the later stages of metastatic spread, tumour nodules can start to develop almost anywhere and it is likely that this happens after pulmonary metastases enter the pulmonary vein and are then distributed through the systemic arterial system.

It is easy to understand how tumours which reach the pleural or peritoneal cavities can drop into the fluid and be disseminated throughout that **coelomic cavity**. Similarly, the **cerebrospinal fluid** provides an easy route of spread for cerebral tumours, which do not generally metastasise outside the central nervous system.

One cubic centimetre of tumour can shed millions of cells into the circulation each day; so why are metastases not inevitable? Let us consider the steps required to produce a metastases. First, the tumour has to grow at the primary site and infiltrate the surrounding connective tissue, which may necessitate breaking through a basement membrane. Then it can reach the lymphatic and blood vascular channels, which are an important route for dissemination. The vessel wall is traversed and the tumour cells must detach to float in the blood or lymph and hope to evade any immune cells which might destroy them. Next they must lodge in the capillaries at their destination, attach to the endothelium and penetrate the vessel wall to enter the perivascular connective tissue where they finally proliferate to produce a tumour deposit.

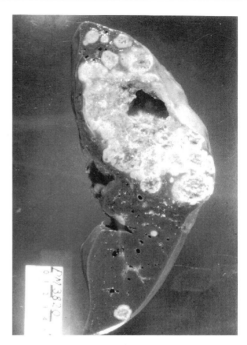

Fig 4.18   Section of the liver showing multiple pale nodules due to metastatic carcinoma.

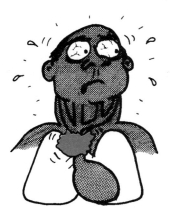

Direct: e.g. Mediastinal tumour surrounding and compressing the superior vena cava. This causes venous engorgement of the head, neck and arms to produce headache and proptosis (bulging eyes due to cavernous sinus distension)

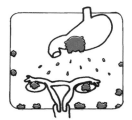

Transcoelomic: e.g. Gastric carcinoma cells seeding through the peritoneal cavity. Krukenberg gave his name to metastatic gastric carcinoma involving the ovaries.

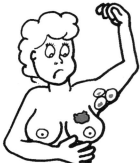

Via lymphatics: e.g. Carcinoma of breast first spreads to the local axillary lymph nodes.

Carcinomas generally first spread via lymphatics.

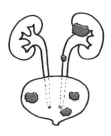

Field change: e.g. Transitional cell carcinoma. Urothelial tumours may synchronously arise at several sites, e.g. renal pelvis, ureter & bladder. This is **not** tumour spread, but a 'crop' of separate primary tumours, thought to arise due to a "field effect", in which several sites are exposed to the same urinary carcinogens.

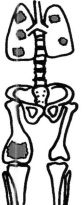

Via the bloodstream: e.g. Osteosarcomas metastasising to the lungs, or gastrointestinal carcinomas spreading to the liver via the portal vein.

Sarcomas generally spread via the bloodstream.

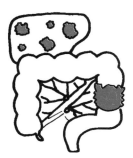

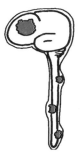

CNS spread: Primary central nervous system tumours will metastasise to brain or spinal cord but appear to be confined by the blood: brain barrier and the dural membranes.

Fig 4.19 Routes of tumour spread

What stands between the primary tumour and the vessel? First, there is a variety of extracellular matrix components to break through for which the tumour may produce a number of enzymes. Loose connective tissue is not much of a barrier but cartilage and dense fibrous areas, such as tendons and joint capsules, can resist tumour spread. There is likely to be a basement membrane so the tumour has to have a type IV collagenase. Tumours often have collagenases to dissolve collagen but are less able to digest elastic tissue. This may be one of the reasons why arterial walls, which contain a lot of elastic, are less readily penetrated than venous walls. Alternatively, it may be because arterial walls are thicker and have protease inhibitors. Once in the vessel lumen, tumour cells are prey to any immune surveillance. Finally, the tumour must attach to the endothelium at its destination which may involve specific adhesion molecules (addressins) that 'home' the metastatic tumour to a particular site, analogous to the 'homing' of lymphocytes.

Figure 4.20 illustrates some of these stages and shows the factors increasing cell mobility, facilitating movement through stroma and improving tumour survival. Most of our discussion about tumour cell biology has concentrated on how genetic changes enhance cell proliferation. However, this figure emphasises the variety of ways in which a proliferating tumour cell differs from a proliferating normal cell. For example, tumour cells may show decreased expression of E-cadherin, which normally acts as an adhesion molecule between epithelial cells, and increased motility influenced by an autocrine motility factor. Tumour cells can also influence the production of stroma so that tenascin may predominate which does not bind readily to tumour cells. This sort of information suggests that it is not only changes in the tumour cells which produce local invasion and metastasis but that interactions between tumour cells, normal cells and stroma are also important. This has been known for a long time as early experiments using *in vitro* cell cultures demonstrated that normal cells would grow to form monolayers and then stop. This is referred to as **contact inhibition**. If some cells from this culture were transferred to a new culture vessel (passaged), they would begin to grow again; however, normal cells would only survive about 30–50 **serial passages**. Cultures of proliferating tumour cells differ in that they lose contact inhibition and so can grow as disorganised multilayers and they are also immortal, i.e. each individual cell does not last forever but the clone of cells can be passaged indefinitely.

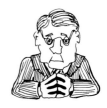

What are the possible routes of tumour spread?

Direct
Lymphatic
Venous
Transcoelomic cavities
Cerebrospinal fluid
Arterial

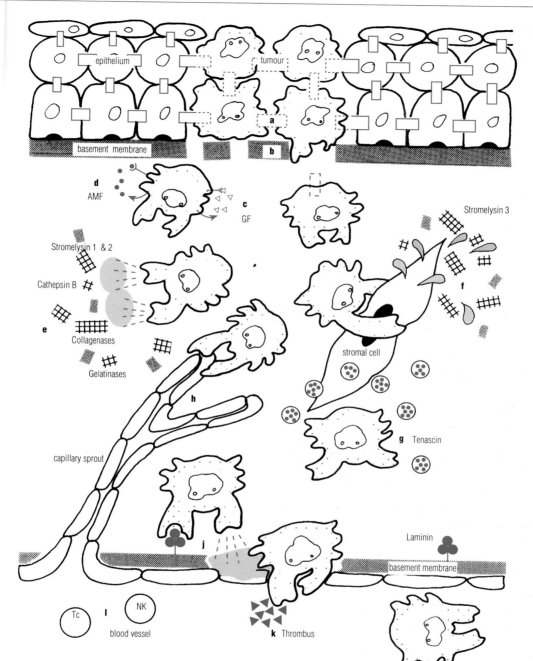

Factors increasing cell mobility:

a. ↓ adherence of tumour cells, e.g. loss of cell-cell adhesion via cadherin

b. Synthesis by tumour cells of defective basement membrane (b.m.) or failure to synthesise b.m.

c. ↑ growth factor secretion, stimulating self and neighbouring tumour cells

d. ↑ motility (secretion of autocrine motility factor)

Facilitation of movement through stroma:

e. by secretion of collagenases, stromelysins 1 & 2, gelatinases and cathepsin B

f. by stimulation of stromal cells to secrete stromelysin 3

g. by stimulation of stromal cells to secrete alternative extracellular matrix, e.g. tenascin instead of fibronectin

Factors improving tumour survival & spread:

h. Tumour angiogenesis factors improve blood supply

j. Laminin receptors facilitate attachment to & penetration of basement membrane

k. Thrombogenesis: thrombus veils tumour cell from surveillance mechanisms

l. Evasion of host immune response by ↓MHC class I receptors and ↓ recognition sites for cytotoxic T lymphocytes and NK cells

Fig 4.20 Factors increasing tumour cell motility and survival

The role of the immune system

We are all aware of the role played by the immune system in defending us against infections, so it is not surprising that questions have been raised as to whether it has any role in protection against cancer. It was Paul Ehrlich, in 1909, who postulated that without the immune system constantly removing the 'aberrant germs', human beings would inevitably die of cancer. Many attempts were made to establish the role of the immune system in cancer, and initial experiments, which transplanted tumours from one animal to another, appeared to support the concept. It was later realised that the destruction of these transplanted tumours was not due to immunity but to transplant rejection. Now, inbred mice can be used experimentally, thus avoiding the factor of transplant rejection. In certain tumours it has been shown that, if the tumour is removed from a mouse and the animal rechallenged with the tumour, the tumour is rejected. This supports the idea that immunity is involved in tumour rejection, but life is not quite so simple as we shall see.

You will recall that the cells of the immune system have to be able to distinguish between 'self' and 'non-self', by identifying specific antigens on the cell surface. Malignant tumours are derived from 'self', so if the immune system is to defend against tumours, the malignant cells must acquire antigens that differentiate them from normal cells. These are termed **tumour specific antigens** and the whole subject is highly controversial.

In man, there is no conclusive proof that tumours carry specific antigens on their cell surfaces that allow a specific immune reaction to be mounted. However, there is evidence from animal experiments that surface antigens are altered in some tumours induced by viruses or chemicals. Viral-induced tumours in animals can display a new surface antigen (T) which is believed to be a viral peptide associated with the major histocompatibility complex (MHC). This provokes a specific cytotoxic T cell response and all tumours induced by a particular virus display the same antigen, regardless of the cell of origin. The obvious potential application for this lies in immunising against tumours.

Chemically-induced tumours in animals (e.g. by benzopyrene) may also display new surface antigens which induce a specific immune response, but these antigens are very varied, with primary tumours in the same animal exhibiting antigenic differences, so there is no cross-resistance through immunisation.

In man, there is a suggestion that immune cells may have some effect, as many tumours have lymphocytic infiltrates and some show signs of regression. A good example of this phenomenon is seen in skin melanomas.

Of course, the immune response need not be antigen-specific. Besides B and T lymphocytes, the body has at its disposal **natural killer cells** (NK cells) and **macrophages**. NK cells have the capacity to destroy cells without prior sensitization as well as the ability to participate in antibody-dependent cellular cytotoxicity (ADCC). Macrophages are also involved, either due to non-specific activation or in

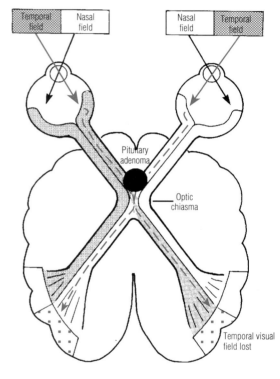

Compression of the optic chiasma by a benign pituitary adenoma damages the optic nerve fibres serving the temporal visual fields, resulting in bitemporal hemianopia.

Fig 4.21 Tumour effects: compression

collaboration with T lymphocytes, and can participate via ADCC or by the release of cytotoxic factors, such as TNF (tumour necrosis factor), hydrogen peroxide and a cytolytic protease.

Do we have an immune surveillance system against cancer, be it specific or non-specific? The answer is we don't know. It is likely that a small number of tumours are influenced by immune activity as it is well known that patients suffering from congenital or acquired immuno-deficiency are at an increased risk of certain cancers. They have a high risk of lymphomas and skin cancers but common cancers, such as breast, colon and lung, do not occur with increased frequency

The clinical effects of tumours

Local effects

The local effects depend on the site of the tumour, the type of tumour and its growth pattern. Some complications, such as haemorrhage, are more common in malignant tumours because of their ability to invade underlying tissues and their vessels. However, it must be remembered that even a microscopically benign tumour (e.g. a meningioma on the surface of the brain) can kill the patient due to its local effects.

Local effects can complicate both benign and malignant tumours. They include:

- compression
- obstruction
- ulceration
- haemorrhage
- rupture
- perforation
- infarction

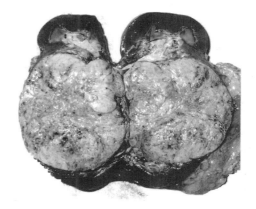

Fig 4.22 Section of the kidney with a large renal cell carinoma compressing the normal parenchyma and obstructing the pelvis.

Compression and obstruction

A patient with any intracranial tumour (e.g. meningioma, astrocytoma, oligodendroglioma) may present with headaches, nausea and vomiting, because the mass growing within the closed cavity of the cranium raises the intracranial pressure. If the tumour is not removed and the pressure continues to rise, the patient will die from pressure effects on the vital respiratory centres.

A more localised example of the effect of compression is when the pituitary gland enlarges in the small cup-shaped space of the sella turcica. Local pressure will cause erosion of the bony sella and compression of the optic chiasma that sits directly above. The patient will then present with visual disturbance, classically a bitemporal hemianopia.

Compression and obstruction have been included in the same section because there is often an overlap. Compression can directly damage normal tissue, as described for the pituitary, or it may cause obstruction. This occurs, for instance, when a tracheal tumour obstructs a normal oesophagus or vice versa. In the brain, compression of the brainstem structures may obstruct the flow of cerebrospinal fluid and a large prostate (benign or malignant) may compress the prostatic urethra. Alternatively, a tumour can grow into the lumen of the gut or into an airway so that it produces obstruction directly.

Ulceration and haemorrhage

An ulcer is defined as a macroscopically apparent loss of surface epithelium and may be benign or malignant. Ulceration of the skin will lead to a crust of dried fibrin and cells covering the area and is unlikely to produce severe haemorrhage. However, ulceration of the gut, particularly the stomach and duodenum, may result in life-threatening haemorrhage or perforation. Here the absence of epithelium means the loss of an important defence mechanism which normally protects the underlying tissue from acid and enzymes. Once the submucosa is exposed to these agents, large vessel walls can be digested resulting in massive bleeding.

Rupture or perforation

Rupture or perforation typically affects tumours of the gastrointestinal tract and will occur if the intraluminal pressure exceeds the strength of the wall or if the wall is eroded or weakened by tumour, ischaemia or enzymic action. Obviously, there is a risk of dilatation and rupture when part of the gut becomes obstructed as the gut contents cannot follow their normal route. Rupture may also occur in closed organs, such as the ovary, because the tumour is stretching the capsule, often because of accumulation of fluid or mucin as well as the proliferation of neoplastic cells.

Infarction

Many malignant tumours will show necrosis and infarction in their central region, which is believed to result from inadequate blood supply. In experimental models, a tumour can only expand to a diameter of 1–2 mm. before it must stimulate new blood vessel formation and, in human tumours, zones of necrosis may be encountered approximately 1–2 mm from a blood vessel. Therefore, it appears that this is the maximum distance for diffusion of nutrients. Tumours attempt to solve this by secreting **angiogenetic factors** which stimulate capillaries to grow into the neoplasm.

Local anatomy influences the likelihood of infarction related to large vessel obstruction. The bowel, ovaries and testes are particularly liable to **torsion**, i.e. twisting on their vascular pedicle which occludes the vessels.

Although we often separate the complications of tumours under the headings of local tumour and metastatic tumour, a metastasis can produce any of the local effects mentioned above. In particular, lymph nodes containing metastases can cause obstruction at crucial sites, such as the porta hepatis or the hilum of the lung.

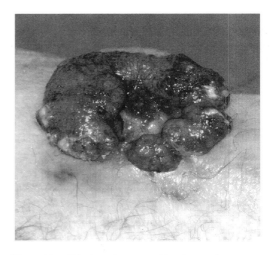

Fig 4.23 Skin from forearm with a large, ulcerated, squamous cell carcinoma.

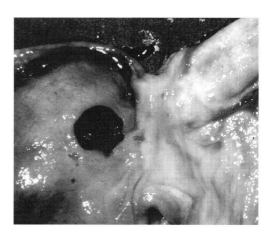

Fig 4.24 Perforated benign peptic ulcer with a regular smooth edge.

Endocrine effects

Well-differentiated tumours not only look like their tissue of origin but can also act like them. Thus tumours of endocrine organs can produce hormones which act on the same tissues as their physiological counterparts but are not under normal feedback control.

Cushing's syndrome provides an interesting example of where different endocrine tumours can produce the same clinical problems. In Cushing's syndrome, the patient suffers from osteoporosis, muscle wasting, thinning of the skin with purple striae and easy bruising, truncal obesity and impaired glucose tolerance. All this is the result of excess glucocorticoids. The same picture can be produced by prolonged administration of steroids to treat diseases (e.g. chronic asthma) but here we are interested in the tumours which can cause it.

The adrenal produces corticosteroids when stimulated by adrenocorticotrophic hormone (ACTH) from the pituitary. The corticosteroids then provide negative feedback to the pituitary and ACTH levels drop. Cushing's syndrome can result from an adenoma in the pituitary gland, which produces ACTH, or a cortical tumour in the adrenal cortex, which secretes corticosteroids. Normal feedback does not operate as the adenoma cells behave autonomously. However, if very high doses of steroid (dexamethasone suppression test) are given, then the pituitary adenoma will reduce its ACTH production and endogenous steroid levels will fall, but excess steroid due to an adrenal adenoma will not be suppressed.

Some non-endocrine tumours can produce substances which have the same effects as hormones, so-called inappropriate production. One of the commonest results is Cushing's syndrome when ACTH is produced by oat cell (anaplastic small cell) carcinoma of the bronchus, carcinoid tumours, thymomas or medullary carcinoma of the thyroid. This inappropriate and autonomous production does not suppress with high doses of dexamethasone.

Paraneoplastic syndromes

This refers to symptoms in cancer patients that are not readily explained by local or metastatic disease. Endocrine effects are generally included as a paraneoplastic syndrome if the production is inappropriate (as above) but not if the tumour arises from a tissue that normally produces that hormone.

Hypercalcaemia is a common, clinically important and complex problem. In a patient with widespread metastases in bone, it may be explained as a local destructive effect of the tumour on bone which releases calcium. However, hypercalcaemia can also occur without metastatic bony deposits and, in some cases, it appears that a parathyroid hormone like peptide or TGF-α is secreted by the primary tumour and this is most likely with bronchial squamous cell carcinoma and adult T cell leukaemia/lymphoma.

Clubbing of the fingers and hypertrophic osteo-arthropathy are also common with lung carcinoma but can

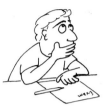

Name some of the paraneoplastic manifestations of tumours.

Endocrine effects
        Cushing's syndrome
        Inappropriate ADH secretion
Hypercalcaemia
Clubbing
Hypertrophic osteoarthropathy
Peripheral neuropathy
Cerebellar degeneration
Skin rash

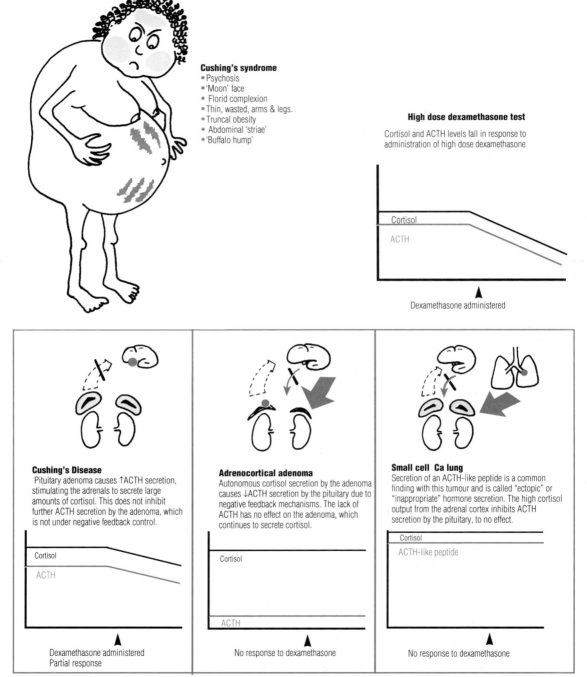

Cushing's syndrome
- Psychosis
- 'Moon' face
- Florid complexion
- Thin, wasted, arms & legs.
- Truncal obesity
- Abdominal 'striae'
- 'Buffalo hump'

High dose dexamethasone test

Cortisol and ACTH levels fall in response to administration of high dose dexamethasone

Cortisol

ACTH

Dexamethasone administered

Cushing's Disease
Pituitary adenoma causes ↑ACTH secretion, stimulating the adrenals to secrete large amounts of cortisol. This does not inhibit further ACTH secretion by the adenoma, which is not under negative feedback control.

Cortisol

ACTH

Dexamethasone administered
Partial response

Adrenocortical adenoma
Autonomous cortisol secretion by the adenoma causes ↓ACTH secretion by the pituitary due to negative feedback mechanisms. The lack of ACTH has no effect on the adenoma, which continues to secrete cortisol.

Cortisol

ACTH

No response to dexamethasone

Small cell Ca lung
Secretion of an ACTH-like peptide is a common finding with this tumour and is called "ectopic" or "inappropriate" hormone secretion. The high cortisol output from the adrenal cortex inhibits ACTH secretion by the pituitary, to no effect.

Cortisol

ACTH-like peptide

No response to dexamethasone

Response to high dose dexamethasone test

Fig 4.23 Distant effects of tumours: e.g. Cushing's Syndrome

occur in non-neoplastic conditions including cyanotic heart disease and liver disease. It is not clear how it develops, nor why sectioning the vagus nerve can lead to its disappearance! Equally mysterious are the skin disorders, peripheral neuropathy and cerebellar degeneration which may also occur.

The **general effects** of tumours are not classed as paraneoplastic syndromes, although they are extremely common and must not be forgotten. These include general malaise, weight loss and lethargy, which are due to a combination of metabolic and hormonal influences exacerbated by any malnutrition or infection. An important chemical factor that may play a role in cachexia is **cachexin**, which is also known as **tumour necrosis factor** (TNF). This molecule is not produced by the tumour cells, but by activated macrophages. Anaemia is also common and can contribute to the general malaise. This may be a direct effect of metastatic deposits in bone marrow or an indirect effect of mediators which suppress haemopoiesis.

Treatment of cancer

We will discuss this under individual headings; however, many patients receive a combination of treatment regimens.

Local excision
Local treatment aims to provide a cure or to provide specific symptomatic relief. Cancers, such as squamous and basal cell carcinomas of the skin and cancers arising within polyps in the colon, can be cured by local excision. In tumours of the bowel, local excision may relieve an obstruction and provide good long-term remission of symptoms.

Radiotherapy
Radiotherapy can be given from an external source or by implanting a small radioactive source into the tissues. Delivery schedules vary from centre to centre but the general idea is to divide, or fractionate, the doses in order to get the maximum kill of tumour cells with the minimum damage to normal tissues. Implanted radioactive sources are very useful for providing high-dose local radiation and are particularly useful in cancers of the head and neck where there are many vital structures close together.

Chemotherapy
Chemotherapy is a relatively new and rapidly evolving form of treatment. In patients suffering from haematological malignancies (e.g. leukaemia) or disseminated disease, surgery and radiation are not realistic options. You cannot excise a leukaemia and you cannot irradiate every single metastasis in the body!

In the 1950s, alkylating agents (e.g. busulphan) and antimetabolites (e.g. methotrexate) were introduced and proved useful in the management of disseminated cancers. The main problem is that all of the body's normal tissues are also exposed to the drug and so the challenge is to deliver enough drug to kill the tumour without killing the patient! The mode of action of some chemotherapeutic agents is discussed in Chapter 3.

Endocrine-related treatment

This often involves giving a drug that inhibits tumour growth by removing an endocrine stimulus. For example, many breast carcinomas have receptors for oestrogen which stimulate tumour growth. A drug such as tamoxifen will block these receptors and reduce progression of the disease. An alternative approach would be to remove the ovaries which produce oestrogen, much as the testes can be removed in males with prostatic adenocarcinoma to reduce the stimulus for tumour growth from androgens.

Immunotherapy

DNA recombinant technology has enabled the production of cytotoxins in sufficient quantities for therapeutic use. The interferons and TNF are of particular interest. α-Interferon and β-interferon have been used to treat a variety of tumours with some good effect, although it appears that they may best be used in combination with other treatments. Renal carcinomas, melanomas and myelomas have shown a 10–15% response, various lymphomas show a 40% response and hairy cell leukaemia and mycosis fungoides have an 80–90% response rate. TNF-α has been used in the treatment of melanoma although, to date, the responses have been disappointing. Lymphokine activated killer (LAK) cells are a subset of NK cells which have been used in combination with IL-2 to treat renal carcinomas and some melanomas and colorectal cancers.

Since tumour cells do not appear to bear specific antigens, the trials to increase specific immunity have, not surprisingly, been a failure. Even so, there is considerable interest in raising monoclonal antibodies to tumour cells. The hope is that it might be possible to attach drugs to these antibodies so that they would be delivered specifically to the tumour cell – the concept of the 'magic bullet'. However, there are still a lot of maybes!

Palliative treatment

The treatment of cancer has a wider role than merely providing a cure, and cancer physicians are not interested in simply achieving a response to the administered treatment. Palliative treatment does not just refer to treatment that is given to patients in order to make them comfortable prior to death. It is and should be part of the oncological support given to all cancer patients and not only includes medication for the control of pain and nausea but also chemotherapy and radiotherapy for the relief of local symptoms. The term 'continuing care' is sometimes used for this multidisciplinary approach starting with diagnosis and extending to the patient's death. The important point is that our knowledge of all modalities of treatment including pain control have advanced considerably in recent years and the

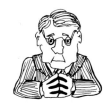

What modes of treatment are available for the management of cancer patients?

Local excision
Radiotherapy
Chemotherapy
Endocrine therapy
Immunotherapy
Palliative treatment

Most patients require a combination of treatments

pessimistic view that, if one has cancer one must pass one's last hours either conscious, but in agony, or pain-free but unconscious, is no longer justified.

Fortunately not all growths are malignant and, in the remainder of the chapter, we will consider the benign disorders of cell growth.

Benign growth disorders

Cells have to adapt to any changes in nutrient supply or workload so as to survive and to continue performing their cellular function. These adaptations take place at both the cellular and subcellular levels. We will discuss these adaptations with an emphasis on the changes that are important in pathology, and, as with the previous section, we will consider the clinical situations in which they are encountered. The changes that we will discuss are:

- neoplasia
- hyperplasia
- hypertrophy
- atrophy
- metaplasia
- dysplasia.

Let us begin by considering a clinical situation in which these adaptive changes may be encountered.

A 70 year old man visited the urology clinic complaining of difficulty with micturition. He passed urine 15–20 times per day and several times during the night (nocturia). The stream of urine was poor and he found that on some occasions it dribbled. The urologist detected an enlarged prostate on rectal examination and the patient had part of his prostate removed to improve the flow.

Some of you may be wondering why an enlarged prostate obstructing urine flow through the urethra should result in increased urinary frequency. The reason is that the enlarged median lobe protrudes into the bladder to produce a dam behind which some urine stagnates. This means that after micturition there is still urine in the bladder and the patient feels the urge to pass urine again. The stagnant urine is also prone to infection or stone formation. The poor urine flow is due to narrowing of the prostatic urethra and the 'ball valve' effect of the median lobe pressing forward on the urethral orifice.

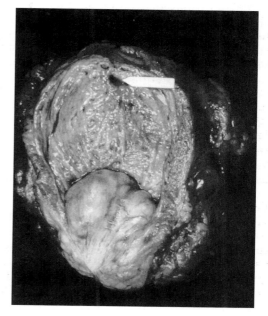

Fig 4.24 Bladder and prostate opened anteriorly. The median lobe of the prostate is markedly enlarged and there is a thickening of the bladder wall with a diverticulum (arrow).

Hyperplasia and hypertrophy

Hyperplasia is defined as an increase in the *number* of cells in an organ or tissue, while hypertrophy is an increase in cell *size*. Often the two co-exist in a tissue because some cell types are incapable of division and so must increase their size (hypertrophy) to cope with any extra work while other cells can proliferate to share their additional work (hyperplasia). In Chapter 1 on healing and repair (page 47), we noted that cardiac and skeletal muscle and nerve cells are unable to replicate whereas epithelial cells and fibroblasts can. Smooth muscle cells can respond by a combination of hyperplasia and hypertrophy. This means that in the prostate the glandular epithelium and the fibroblastic stroma will show hyperplasia and the smooth muscle is hypertrophic and hyperplastic. Why should the prostate enlarge with age, since its workload does not increase? Presumably there is an over-reaction to years of androgen stimulation but nobody really knows.

When the hypertrophy or hyperplasia is useful, i.e. it allows the organ to cope with extra work, it is called **physiological**. If the enlargement does not appear to serve a purpose, then it is termed **pathological**. Thus the prostatic changes would be pathological.

Physiological hyperplasia and hypertrophy may be mediated through hormonal changes or growth factors. Pregnancy is an example of hormone-induced hyperplasia and hypertrophy that allows an organ the size of a pear to enlarge to accommodate a full term baby and prepares the breasts for lactation. The smooth muscle cells of the uterus enlarge (hypertrophy and hyperplasia) ready for the work of pushing the baby into the world (aptly named 'labour') and the number of glandular milk-producing cells in the breast increases (hyperplasia).

A fascinating example of physiological hyperplasia that occurs in the body is the regeneration of the liver following partial hepatectomy. If you chop off half the liver, in time the liver will completely regenerate to its normal size! It is not recommended that you try this on your colleague – a rat perhaps – but not your colleague! The experimental evidence suggests that the remaining liver produces a growth factor, TGF-α, which causes an increase in mitotic activity and hence an increase in the cell number. What is remarkable is that it knows when to stop! It is believed that a growth inhibitor, TGF-β, is involved in this process.

Atrophy

The hypertrophic and hyperplastic changes are confined to a specific time and situation and regress once the functional need has been fulfilled. Extra cells are lost through the process of apoptosis described in Chapter 3. This reduction in size is called **atrophy.** It is similar to the changes taking place after the menopause when there is no further use for the reproductive organs and so they atrophy through a

Physiological   **Pathological**

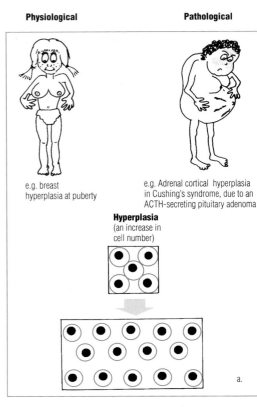

e.g. breast hyperplasia at puberty

e.g. Adrenal cortical hyperplasia in Cushing's syndrome, due to an ACTH-secreting pituitary adenoma

Hyperplasia
(an increase in cell number)

a.

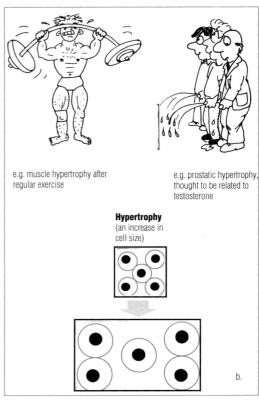

e.g. muscle hypertrophy after regular exercise

e.g. prostatic hypertrophy, thought to be related to testosterone

Hypertrophy
(an increase in cell size)

b.

combination of reduction in cell size and cell number. Since this is part of normal development, it is termed **physiological atrophy** to distinguish it from **pathological atrophy** which results from an abnormal state. An example of pathological atrophy is the severe muscle wasting that may follow an episode of poliomyelitis or the muscle wasting that is commonly observed in limbs immobilised in plaster following a fracture.

Hyperplasia versus benign neoplasms

Malignant neoplasia has been discussed in detail in the first half of this chapter and the classification of benign neoplasms included in Fig 4.8 page 163. A benign neoplasm, such as an adenoma in the colon, is an uncontrolled focal proliferation of well-differentiated cells which does not invade or metastasise. Unfortunately, the term is sometimes used inaccurately and some tumours do not quite fulfil these criteria, but it will serve as a working definition. The difference between a benign neoplasm and hypertrophy/hyperplasia is that the neoplasm will not atrophy when the workload or stimulus is reduced. Although benign, these tumours can cause many clinical problems as discussed in the section on the local effects of tumours (page 183). One of the commonest benign tumours necessitating removal is the leiomyoma (fibroid) of the uterine myometrium which may contribute to heavy and painful menstruation. Benign melanocytic tumours of the skin are removed for cosmetic reasons or fear of malignant change. Endocrine tumours are generally benign but can cause dramatic systemic problems through excessive production of hormones (page 185) and some 'benign' intracranial tumours like meningiomas can kill the patient because the skull cannot stretch to accommodate the 'benign' expansion. Remember that something which is 'benign' to the pathologist may appear 'malignant' to the patient!

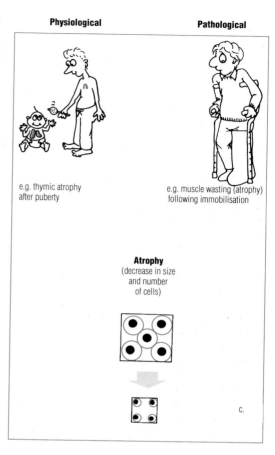

Fig 4.27 (a,b,c) Physiological and pathological examples of hyperplasia, hypertrophy and atrophy.

Metaplasia and dysplasia

The uterine cervix serves as a useful model for this discussion of **metaplasia and dysplasia**. The changes in the cervix are now well documented because of the national programme designed to screen women of reproductive age to detect early changes associated with cancer. Screening involves scraping some cells from the junctional zone of the cervix using a spatula. These are spread onto a glass slide, fixed and stained by the Papanicolaou technique.

The cervix has a transitional zone between the squamous epithelium of the ectocervix and the columnar epithelium of the endocervix. If there is chronic inflammation of the cervix, the columnar epithelium may be replaced by squamous epithelium – so-called squamous metaplasia.

Metaplasia is the *conversion of one type of differentiated tissue into another type of differentiated tissue*. This is most common in epithelial tissue although it can occur in other types of tissues such as mesenchymal tissues. Generally it is a response to chronic irritation and is a form of adaptation which involves, for example, replacing a specialised glandular or respiratory epithelium with a more hardy squamous epithelium.

Metaplasia is benign and reversible but its importance lies in the fact that the stimulants and irritants causing the metaplasia may persist and play a role in carcinogenesis.

The exfoliated cervical cells may show dysplasia, which is more worrying because it is a step on the road to an invasive tumour. The term **dysplasia** was originally used to mean an abnormality of development. Unfortunately, it is a term that is used too loosely and this causes confusion. In pathology reports concerning the microscopy of tissues, dysplasia refers to a combination of abnormal cytological appearances and abnormal tissue architecture. Its importance lies in its precancerous association. However, the term is still used to describe some gross abnormalities of development encountered in neonatal pathology, such as renal dysplasia and bronchopulmonary dysplasia, which have no precancerous association.

Dysplasia in the cervical squamous epithelium involves an increased cell size, nuclear pleomorphism, hyperchromatism, loss of orientation of the cells so that they are arranged rather haphazardly and abnormally sited mitotic activity (Fig 4.29). Of course, these appearances are the same as those described in malignant change but they differ in extent. When the full thickness of the epithelium is involved, it can be called 'carcinoma in situ' while involvement of only the lower third is 'mild dysplasia'. Many pathologists and clinicians felt that it was inappropriate to have different names for various stages of the same process and so the term 'cervical intraepithelial neoplasia' (CIN) was introduced. CIN I is the equivalent of mild dysplasia and describes abnormalities affecting the lower third of the epithelium; CIN II (replacing moderate dysplasia) is used for changes reaching the middle third; and CIN III (replacing severe dysplasia or carcinoma in situ) refers to full thickness involvement. Similar terminology can be used for changes in the squamous epithelium of the vulva (VIN) and larynx (LIN), although *glandular* epithelial changes (e.g. stomach or large bowel) are subdivided into mild, moderate or severe dysplasia.

It should not be assumed that dysplasia is irreversible. It is believed that early stages of dysplasia may revert to normal if the stimulus is removed. However, severe dysplasia will often progress to cancer if left untreated and, for this reason, it is sometimes referred to as carcinoma in situ. If severe dysplasia is cancer confined to the epithelium, what are moderate and mild dysplasia? Fortunately, terminology like intraepithelial neoplasia helps clarify our thinking and, in practice, severe dysplasia is treated as a favourable type of cancer, while milder degrees of dysplasia

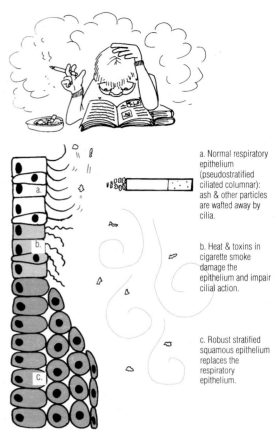

a. Normal respiratory epithelium (pseudostratified ciliated columnar): ash & other particles are wafted away by cilia.

b. Heat & toxins in cigarette smoke damage the epithelium and impair cilial action.

c. Robust stratified squamous epithelium replaces the respiratory epithelium.

Fig 4.28 Metaplasia e.g. squamous metaplasia of bronchial respiratory epithelium in smokers

can be managed slightly less aggressively but followed to ensure that they do not progress to more severe disease.

The concept of dysplasia fits with our current multistep theory of neoplasia in that it represents a stage between benign hyperplastic proliferation and overt cancer. The concept of dysplasia as a cancer in its early stages has also led to the institution of screening programmes for cervical and breast carcinoma. The logic behind this is that if dysplastic changes precede carcinoma by several months or years and patients with dysplasia can be identified and treated we can reduce the death toll from that cancer. Obviously, deaths from that cancer must be fairly common to make this worthwhile and we must be confident that the 'at risk' group are being screened sufficiently often to detect the early changes. For example, if the progression from CIN II to invasive tumour took only one year, then it would be of limited value to screen patients every three years. Much of the interest in genetic and immunocytochemical markers of malignancy lies in the hope that they will be able to detect ever earlier precancerous changes to increase the potential benefits of such screening programmes.

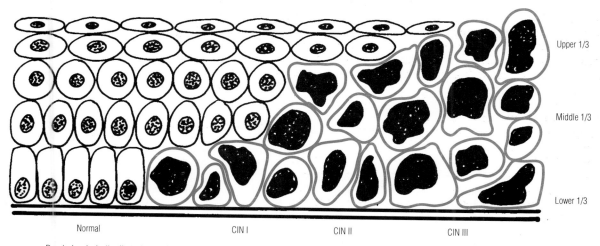

Upper 1/3

Middle 1/3

Lower 1/3

Normal   CIN I   CIN II   CIN III

Dysplasia principally affects the transformation zone of the cervix, i.e. the junction between the columnar epithelium of the endocervix and the squamous epithelium of the ectocervix. It is graded CIN I, CIN II, CIN III, depending on the layers of the epithelium involved. It starts in the basal layer. Dysplastic cells fail to mature and show the nuclear features of malignancy, e.g. ↑ nuclear:cytoplasmic ratio and nuclear pleomorphism and mitoses occur above the basal layer.

Fig 4.29 Dysplasia e.g. uterine cervix

Clinicopathological summary

Clinical

A 38 year old lady came to the surgery for a cervical smear.

She was single and had been living with her boyfriend for the last six months. She had divorced her husband two years ago and since then had had a number of casual relationships. Her first sexual contact was at the age of sixteen.

Four years ago her smear showed warty change and the last one, one year ago, again showed extensive warty change with possible dyskaryosis. The hospital had asked for a repeat smear as the epithelial cells were obscured by inflammatory debris.

She initially ignored the recall due to social problems.

The result of the repeat smear showed warty change and severe dyskaryosis and she was referred for a colposcopic biopsy.

The cervical biopsy confirmed the above findings and she was booked in to have a cervical cone biopsy.

The results of the cone biopsy came as a shock. The report read that she had extensive **squamous metaplasia** with **wart virus** change together with **severe dysplasia** between 3 o'clock and 5 o'clock and a **focus of invasive squamous cell carcinoma** which was completely excised. Invasive tumour did not involve deep tissues or invade blood vessels. The dysplastic epithelium extended to the endocervical excision margin and was therefore not completely excised.

The report was discussed with the patient and she was advised to have a hysterectomy.

The examination of the hysterectomy specimen showed residual foci of severe dysplasia but no invasive carcinoma. The excision was complete and she was discharged after an uneventful recovery.

Pathology

Carcinoma of the cervix is an important cause of death and the cervical screening programme has been instituted to try and reduce this toll. The idea is that, if the disease can be picked up at an early stage, it should be possible to cure it.

The risk factors for cervical cancer include: smoking, early onset of sexual intercourse, multiple sexual partners, a sexual partner with a history of promiscuity and infection with the human papilloma virus (HPV).

Her history reveals that she had a number of risk factors including wart virus change on her previous cervical smears.

The normal routine recall for cervical smears is three years, but early recall is instituted for suspicious or abnormal smears.

Severe dyskaryosis is the cytological equivalent to severe dysplasia on histological examination. Dysplasia is a premalignant condition in which there are cytological features of malignancy, i.e. increased nuclear : cytoplasmic ratio, nuclear pleomorphism, hyperchromatism, loss of maturation and mitotic activity. Dysplasia can be graded into mild, moderate or severe. Severe dysplasia implies a full thickness abnormality and the feature distinguishing this from carcinoma is the absence of invasion through the basement membrane. Metaplasia, on the other hand, is entirely benign. It is a form of adaptation to injury, where one type of epithelium is replaced by another. In the cervix, the glandular epithelium, after repeated bouts of inflammation, changes to a more resistant squamous epithelium.

The cone biopsy is a way of performing a local excision of the cervix: the tissue removed is in the form of a cone. A suture is usually put at 12 o'clock i.e. anterior, to orientate the specimen. The role of the pathologist is to map the abnormal areas, to assess the abnormality in terms of severity and to comment on completeness of excision.

She was 38, and still capable of having children. The decision to have a hysterectomy can be a difficult one, although she had very little choice.

The hysterectomy specimen did not reveal any more areas of carcinoma and the single focus of carcinoma was completely excised, so she should be cured.

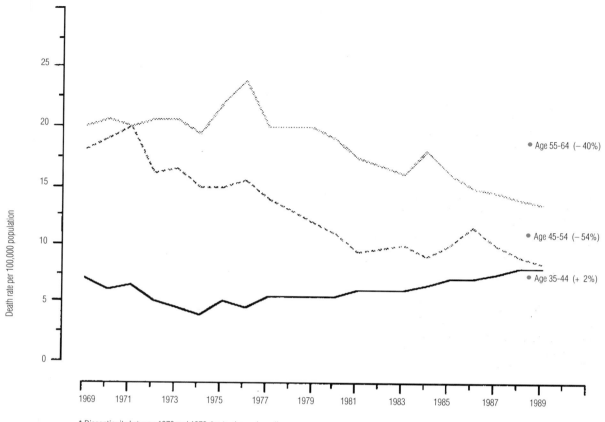

* Discontinuity between 1978 and 1979 due to change in coding
● Percentage change from 1969 to 1989

Source: OPCS (ICD 80)

4.30 Trends in death from cancer of the cervix, England females 1969–1989 * (from *The Health of the Nation*, London: HMSO)

In conclusion: science, like most aspects of life, has its fashions. Much of this chapter has concentrated on our evolving understanding of the role of the genetic code in producing cancer. Earlier workers have emphasised the importance of the interaction between cells and their environment, eloquently expressed by Sir David Smithers in 1962. Perhaps the truth lies in some combination of the two theories.

"Cancer is no more a disease of cells than a traffic jam is a disease of cars. A lifetime of study of the internal combustion engine would not help anyone to understand our traffic problems. A traffic jam is due to a failure of the normal relationship between driven cars and their environment and can occur whether they themselves are running normally or not."

– Sir David Smithers

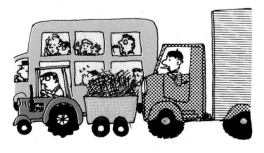

Further reading ———————————————————————————

A.D. Wyllie. (1992). Growth and neoplasia. Ch 10. *Muir's Textbook of Pathology*. Ed. R.N.M MacSween & K. Whaley. 13th Edition. Edward Arnold. London.

R.S. Cotran, V. Kumar & S.L. Robbins. (1989). Neoplasia. Ch 6. Robbins *Pathologic Basis of Disease*. 4th Edition. W.B. Saunders Company. Philadelphia.

D. Carney & K. Sikora. (1990). *Genes and Cancer*. John Wiley & Sons. Chichester.

L.M. Franks & N.M. Teich. (1991). *Introduction to the Cellular and Molecular Biology of Cancer*. 2nd Edition. Oxford University Press. Oxford.

R. Doll. (1992). Epidemiology of human neoplasms. *Oxford Textbook of Pathology*. Ed. J. McGee, P.G. Isaacson & N.A. Wright. Oxford University Press. Oxford.

Chapter 5

Genes and Disease _____

Introduction and Clinical History

It is a common misconception amongst medical students that pathology is an exact science. It is sometimes difficult to see why the examination of tissues at postmortem, both grossly and microscopically, cannot give a precise answer. Yet a short time in a laboratory will reveal that the terms 'possibility' and 'probability' are well known to the pathologist. If you encounter a patient with metastatic tumour in the liver, it is *possible* that the primary tumour may have arisen in the nose, but it is much more *probable* that it arose in the colon! The study of genetics involves appreciating how the inheritance of genes produces diseases so that the *probability* of a particular individual developing a disease can be calculated.

Most of us take our existence for granted but life really is a source of constant wonder and it has occurred against probability. Let us begin when there was no life on earth. At some stage, molecules must have come into existence that were capable of self-replication and these molecules multiplied. Ironically, if you have two molecules, one that manages to replicate and make copies without any mistakes while the other makes a lot of mistakes each time it is copied, then the correctly copied molecule is more likely to increase in number. However, the molecule that copies perfectly will never change and it will still be the same molecule after one year, after 50 years and after a billion years. If a random mistake happens in the copying then there is the opportunity for change; possibly for the better, probably for worse. This is the basis for evolution recognised by Darwin in 1838. The other important factor is that there should be a 'struggle for survival', an evolutionary pressure that gives an advantage to the molecules or animals best adapted to the prevailing conditions.

The probability of inheriting characteristics from parents was studied by Gregor Mendel. Mendel took garden peas with contrasting characteristics, seven to be exact, and bred from the plants which differed in only one characteristic. For the sake of discussion, let us consider violet and white flowers. He crossed plants with violet flowers with those bearing white flowers to produce the next generation, called the F1 generation. He found that the F1 generation plants all had the same colour flowers. Let us say that they were all violet. The F1 plants were then self-pollinated (inbred) to produce the next generation, called F2. Interestingly, there were three plants with violet flowers for every one plant with white flowers. He took this one step further and self-pollinated the white plants which gave rise to an F3 generation of plants that all had white flowers.

SHE HAD ONE MAD CAT AND ONE SAD RAT
SHE HAD ONE **B**AD CAT AND ONE SAD RAT
THE MAD BAD CAT ATE THE ONE SAD RAT
THE MAD SHE CAT ATE THE ONE SAD RAT
THE MAD HEC ATA TET HEO NES ADR AT

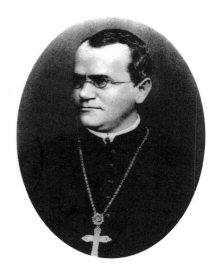

Fig 5.1 Gregor Mendel was born in Heizendorff, Moravia on 22nd July 1882. He joined the Augustine order in 1843 and ten years later, after studies at the University of Vienna, he went to the monastery at Brünn. His famous work with the peas began in 1856 but it was not until 1865 that he communicated the results to the Brünn Society of Natural Science. They remained in the archives until they were discovered in 1900, 35 years after publication, by three botanists pursuing a similar path. Mendel died in 1884.

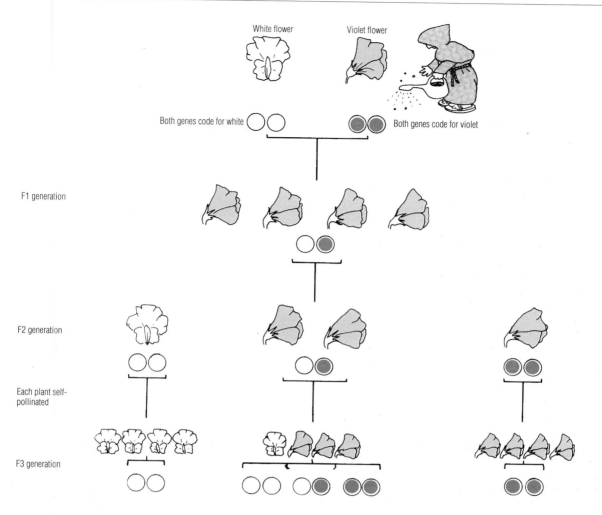

White flower

Violet flower

Both genes code for white

Both genes code for violet

F1 generation

F2 generation

Each plant self-
pollinated

F3 generation

Self-pollination of the violet plants produced an intriguing result; some plants produced only violet plants while others produced a mixture of white and violet plants in the ratio of 1:3. As Mendel correctly deduced, although the violet plants in the F2 generation all looked the same, they had different inheritance factors. He postulated that each plant must possess two factors which determine a characteristic, such as colour of the flower. If two plants are crossed, each will contribute one factor to the next generation and it is purely random as to which factor is passed on. This is the **law of segregation**, also known as Mendel's first law.(Fig. 5.2). We now know that these 'factors' are on chromosomes which are paired and the two genes on the two chromosomes are **alleles** of each other. In Mendel's experiment, violet is the **dominant** allele and white is the **recessive** allele. The F1 generation has one white plant, which is **homozygous** for the white allele, one violet plant which is homozygous for the violet allele and two violet plants which are **heterozygous**, i.e. they have one white and one violet allele but the violet one dominates. In simple examples like this,

Fig 5.2 Mendelian inheritance

one allele dominates, i.e. if the plant has at least one violet allele then all the flowers will be violet. Sometimes the situation is more complicated as there will be **variable penetrance,** i.e. the 'dominant' allele only dominates in a percentage of cases. It was later appreciated by Morgan (1934) that cell differentiation might depend on the variation in the action of genes in different cell types. In the later part of the nineteenth century, DNA, RNA and histones were discovered and it was originally believed that the histone proteins were genes. However, in 1944, Avery, MacLeod and McCarty recognised that DNA was the structural component of the gene. In 1953, Watson and Crick elucidated the double helical structure of DNA that provides the basis for its ability to replicate.

Obstetrics forms a major part of the medical curriculum, and during your training you will meet pregnant women who are naturally concerned about their unborn baby. Let us briefly consider a clinical scenario to illustrate a possible problem you might encounter.

A 34 year old lady was seen in the antenatal clinic complaining of abdominal pain and 'spotting' of blood. This was her first pregnancy and examination revealed a uterus of approximately 20 weeks size. The gestation should have been 22 weeks according to her estimated date of delivery. The doctor failed to hear a fetal heart sound and he arranged an ultrasound scan. This revealed an intrauterine death and a termination was carried out to evacuate the dead fetus.

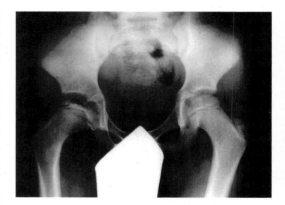

Fig 5.3 Pelvic X-ray with avascular necrosis of the right femoral head in a patient with sickle cell disease.

Post mortem examination showed a male fetus of 20 weeks gestation without external or internal abnormalities. Chromosomal studies carried out on fetal skin and muscle, however, revealed Down's syndrome (47,XY: +21).

Let us consider some of the questions you may be faced with; after all, you will need to be able to answer them!

- What are the risks of having an abnormal baby?
- How soon can any abnormality be detected?
- What are the commonest genetic diseases?
- How are they caused?
- Are all inherited abnormalities apparent in infancy?
- Can the genes change after birth?

What are the risks of having an abnormal baby?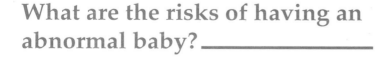

Family history

Here we are concerned principally with inherited diseases, so any family history of abnormality will be important. The problem is to decide which of the enormous range of diseases is due to a genetic abnormality that can be transmitted to the offspring. This requires careful observation of the incidence of a disease in the general population and within a family group. Many disorders, however, are multifactorial in nature, with both genetic background and environmental agents influencing the outcome. We have already encountered this in our discussion on breast cancer. In many cancers, there is an increased risk in close relatives but, at least in the antenatal clinic, the main concern will be conditions which are known to be inherited in a Mendelian fashion. Although many of these conditions are rare, over 4000 separate types have been identified.

We will illustrate the importance of family history by considering the example of sickle cell disease.

Sickle cell disease

Patients may present with abdominal pain, joint pains, cerebral symptoms, renal failure and cardiac failure, which result from ischaemic and thrombotic damage. This occurs because the red cells 'sickle' so altering their shape and occluding capillaries. The red cells have an abnormal haemoglobin which, under hypoxic conditions, polymerises and alters the cell's shape.

In 1949, Pauling analysed the haemoglobin from patients with sickle cell anaemia and discovered that its mobility on electrophoresis differed from normal haemoglobin. He called it haemoglobin S (HbS). Later, family studies suggested that the gene for sickle cell haemoglobin was an allele of the normal gene on chromosome 11 for the beta chain of the haemoglobin molecule, i.e. an alternative gene at the same locus on the chromosome. The difference between the normal haemoglobin gene and the sickle cell gene is a change in one base pair: GAG becomes GTG. This causes valine to replace glutamic acid in position 6 of the beta chain. That's it – a **point mutation** changing just one nucleotide leads to the translation of one different amino acid, which entirely changes the property of the molecule!

Fortunately, genes are paired and people who are heterozygous (i.e. one normal gene, one sickle gene) do not usually have any problems unless they become unusually hypoxic (e.g. possibly at operation). They have a mixture of the normal and abnormal haemoglobin. For practical purposes, we can regard sickle cell disease as an **autosomal recessive** disorder. How should we counsel a healthy pregnant woman who has a family history of sickle cell disease? The problem lies in deciding which members of the family are carriers of the gene because two people with sickle cell trait (heterozygotes) are likely to produce one healthy child, one sick child and two carriers. Carriers of the sickle cell gene can be identified by adding a reducing agent to the blood *in vitro* which induces the red cells to sickle. More recently, techniques have been developed to analyse the DNA itself. This is particularly useful in prenatal diagnosis for testing the fetus before it has switched on to full production of the beta chains. You cannot detect the abnormal beta chains in foetal red blood cells because the

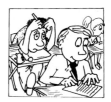

Describe the normal and abnormal forms of haemoglobin

Normal

HbA	$\alpha_2\beta_2$	96% in adult
HbA2	$\alpha_2\delta_2$	3% in adult
HbF	$\alpha_2\gamma_2$	1% in adult

large amounts in foetus/neonate

Abnormal

HbS	sickle cell disease
	βchain position 6 has val

Thalassaemias

α
Genotype

$-\alpha/\alpha\alpha$	silent carrier
$-\alpha/-\alpha$	α trait
$--/\alpha\alpha$	
$--/-\alpha$	HbH β4
$--/--$	Hydrops fetalis with HbBarts γ4

generally due to gene deletion

β

β^0	complete absence of β chains chains – has α_4 haemoglobin
β^+	reduction in β chains

Thalassaemia major = homozygous
Thalassaemia minor = heterozygous

β thalassaemia is generally due to defects in transcription, processing or translation of the genes

fetus is relying on haemoglobin produced from alpha and gamma chains, i.e. HbF. Instead you can remove a small piece of placenta (chorionic villus sampling) for DNA analysis relying on the point mutation to alter the binding of specific oligonucleotide probes or interfere with restriction enzyme digestion (see later).

Let us digress to consider the evolutionary aspects of sickle cell disease. If two hypothetical parents with sickle cell trait have four children, one should die before being able to reproduce. That child will be homozygous for the abnormal gene and so we might expect the incidence of that gene to reduce in the population because of its disadvantage for survival. However, the gene has not died out but is very common in areas where malaria is endemic. This suggests that the sickle cell carriers have a survival advantage in malarial-infected areas. How would this operate? Let us consider the life cycle of malaria.

The malarial parasite has to transfer from a mosquito into a human's blood stream and then invade the red blood cells to complete its reproductive cycle. The infected red cell has a lower oxygen tension so, if the patient has sickle cell trait (i.e. some HbS), the cell will collapse and the parasite will suffer. The fascinating thing is that when this mutation first appeared in one gene, the corresponding allele would have been normal and the patient would have a 'perfect' genetic combination that protected against malaria and left the person in good health. As the survival of these patients was enhanced, so was the spread of this new gene, and the geographical distribution of sickle cell disease correlates with the distribution of malaria, after allowing for the effects of emigration. Sickle cell trait is not the only method that evolution has devised for defending against malaria. There are other haemoglobinopathies, such as thalassaemia, and conditions where the red cell surface markers, necessary for entry of the parasite, are altered.

Maternal age

There is a dramatic increase in the number of chromosomally abnormal fetuses in women over the age of 35 years. This affects a wide variety of disorders with the commonest being trisomy 21 or Down's syndrome.

People with **Down's syndrome** are mentally retarded, may have congenital heart disease and an increased incidence of infections and leukaemia. In 1959, Lejeune and his colleagues showed that these patients have an extra chromosome 21. This most commonly arises because of **non-disjunction** of chromosome 21 during meiosis in one of the parents, so that either the egg or the sperm carries two copies of chromosome 21. In about 5% of cases, there is a translocation of chromosome 21 to 14 and occasionally translocations of 21 to 22, or 21 to 21. A **translocation** is the transfer of part of one chromosome to another chromosome. Translocations occur because the repair mechanism for breakages in the chromosomes can join the wrong pieces

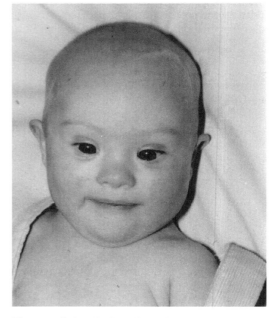

Fig 5.4 Baby with Down's syndrome exhibiting the prominent epicanthic folds and oblique palpebral fissures.

together. If this results in pieces of chromosomal material being exchanged between chromosomes with no loss of genetic material, or joining of one entire chromosome with another, then the individual is said to have a **balanced translocation** and is clinically normal. However, the genes are only 'balanced' in diploid cells and the haploid gametes will have an abnormal amount of the translocated segment. Therefore, sperm or ova from individuals with balanced translocations have a high risk of producing an abnormal child. For Down's syndrome, the risk is 10% when the mother is the carrier of the translocation and 2.5% if the father is the carrier. Obviously, it is important to investigate the parents of children with such inherited disorders to look for balanced translocations, although non-disjunction is the commonest cause.

About half of fetuses affected by Down's syndrome do not survive to term. The incidence in live births is 1 in 650; however, that is an average figure for all ages. The risk at age 30 is 1 in 900, which doubles by age 35, stands at 1 in 100 at age 40 and 1 in 40 at age 44. This age distribution makes it sensible to screen women over 35 years by examining chromosomes cultured from amniotic cells and measuring α-fetoprotein levels which are *lowered* in Down's. (N.B. they are *raised* in many other abnormalities, e.g. neural tube defects.)

Infective and environmental hazards during pregnancy

Infections during the first trimester may cause intrauterine death or a variety of abnormalities. The most important are rubella, cytomegalovirus and toxoplasma. Environmental hazards, such as radiation, industrial chemicals, alcohol and tobacco, may retard growth and predispose to spontaneous abortion. Neither infections nor environmental agents induce transmissible changes in the parent's genome and so there is no risk of recurrence, provided that the agent is not encountered in future pregnancies.

How soon can any abnormality be detected? _____

Fortunately, most pregnancies progress without any problems to produce a normal healthy baby after 40 weeks' gestation. It would be unreasonable to subject all pregnant women to the stress and possible hazards of the many investigations that are available to detect fetal abnormalities. Instead, it is sensible to make only simple observations on those women who are expected to have a trouble-free pregnancy. These include recording the size of the uterus at each visit as an indicator of fetal growth, listening to the

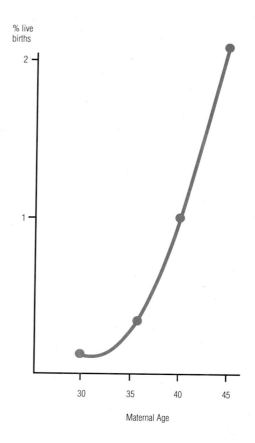

Fig 5.5 Incidence of Down's Syndrome with increasing maternal age

fetal heart and enquiring about fetal movements. In recent years, the quality of **ultrasound scanning** has achieved a standard that makes it useful for detecting internal and external fetal malformations as well as giving accurate information on the rate of fetal growth through head circumference and body length measurements. For detecting fetal abnormalities, it is best performed between 17 and 20 weeks' gestation. All of the tests that we have mentioned so far are non-invasive and free of any risks to mother or baby.

There are also invasive tests, one of the simplest of which is to measure the **mother's serum α-fetoprotein** (AFP) concentration. This is most important as a screening test for neural tube defects (e.g. spina bifida and anencephaly). It is measured at about 16–18 weeks' gestation and will be raised in 90% of mothers bearing children with open neural tube defects and 95% of anencephalic cases. Obviously, this means that 5–10% of cases will remain undetected so it is essential to offer more sensitive techniques to mothers at particularly high risk. AFP is also increased in multiple pregnancies, threatened abortions and a variety of fetal malformations. Its level is lowered in Down's syndrome.

Amniocentesis can be performed between 15 and 16 weeks' gestation and involves removing about 20 ml of amniotic fluid, which contains small numbers of amniotic cells that can be cultured. The fluid can be tested for AFP and acetylcholinesterase activity to detect neural tube defects or more specialised tests for detecting rare inborn errors of metabolism. The cells are cultured and used for chromosome analysis.

Chromosomal analysis

The human nucleus contains 23 pairs of chromosomes: 22 pairs of autosomes and one pair of sex chromosomes. It has been apparent for some time that certain diseases are associated with specific chromosomal abnormalities and it is logical to divide these into those affecting the *autosomal chromosomes* and those affecting the *sex chromosomes*. As we shall see, these groups can also be divided into abnormalities affecting *numbers* of chromosomes and those affecting the *structure* of chromosomes.

Disorders affecting the number of chromosomes are most commonly **aneuploid**, i.e. the chromosome number is not an exact multiple of the haploid set. This may involve extra chromosomes or loss of chromosomes. Structural changes to individual chromosomes can be deletions, inversions, duplications, translocations, ring chromosomes or fragile sites (Fig. 5.7).

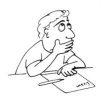

Discuss the significance of changes in maternal serum AFP level

Raised in:	Multiple pregnancies
	Threatened abortion
	Anencephaly
	Open neural tube defects
	Anterior abdominal wall defects
	Skin defects
	Turner's syndrome
	Placental haemangioma
Lowered in:	Down's syndrome

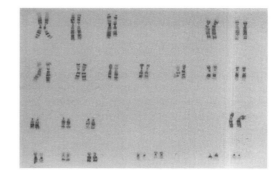

Fig 5.6   Normal chromosomal spread.

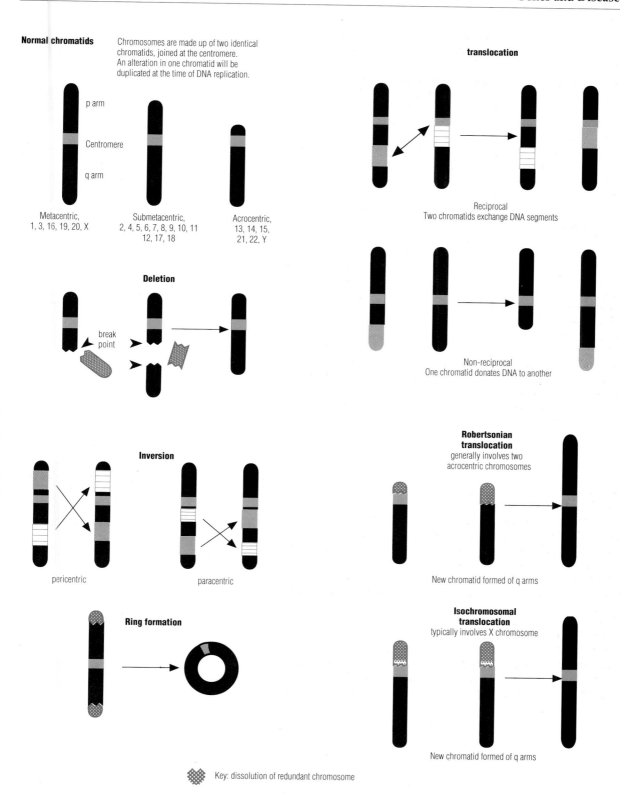

Fig 5.6 Structural chromosomal abnormalities

Chromosomal analysis is most commonly performed on cells from the skin, bone marrow or peripheral blood in postnatal life but, prenatally, cultured amniotic cells or samples of chorionic villi can be used. Colchicine is added to arrest the cells in metaphase and hypotonic saline causes the cells to swell and disperse the chromosomes. Analysis involves staining the chromosomes to show up the bands as alternating light and dark areas and then photographing them under a light microscope. The photographs of the chromosomes are cut up and the chromosomes rearranged in pairs. This simple method allows identification of the individual chromosomes and will reveal gross changes, such as loss or addition of whole or large parts of chromosomes.

At metaphase, the two chromatids of each chromosome are joined by a centromere and the long arm is termed 'q' and the short arm is 'p'. There is a convention for reporting karyotypes so that the total number of chromosomes is given first followed by the sex chromosomes, e.g.

46,XY   normal male
47,XXY   male with Klinefelter's syndrome

If there is a change in chromosomal number, then the affected chromosome is indicated with a + or −
47,XX +21   female with Down's syndrome

If there is a structural rearrangement, the karyotype indicates the precise site affected and the nature of the abnormality
46,XX del7(p13–ptr)   deletion of the short arm of chromosome 7 at band 13 to the end of the chromosome
46,XY t(11;14) (p15.4;q22.3)   a translocation between chromosome 11 and 14 with the break points being band 15.4 on the short arm of chromosome 11 and band 22.3 on the long arm of chromosome 14

Mosaicism indicates that two different cell lines have derived from one fertilised egg and the karyotype specifies both cell lines
46,XX / 47,XX + 21   Down's mosaic
46,XX / 45,X   Turner's mosaic

The child with mosaicism has two genetically different cell types distributed in its tissues. These are not distributed evenly and some affected individuals may demonstrate only a normal phenotype in their peripheral blood lymphocytes. Therefore, it may be necessary to culture from other organs, such as skin, to confirm a suspected abnormality. Patients with mosaicism are generally less severely affected than those with the full disorder. This makes prenatal counselling difficult if mosaicism is detected in a fetus, as the clinical effects could be mild. There is also the complication that any mosaicism detected in chorionic villus samples may only indicate an abnormal genotype in some placental cells and the fetus need not be affected.

Define haploid, diploid, polyploid and aneuploid

Haploid: cells have only one set of chromosomes i.e. "n" – as occurs in gametes.
Diploid: cells have the normal number of chromosomes i.e. 46=2n as occurs in somatic cells.
Polyploid: possession of complete extra sets of chromosomes, i.e. xn
Aneuploid: an abnormal number of chromosomes that is not an exact multiple of the haploid number.

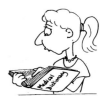

Mosaicism-
the presence of two or more cell lines that are both karyotypically and genotypically distinct but derived from the same zygote.

Chorionic villus sampling has some advantages over amniocentesis in that it can be performed between 8 and 12 weeks' gestation so that a diagnosis can often be made by 12–14 weeks' gestation when termination is easier. It also provides material suitable for DNA analysis which is necessary when the genetic changes are too small to be seen on light microscopical chromosomal preparations.

DNA analysis

First, let us remind ourselves of some basic facts about DNA (deoxyribonucleic acid). DNA consists of two antiparallel strands which have a backbone of deoxyribose sugars from which project **purine** and **pyrimidine** bases. The sequences of these bases determines the genetic code. It is estimated that there are approximately 6 billion bases in the human genome. The purine bases are adenine (A) and guanine (G) and the pyrimidine bases are cytosine (C) and thymine (T). The two strands form a right-handed double helix with about ten nucleotide pairs per helical turn. They are linked through these purine and pyrimidine bases with G always pairing with C and A pairing with T. This point is fundamental to the use of probes for analysing DNA.

The binding of complementary purine and pyrimidine bases also allows DNA to act as a template for the production of mRNA. This process is called **transcription**. The mRNA moves to the cytoplasm, attaches to a ribosome and is then used for protein production. This is termed **translation** and involves binding of transfer RNAs (tRNA) carrying a specific amino acid. The amino acids then combine to form a polypeptide chain and are released (see Fig. 5.8). RNA differs from DNA in three respects: it is a single-stranded molecule, it contains ribose sugar instead of deoxyribose and the base thymine (T) is substituted by uracil (U).

Registration fragment analysis

There have been two major advances that have made DNA analysis possible: the ability to cut DNA and the ability to sort the resulting fragments. It was discovered that bacteria produce enzymes that are capable of cutting DNA at specific sites and only at those sites. These enzymes are called **restriction endonucleases** and the DNA fragments are known as **restriction fragments**. Different bacteria produce enzymes that cut DNA at different sites. How is this useful in diagnosis? If you consider the sentence on the right, there are two identical sentences. One has been cut whenever a 'be' appears and the other whenever 'is' appears. You can see that the fragments produced are of different lengths. In the first case, there are three fragments with the smallest composed of 'no music'. In the second case, there are two large fragments. The same principle applies to the endonucleases. Once fragments of different sizes are

The capacity to blunder slightly is the real marvel of DNA, without this special attribute, we would still be anaerobic bacteria and there would be no music.

The capacity to blunder slightly is the real marvel of DNA, without this special attribute, we would still be anaerobic bacteria and there would be no music.

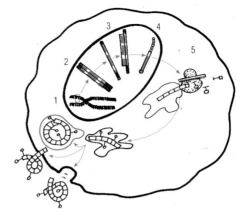

1. Gene
2. Activation of promotors & enhancers
3. Separation of DNA strands; synthesis of m-RNA (TRANSCRIPTION)
4. Capping, splicing & tailing; export from nucleus
5. TRANSLATION: protein synthesis on ribosome
6. New protein modified in golgi zone, e.g. glycosylation

Transcription:
Promotors and enhancers help RNA polymerase attach to DNA, to catalyse m-RNA formation. Transcription begins at a 'start' sequence in the flanking region adjacent to the gene and continues in a 5' → 3' direction.

The penultimate base sequence signals an adenine-rich 'poly-A' tail. Transcription ceases when a 'stop' signal is reached.

Capping, tailing and splicing of m-RNA:
The poly-A tail and a 7 methylguanine cap are added, facilitating transport from the nucleus to the cytoplasm. The introns are removed when the RNA is cleaved at splicing sequences encoded at the intron/exon borders.

Translation: m-RNA is translated on the ribosome. Each base triplet (codon) binds complementary base triplets on a t-RNA molecule, whose amino acid is then detached and added to the growing protein molecule. This may later be modified in the golgi apparatus to attain its final configuration.

Key:
base pair: complementary nucleotides on opposite DNA strands, e.g. G:C or A:T
The unitary measurement of DNA is the base pair.
gene: group of base pairs encoding one protein molecule.
exon: protein-encoding segment.
intron: non protein-encoding segment.
codon: base triplet, i.e. group of 3 nucleotides which encode one amino acid.

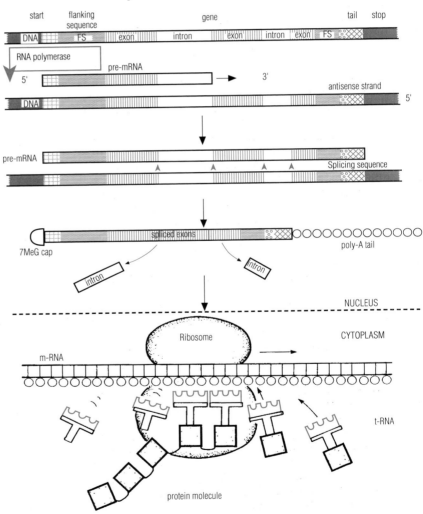

Fig 5.8 Gene expression

produced, they are run on an electrophoretic strip, which separates the fragments according to their size, and then 'stained' with a DNA probe. The details of these electrophoretic methods are not important, suffice it to say that the method used for DNA fragments is called **Southern blotting**, after its inventor, and the corresponding technique for RNA is **Northern blotting**. The binding of the probe to its complementary sequence is called **hybridisation**. The **DNA probe** or **oligonucleotide** is a short length of DNA whose nucleotide sequence is known. These are labelled, e.g. with a radioactive element, so that their position on an electrophoretic strip can be identified by autoradiography. Their importance lies in their ability to bind only to a specific section of the patient's DNA, i.e. to a piece with an identical sequence of complementary bases.

The restriction endonuclease technique can be used for detecting heterozygous and homozygous carriers of the sickle cell gene, which we mentioned was due to a point mutation changing GAG to GTG. There is a restriction enzyme called Mst II which recognises the area including GAG in the normal genome and will digest the DNA at this point. As the diagram shows, those with the normal gene will produce a fragment 1.1 kilobases long, while those with the abnormal gene will not digest at that position and the fragment will be longer. To 'stain' these on a strip requires a probe that will bind anywhere on this fragment. In practice now, it is more common to look for the sickle cell gene by the polymerase chain reaction (see later).

This use of restriction endonucleases relies on the enzyme digesting at exactly the point that mutates to cause the disease. Often we do not know the precise mutation responsible for an inherited disease, but it may be possible to identify which section of DNA it is in by comparing the DNA of affected family members with healthy family members. The human genome has approximately 6 billion bases, so how do we start looking for differences? We can look for **restriction fragment length polymorphisms**. These are variations in DNA fragment lengths that can be produced by using a restriction endonuclease and probe appropriate for detecting a particular disease. For example, the DNA from family members with Huntington's disease was investigated with an enormous range of enzymes and probes. It was discovered that digestion with an enzyme called Hind III, combined with hybridisation with a probe called G8, identified variations in the short arm of chromosome 4 that segregated with the disease. What is the principle behind this technique? It relies on variations in the genetic code that influence restriction endonuclease digestion but do not cause any clinical problems. We have already seen that a change of just one base causes sickle cell disease, so why do other common mutations have no effect? It is because only about 10% of DNA codes for proteins while the rest have no clearly defined function. The coding regions (structural genes) are fairly constant from person to person and mutations in these regions generally cause disorders. The non-coding regions can vary from person to

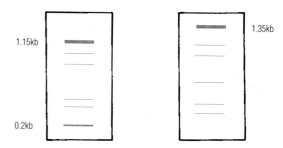

The DNA fragments are digested by endonucleases and separated by gel electrophoresis

The DNA bands are transferred to a DNA membrane

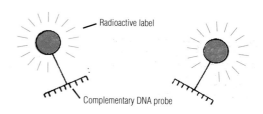

Radioactive probes to part of the globin gene are added

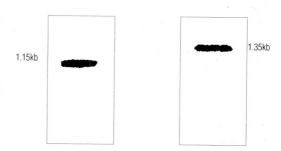

The autoradiograph reveals which fragment contains the probe binding site

Fig 5.9 Gel electrophoresis following restriction endonuclease digestion to detect abnormal globin gene

person and this diversity is useful for producing the 'DNA fingerprint'.

If a mutation has occurred in a non-coding region that is fairly close to the gene responsible for a disease, then it will be inherited with the disease gene. Obviously, the same mutation must not have occurred near to the normal gene or no difference will be detected. Provided that an enzyme exists which digests at the altered non-coding area, then the disease gene can be tracked. There is the inevitable problem of new mutations or cross-over of chromosomal material that might 'unlink' the mutant non-coding region from the disease gene, but this technique is useful for counselling families for future pregnancies *after* an affected child is born.

So far, we have only mentioned the use of oligonucleotide probes as 'stains' for the altered fragment produced by restriction endonuclease digestion. They can also be used on DNA without digestion to demonstrate **deletions** that are too small to see on light microscopical chromosomal preparations. Haemophilia A, Duchenne muscular dystrophy, α-thalassaemia and some cases of β-thalassaemia can be detected in this way.

Their most sophisticated use, however, is for 'staining' the gene that causes the disease. Provided that the same genetic change is always responsible for the disease, then this approach can be used without the need for family studies. In sickle cell disease, an oligonucleotide probe has been produced that detects the normal β globin gene sequence and another probe detects the mutant sickle gene. Each probe binds only to its specific complementary nucleotide sequence so the 'normal' probe binds to the normal gene, the 'sickle' probe binds to the mutant gene and, in heterozygous people, both probes will bind – one to each chromosome 11. How do the oligonucleotide probe sequences differ? Since we know that sickle cell disease involves a change from GAG to GTG, then the probes must be:

Normal probe •••••• CTC ••••••
Sickle probe •••••• CAC ••••••

Polymerase chain reaction

One of the problems of analysing DNA is that a relatively large amount of material is required. Since DNA's normal role is to act as a template for producing complementary DNA or RNA strands, this approach can also be used diagnostically. It is called the **polymerase chain reaction** (PCR) and involves amplifying a specific segment of DNA through successive rounds of replication (Fig. 5.10). This amplified segment, which should contain the area suspected of containing the mutant code, is then cut with the appropriate restriction enzyme and run on an electrophoretic agarose gel. It is not necessary to use a specific probe to stain the digested fragments because it is the relevant area that has been amplified. Instead it can be

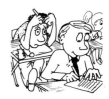

Describe the techniques available for ante-natal investigation

Method	Use
Ultrasound screening	Structural abnormalities
Maternal serum AFP screening	Neural tube defects
Amniocentesis	Chromosomal analysis Biochemical analysis, e.g. AFP
Chorionic villus sampling	DNA analysis Chromosomal analysis Biochemical analysis
Fetoscopy	Fetal material sampling Direct examination

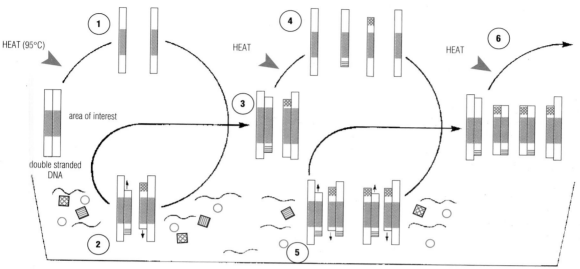

Medium contains oligonucleotide primers which will flank the area of interest by binding adjacent complementary sequences in the DNA molecule, thermostable DNA polymerase and the four deoxyribonucleoside triphosphates.

1 Heat-denatured DNA strands separate; each becomes a template

2. The two oligonucleotide primers anneal to the DNA adjacent to the area under investigation. DNA replication occurs, in which complementary bases extend in a 5' to 3' direction along each DNA strand, spanning distances of up to 10 kb.

3. Two new, shorter, DNA strands have been formed. The cycle begins again when the DNA is again denatured by heating.

4. Old and new DNA strands become templates for replication.

5. This time, DNA replication along the strands formed in steps 2 & 3 can proceed only as far as the primer, producing 'short products' whose primary content is the region under study.

6. The cycle is repeated 20-30 times. This technique permits the study of DNA from one target molecule in a single cell, with an amplification factor of up to 10^{12}.

Fig 5.10 Polymerase chain reaction (PCR)

viewed under ultraviolet light after staining with ethidium bromide. This is much faster than using autoradiography and can provide a result within two days of taking the sample. PCR is also used in forensic work to produce the 'DNA fingerprint' from small samples of blood, semen or hair left at the scene of a crime.

Finally, let us summarise the methods for detecting abnormalities and their risk of accidentally damaging the fetus:

Technique	Risk	Performed in:
Maternal blood sampling	Safe	2nd trimester
Ultrasonography	Safe	2nd trimester
Amniocentesis	0.5%	2nd trimester
Chorionic villus sampling	2%	1st trimester
Fetoscopy	3%	2nd trimester

What are the commonest genetic disorders and how are they caused?

Table 5.1 lists the incidence per 1000 live births of the commonest genetic disorders. It is helpful to subdivide them into **single gene disorders**, which will be inherited in a Mendelian fashion, and **chromosomal disorders**.

There are several points to highlight. The first is that the incidence relates to live births, which means that genetic abnormalities causing intrauterine death will be under-reported. This principally influences the figures for the chromosomal abnormalities, as their incidence in spontaneous abortions and stillbirths is 50% while the incidence in live births is 6.5 per 1000. In spontaneous abortions with chromosomal abnormalities, around 50% will have a trisomy, 18% will be Turner's syndrome (XO) and 17% will be triploid.

The commonest condition is X-linked red-green colour blindness which, fortunately, is only a very minor handicap (and is not an excuse for avoiding histology sessions!). **Klinefelter's syndrome** is due to an extra X chromosome in males (47,XXY). Affected individuals are generally of normal intelligence and are tall with hypogonadism and infertility. **XYY syndrome** also produces tall males. They may have behavioural problems, especially impulsive behaviour.

In **familial hypercholesterolaemia** patients have increased plasma low density lipoprotein (LDL) levels and a predisposition for developing atheroma at an early age which gives them an eight-fold increased risk of ischaemic heart disease. The primary defect is a deficiency of cellular LDL receptors so that the liver uptake is reduced and plasma levels are two to three times normal. Around 30 different mutations of the LDL receptor gene have been identified. About 1 in 500 people are affected and they are heterozygotes that have half the normal number of LDL receptors. One in a million people are homozygotes and they usually die from cardiovascular disease in childhood.

Adult polycystic kidney disease is due to a defect on the short arm of chromosome 16 that is inherited in an autosomal dominant fashion. Both kidneys are enlarged with numerous fluid filled cysts and may weigh a kilogram or more (normal = 150 g). The patients develop symptoms of renal damage and hypertension in their third or fourth decade.

Triple X syndrome produces tall girls who may have below average intelligence and, although gonadal function is usually normal, there may be premature ovarian failure. **Fragile X syndrome** was first described in 1969 and is now recognised as the second commonest cause of severe mental retardation after Down's syndrome. Affected males have a reduced IQ, macro-orchidism and a prominent forehead and jaw. Heterozygote females can show mild retardation but

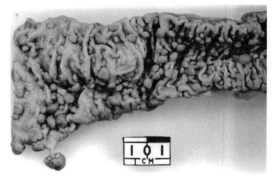

Fig 5.10 A section of colon from a patient with polyposis coli showing numerous polyps.

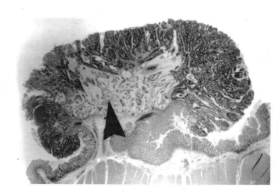

Fig 5.11 Photomicrograph of a colonic adenomatous polyp with early invasion and malignant change (arrow).

Table 5.1 Common genetic disorders

Condition	Estimated frequency per 1000 live births	Abnormality
Red–green colour blindness	80*	X
Total autosomal dominant diseases	10	AD
Dominant otosclerosis	3	AD
Klinefelter's (XXY)	2*	C
Familial hypercholesterolaemia	2	AD
Total autosomal recessive diseases	2	AR
Trisomy 21 (Down's)	1.5	C
XYY syndrome	1.5*	C
Adult polycystic kidney disease	1	AD
Triple X syndrome	0.6†	C
Cystic fibrosis	0.5	AR
Fragile X-linked mental retardation	0.5*	X
Non-specific X-linked mental retardation	0.5*	X
Recessive mental retardation	0.5	AR
Neurofibromatosis	0.4	AD
Turner's syndrome (XO)	0.4†	C
Duchenne muscular dystrophy	0.3*	X
Haemophilia A	0.2*	X
Trisomy 18 (Edwards's)	0.12	C
Polyposis coli	0.1	AD
Trisomy 13 (Patau's)	0.07	C

AD, autosomal dominant; AR, autosomal recessive;
X, sex-linked disorders; C, chromosomal disorders.
* per 1000 male births.
† per 1000 female births

counselling is difficult because not all female carriers show the chromosomal abnormality on testing. **Turner's syndrome** (monosomy X, i.e. 45,X) is a common cause of fetal hydrops and spontaneous abortion. About 95% of affected pregnancies will abort. Those surviving to delivery will be less severely affected and generally show short stature, webbing of the neck, normal intelligence, infertility, aortic coarctation and altered carrying angle of the arm (cubitus valgus).

Although, we have listed the common genetic disorders and their karyotype, this does not answer the question: 'How are they caused?' This is really two questions:

- How does the genetic abnormality produce disease?
- How does the genetic abnormality arise?

How does genetic abnormality produce disease?

From our list so far, we have only explained the pathophysiology of familial hypercholesterolaemia. Now we shall discuss the recent discoveries that have increased our understanding of cystic fibrosis. Patients with **cystic fibrosis** present in infancy with pancreatic insufficiency, malabsorption and lung damage. These result from thickened secretions that lead to obstruction, inflammation and scarring. The tenacious secretions are an indicator of a fundamental problem in water and electrolyte handling. This has been recognised for a long time and used as a diagnostic test – the **sweat test** – that looks for elevated levels of sodium in the sweat.

The reason for the increased electrolytes in sweat is that there is defective cyclic-AMP-mediated regulation of chloride channels. The gene has now been identified on the long arm of chromosome 7 (7q31) and called the **cystic fibrosis transmembrane conductance regulator** (CFTR). The CFTR gene codes for a protein of 1480 amino acids and the structure of this protein is similar to the family of ATP-binding proteins. It is not clear yet whether the CFTR protein transports chloride directly or regulates chloride indirectly via another protein, but it is clear that a change in CFTR protein would affect electrolyte transport.

In about 70% of cases of cystic fibrosis, there is a mutation referred to as the delta F508 mutation. This is a deletion in the codon at position 508 that leads to loss of a phenylalanine molecule in a highly conserved region of the CFTR protein. This is thought to alter the folding of the protein. The abnormal protein that is produced is unable to respond to cyclic AMP. In the pancreas and lungs, this leads to reduced chloride and water secretion so the mucus is thick. In the sweat test, the sweat glands secrete water and chloride normally but the secretory coil does not respond to β-adrenergic stimulation and does not reabsorb the chloride ions, hence allowing increased chloride and sodium in the sweat.

How does the genetic abnormality arise?

We need to consider abnormalities of chromosome number separately from abnormalities in chromosome structure or single gene disorders, as different mechanisms operate.

Normal (diploid) cell

Duplication of chromosomes and cross-over of material

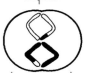

Anaphase I

Two diploid cells produced

Anaphase II may be several years delayed

Four haploid gametes form

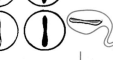

Fertilization generates diploid cells

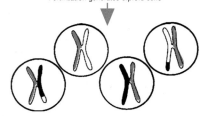

Fig 5.13 Meiosis

Abnormal chromosome number

This occurs because of problems at the anaphase stage of meiosis leading to unequal sharing of the chromosomes so that one daughter cell will have an extra chromosome (trisomy) while the other is missing a chromosome (monosomy). A pair of chromosomes or sister chromatids may fail to separate, so-called **non-disjunction**, or there may be delayed movement (**anaphase lag**) of chromosomes so that one is left on the wrong side of the dividing wall. The cause is unknown but the incidence increases with maternal age as we have discussed when considering Down's syndrome. It may also be associated with irradiation, viral infection or familial tendencies.

Polyploidy means that the cell contains at least one complete extra set of chromosomes. Most commonly, this is one extra set, i.e. 69 chromosomes or triploidy. Affected fetuses usually die *in utero* or abort in early pregnancy. It can result from fertilisation by two sperm (dispermy) or from fertilisation in which either the sperm or ovum is diploid because of an abnormality in their maturation divisions.

Abnormal chromosome structure

Abnormalities in chromosome structure occur when chromosomes are inaccurately repaired after breaks have occurred. **Chromosomal breakage** can happen randomly at any gene locus but there are some areas that are particularly liable to breakage. The rate of breakage is markedly increased by ionising radiation, certain chemicals and some rare inherited conditions. Structural abnormalities, such as translocations, deletions, duplications and inversions (see Fig. 5.7, page 205), occur when two break points allow transfer, loss or rearrangement of chromosomal material.

Single gene disorders also can result from structural abnormalities involving minute areas of the chromosome. These are produced by the same mechanism, i.e. breakage resulting in deletions, etc. Alternatively, single gene disorders are due to a **point mutation** at the gene site. Point mutations are usually spontaneous and of unknown cause, but are probably mostly due to copying errors. Substitution of one base within a codon may lead to a different amino acid being inserted into the protein and major pathological effects, e.g. sickle cell disease. However, this is not inevitable because there are only 20 amino acids but 64 possible codons (4×4×4), which is the basis of '**degeneracy of the genetic code**'. For example, an mRNA sequence of GAA or GAG will code for alanine, thus some point mutations can alter the codon but have no effect on the amino acid sequence. Approximately 25% of point mutations have no effect.

As well as coding for amino acids, codons also act as start and stop instructions. mRNA employs UAA, UAG or UGA as stop codons. If a point mutation produces a **stop codon**,

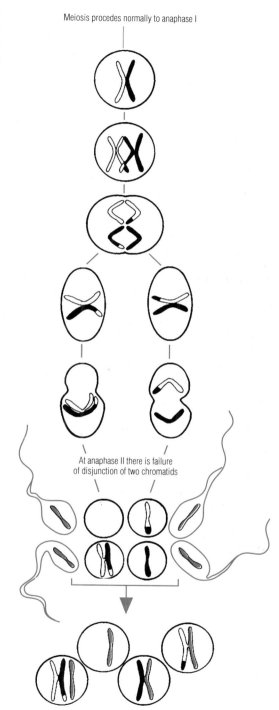

Meiosis procedes normally to anaphase I

At anaphase II there is failure of disjunction of two chromatids

Trisomy and monosomy will result if affected gametes are fertilised

Fig 5.14 Chromosomal non-disjunction

then the amino acid chain will terminate too early and this is the effect of about 5% of point mutations. The ultimate problem is a **frameshift mutation** where gain or loss of one or two bases produces a nonsense message because it alters every codon.

Let us look back at the 'cat and rat' sentences that started this chapter. Hopefully, their significance is now clear.

- The first sentence is the normal code.
- The second has a point mutation without a frameshift so there is a 25% probability that it will not have any effect.
- The third sentence has a length mutation, possibly a translocation.
- The fourth sentence is a mutation of the third where SHE represents a premature stop codon.
- The fifth sentence changes the sex of the cat and makes nonsense.

SHE	HAD	ONE	MAD	CAT	AND	ONE	SAD	RAT
SHE	HAD	ONE	BAD	CAT	AND	ONE	SAD	RAT
THE	MAD	BAD	CAT	ATE	THE	ONE	SAD	RAT
THE	MAD	SHE	CAT	ATE	THE	ONE	SAD	RAT
THE	MAD	HEC	ATA	TET	HEO	NES	ADR	AT

Multifactorial inheritance ———

Every new patient is asked about their 'family history'; the idea being that if their parents and siblings suffer from a particular disease then they are at increased risk. Unfortunately, for most diseases it is not known how great that increased risk may be because the inheritance does not follow simple Mendelian principles but is multifactorial. It is likely that there will be a variety of genes involved which interact with a number of environmental factors. Research into multifactorial disorders adopts a similar approach to single gene problems. First, it is necessary to identify the diseases with a significant genetic component by comparing the incidence in family groups with the general population. This genetic contribution is termed **heritability** and some examples are listed opposite.

The next step is to look for genetic, biochemical and immunological features that affected individuals have in common. It is well established that certain HLA types are associated with particular diseases and this may be helpful in counselling affected families. For example, in a family with ankylosing spondylitis, a first degree relative has a 9% risk of developing the disease if HLA-B27 positive but less than a 1% risk if HLA-B27 negative.

The ultimate goal it to identify the gene or genes and the environmental factor(s), so that those at particularly high genetic risk could attempt to avoid the relevant environmental hazard. At a simple level, this would mean giving folate supplements to pregnant women at risk of producing babies with neural tube defects, or advising potential

Heritability = genetic contribution to the aetiology of a disorder

Disease	Estimate of heritability (%)
Schizophrenia	85
Asthma	80
Cleft lip & palate	76
Coronary heart disease	65
Hypertension	62
Neural tube defect	60
Peptic ulcer	35

Calculated from incidence of disease in general population compared with incidence in relatives of an affected subject

'arteriopaths' to modify their diet and not smoke.

Diabetes is a disease where the genetic predisposition is beginning to be better understood. The insulin-dependent (type 1) form was known to be associated with certain HLA types and thought to involve a viral infection in susceptible individuals. Although HLA association need not mean that the HLA genes are involved, in this case study of the histocompatibility areas of chromosome 6 revealed that amino acid 57 in the DQ gene cluster was altered in susceptible individuals. Individuals with aspartate at position 57 had resistance to the disease, whereas mutations substituting alanine, valine or serine increased susceptibility.

Can genes change after birth? ___

The genes can change after birth, both by accident and by design. We have already discussed the accidents that can occur in the production of gametes or in the early divisions of the fertilised egg and these will affect all of the daughter cells, i.e. the whole individual. Now we shall consider the accidents that affect somatic cells after birth and are important in the aetiology of cancer, and the deliberate changes that occur in the genetic code of immune cells to allow them sufficient diversity to tackle the enormous range of potential antigens.

Generation of diversity in the immune system

B and T cells have surface structures that recognise foreign antigens as the first step in mounting an immune response (see page 29). These surface structures are immunoglobulin molecules on B cells and the T cell receptor (TCR) on T cells. They have some structural similarity to each other and to other members of the so-called immunoglobulin gene superfamily, e.g. CD4, CD8, class I and II MHC. It would have been possible to produce millions of subtly different receptors by joining polypeptide fragments in different combinations after translation, but nature has elected to alter the genetic code within lymphocytes and then translate each chain from the mRNA as a continuous polypeptide (possibly because it makes deletion of autoreactive lymphocytes easier). The system is broadly similar for the immuno-globulin light chains and heavy chains and for the α, β, γ and δ chains of the TCR. The genes for each chain are not a continuous structure in non-lymphoid cells but are groups of exons separated by long non-coding introns. There are four groups of exons and, in lymphoid cells during maturation, one gene from each of three of the groups is rearranged so that they lie adjacent to each other. The four groups encode for variable (V), diversity (D), joining (J) and constant (C) regions. There is great diversity within the V, D

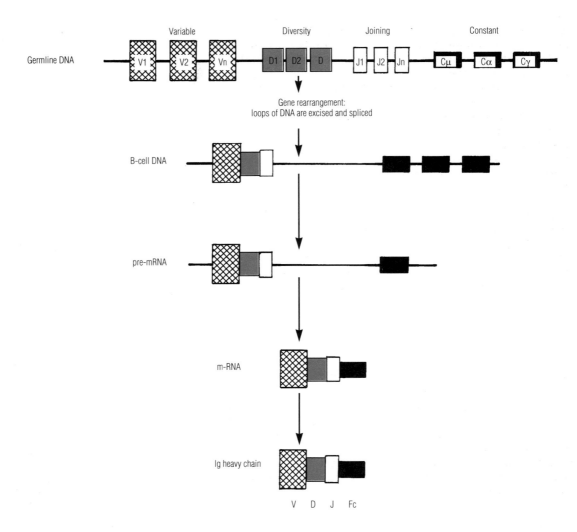

Fig 5.15 Gene rearrangements in the immunoglobulin heavy chain

Diagram showing the pathway leading to the rearrangement of the V,D,J and C genes to produce the final immunoglobulin molecule.

and J groups but the constant region genes are limited in number with only a single gene for each subclass of molecule, e.g. for heavy chains $C\mu$, $C\gamma$, $C\alpha$, $C\delta$, $C\varepsilon$.

It is easy to see how an enormous variety of molecules can be produced in this way. For example, the mouse immunoglobulin heavy chain molecule genome is produced from a choice of 500 V gene segments, 15 D gene segments and 4 J gene segments. Without further mutation, this gives a repertoire of 500×15×4 combinations. That chain will be combined into an immunoglobulin molecule and, in humans, approximately 10^8 different immunoglobulins are produced in this way. Only the V, D and J region genes are rearranged to lie together in the DNA with the C region genes remaining separate. This means that the transcribed RNA in the *nucleus* has a VDJ section distant from the C section so the remaining intron has to be excised to produce mRNA with consecutive V, D, J and C areas. Why is the C region treated differently? Probably because a lymphocyte that has recognised an antigen with the variable region on its surface molecule may need to produce molecules with different constant regions. This occurs in plasma cells that switch their immunoglobulin production from IgM to IgG; the antigen is the same and the variable regions are the same but the constant region has changed. If the alternative C region genes had been removed by the gene rearrangement that occurs in early B cell maturation, this would not be possible.

It must be emphasised that the V, D, J and C groups of genes are different for each type of molecule (i.e. heavy chain, light chain, TCR-α, TCR-β, etc.) so the genes for each chain are rearranged independently. Only the genes on one of a pair of chromosomes is completely rearranged so that it can produce the functional polypeptide.

Use in diagnosis of lymphoid malignancy

Rearrangement of the immunoglobulin and TCR genes occurs early in the maturation of lymphocytes, after which the nuclear DNA sequence in daughter cells will be identical. This can be helpful for distinguishing benign proliferations of lymphocytes from malignant proliferations, i.e. malignant lymphoma. Although most malignant lymphomas can be diagnosed with routine light microscopical sections, some malignant proliferations may mimic reactive collections of lymphocytes. Then DNA analysis of the immunoglobulin and TCR gene regions may be useful as malignant lymphomas often have a detectable rearrangement. Unfortunately, this is not always the case and it is not possible to classify lymphomas as B or T cells by this method because B cell lymphomas can rearrange their TCR genes and vice-versa. In reactive populations of lymphocytes, there are a variety of lymphocyte clones which have proliferated in response to different antigens.

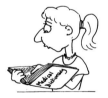

Monoclonal – a population of cells derived from the same parent cell and, hence, genetically similar. Tumours are monoclonal or oligoclonal and demonstrating monoclonality in a lymphoid population suggests that they are malignant.

Polyclonal – cells derived from a variety of parent cells.

Oligoclonal – cells derived from a limited number of parent cells.

Genes and cancer

In the last decade, our understanding of the link between genes and cancer has advanced considerably. It has become apparent that radiation, chemicals, viruses and familial factors may be operating through common genetic pathways to produce a transformed malignant cell. First, we shall look at the knowledge that has been gained from studying familial cancers.

Familial cancers

Familial adenomatous polyposis, retinoblastoma and neurofibromatosis have already been discussed in chapter 4 (page 174). In each of those conditions, affected individuals have a predisposition for producing tumours because they lack the gene for a tumour suppressor substance. The genetic area affected is usually small and consists of either a point mutation or a microdeletion, which would not be apparent on routine chromosomal analysis. This is regarded as the first 'hit', and a second 'hit' is required before the cell is transformed. The second hit removes the normal allele for the tumour suppressor on the paired chromosome. Often this involves a structurally obvious change, such as a translocation or deletion of a large part of a chromosome. Table 5.2 lists some of the tumours that can be inherited with their mode of inheritance and the probable genetic locus involved.

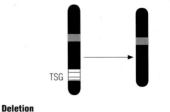

Deletion
e.g. RB gene in retinoblastoma (TSG = Tumour Suppressor Gene)

Table 5.2 Inherited tumours

Syndrome	Principal tumour types	Inheritance	Genetic locus
Familial adenomatous polyposis	Large bowel carcinoma	AD	5q21
MEN I	Pituitary, parathyroid, thyroid, adrenal cortex and pancreatic islet cell	AD	
MEN IIa	Medullary carcinoma of thyroid, phaeochromocytoma of adrenal medulla parathyroid tumours	AD	10
MEN IIb	Medullary carcinoma of thyroid phaeochromocytoma and mucosal neuromas	AD	
Von Hipple–Lindau syndrome	Haemangioblastoma of cerebellum and retina, renal cell carcinoma, phaeochromocytoma	AD	3p25
Retinoblastoma	Bilateral retinoblastomas, osteosarcoma	AD	13q14
Neurofibromatosis type 1	Neurofibromas, neurofibrosarcomas, gliomas, meningiomas, phaeochromocytomas	AD	17q
Dysplastic naevus syndrome	Malignant melanomas		1p11–22
Wilms' tumour	Nephroblastoma	AD	11p13
Li–Fraumeni syndrome	Breast cancer, soft tissue sarcoma	AD	17p13 (p53 gene)

AD, autosomal dominant.

Recognising the link between a gene and a predisposition for a cancer is much more difficult than associating a gene with a disease, such as Down's syndrome. The geneticist needs to analyse the family pedigree and look for differences between 'affected' and 'unaffected' family members but a problem arises because an 'affected' person (i.e. a carrier of the gene) need not have the tumour. This may occur because the gene carrier is still young, is the wrong sex (i.e. male carriers will not produce ovarian tumours) or because, although they have an increased risk, they have been lucky and remained tumour-free. The scientist needs some clues as to which genetic loci may be important because the search through all 23 chromosomes would be too difficult. These clues may come from assessment of large numbers of sporadic tumours to look for chromosomal alterations. It is relatively easy to identify structural changes in chromosomal preparations from tumours and any alterations common to tumours from different patients may be the genetic basis for the malignancy.

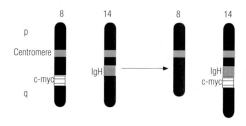

Translocation
e.g. c-myc in Burkitt's lymphoma

Chromosomal abnormalities in sporadic tumours

The **Philadelphia (Ph1) chromosome** is present in 90% of cases of **chronic myeloid leukaemia** and can be used as a diagnostic marker. It is produced by a reciprocal and balanced **translocation** between chromosomes 22 and 9. The breakpoint on chromosome 9 occurs at the locus of the *abl* proto-oncogene and the breakpoint on chromosome 22 is in the region termed the breakpoint cluster region (bcr). Some recent work suggests that the bcr genes code for a protein kinase that could have oncogenic potential. The *abl* proto-oncogene has sequence homology with the tyrosine kinase family of oncogenes but it is only after translocation to chromosome 22 that it produces a mutant protein with tyrosine kinase activity. This particular tyrosine kinase activity is located in the nucleus where it is believed to influence transcription of DNA.

Burkitt's lymphoma cells also show a **translocation**, which is usually between chromosome 8 and 14 but can also occur between 8 and 2 or 22. The breakpoint on chromosome 8 is near the cellular oncogene *myc* which is moved adjacent to the immunoglobulin heavy chain joining or constant region on chromosome 14. Alternatively, the light chain constant regions for lambda light chains (chromosome 22) or kappa light chains (chromosome 2) may move to chromosome 8 near *myc*. Any of these changes is thought to increase transcription of the genetically normal *myc* gene. The *myc* gene product is a nuclear protein that appears to act as a 'competence' factor. 'Competence' factors do not make cells proliferate but allow them to respond to growth signals from 'progression' factors (page 54). Thus, they have an important role in the regulation of the cell

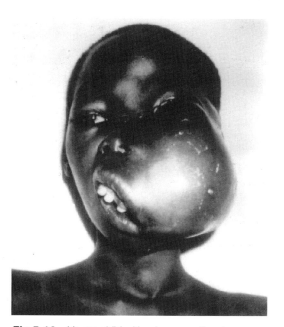

Fig 5.16 Young child with a large maxillary tumour distorting the face. This is a classical presentation of Burkitt's lymphoma.

cycle. The incidence of translocations is highest in lymphomas and leukaemias which may be related to their normal
necessity for rearranging genes during maturation.

Chromosomal deletions have been mentioned when
discussing familial tumours and tumour suppressor genes.
Although they can occur in leukaemias, they are more
common in solid non-haemopoietic tumours. The action of
many are unclear but it is likely that in most cases the
normal gene would code for a tumour suppressor molecule.

Table 5.3 Human tumour chromosomal alterations

Tumour	Chromosomal change	Possible action	Cellular oncogene	Location
Haemopoeitic tumours with translocation				
Chronic myeloid leukaemia	t(9;22) (q34;q11)	Nuclear tyrosine kinase activity altering transcription	c-*abl*	9q34
Burkitt's lymphoma	t(8;14) (q24;q32) t(2;8) (p12;q24) t(8;22) (q24;q11)	Cell cycle regulation	c-*myc*	8q24
Acute myeloid leukaemia	t(8;21) (q22;q22)		c-*mos*	8q22
Solid tumours with deletions				
Retinoblastoma	del13q14	Loss of oncosuppression	RB	
Renal cell carcinoma	del3p	Loss of oncosuppression	?	
Wilms' tumour	del11p13	Loss of oncosuppression	Wilms' gene	
Bladder cancer	del11p13	Loss of oncosuppression	?	
Malignant malanoma	del1p11–22	Loss of oncosuppression	?	
Small cell lung cancer	del17p del13q14 del3p14–23	Loss of oncosuppression	p53 RB ?	
Colorectal cancer	del17p13 del5q21	Loss of oncosuppression	p53 APC	
Breast cancer	del17p13 del13q14 del11p13	Loss of oncosuppression	p53 RB ?Wilms'	
Solid tumours with translocations				
Malignant melanoma	t(1;19) (q12;q13)		?	
Salivary adenoma	t(3;8) (p21;q12)		?	
Solid tumours with amplifications				
Neuroblastoma		Control of cell cycle	N-*myc*	2p24
Breast carcinoma		Increased growth factor receptor activity	c-*neu* c-*myc*	

Gene amplification can alter the karyotype in two different ways. There can be **homogeneously staining regions** (HSRs) added to a particular chromosome, which represent numerous repeats of the same genetic sequence, or there can be **double minutes** that are small paired fragments of chromatin seperate from chromosomes. In neuroblastomas, the oncogene N-*myc* on chromosome 2 is amplified and the extra chromosomal material can become integrated as an HSR in chromosomes 4, 9 or 13.

Point mutations particularly affect the *ras* oncogene family. These code for proteins that bind guanine nucleotides (GTP and GDP) on the inner aspect of the nuclear membrane. Their role is in the transduction of messages from the cell surface to the interior and mutant forms can result in excessive cell stimulation. *ras* mutations commonly occur in pancreatic adenocarcinomas, thyroid carcinomas, colorectal and lung tumours. Although there is no example in human cancer, it is known that chemical carcinogens given to rodents can produce point mutations in *ras* oncogenes.

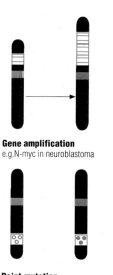

Gene amplification
e.g.N-myc in neuroblastoma

Point mutation
e.g. ras oncogene family in Ca colon

The importance of recognising chromosomal abnormalities in tumours is that it can give insights into the positions of proto-oncogenes and the mechanisms that activate them. We have described activation of proto-oncogenes that occurs through translocation enhancing the rate of transcription, gene amplification that increases the number of transcripts produced, and point mutations that alter the protein product. Theoretically, all of these changes can be produced by chemical carcinogens, radiation or viruses. Viruses, however, are in the unique position of carrying their own genetic information which may alter the infected cell's activities.

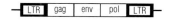

Replication competent:
Viral genome encodes core protein (gag), reverse transcriptase (pol) & envelope glycoproteins (env). LTR sequences contain promoters and enhancers of transcription.

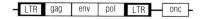

Slow-transforming RNA oncogenic viruses:
If the viral genome is incorporated adjacent to a cellular oncogene (c-onc) or proto-oncogene (p-onc) in the host cell, the presence of viral promoters and enhancers of transcription may lead to over transcription of the oncogene and hence cell transformation, i.e. uncontrolled cell proliferation.

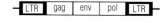

Acutely transforming RNA oncogenic viruses:
Incomplete oncogenic virus:
A viral oncogene (v-onc) has replaced one of the essential genes, here env. The v-onc confers the ability to 'transform' the host cell, i.e. cause uncontrolled proliferation, but the virus cannot replicate unless there is co-infection with another virus which can supply the missing gene.

v-oncs are thought to represent altered cellular oncogenes picked up in the genome incidentally, a kind of 'souvenir' of a previous visit by an ancestor.

Fig 5.17 Types of retrovirus

Viruses and human DNA

The study of viruses has helped enormously in unravelling the relevance of genes in human cancer. Of particular use are the retroviruses, which normally contain just three genes: two coding for structural proteins (*gag* and *env*) and one (*pol*) for the enzyme reverse transcriptase, which produces DNA from RNA. The addition of a fourth gene can often give the virus acute transforming properties, i.e. infection with the altered virus can produce tumours under experimental conditions, so-called **transfection** experiments. These viruses acted as tools to enable scientists to identify the genetic sequences that could transform cell lines. Many of the viral oncogene sequences were recognised as variants of cellular genes that the retrovirus had acquired from the human genome. This focussed attention on the human cells' proto-oncogenes and led to an understanding of the mutations and translocations that can lead to their activation.

Oncogenic RNA viruses

Oncogenic RNA viruses are all retroviruses, i.e. they contain reverse transcriptase, and they can be divided into acute transforming viruses, slow transforming viruses and transactivating viruses. The **acute transforming viruses** produce tumours within a few weeks in infected animals and often are capable of transforming cell cultures. The **slow transforming viruses** take months to produce tumours, which are frequently forms of chronic leukaemia. These two groups of viruses alter the infected cell in different ways. The acute transforming viruses are usually incapable of normal replication because they have lost some genes related to replication but gained genes which confer their transforming capabilities. These additional genes are variants of their host's genes: genes that are called proto-oncogenes when in the host, and viral oncogenes when in the virus. The viral oncogene is not identical to the proto-oncogene, although there is quite extensive sequence homology. The proto-oncogene is a normal cell gene that is normally involved in growth or differentiation. The viral oncogene is structurally altered which, in some way, deregulates cell growth. Alternatively, the proto-oncogene may be inserted near a potent viral promoter resulting in increased expression. In some cases, acute transforming viruses and normal retroviruses co-infect cells so that the non-transforming retrovirus can provide the replication information that the transforming virus lacks.

Slow tranforming retroviruses do not contain oncogenes, have the normal three gene structure to their genome and are capable of replication. They alter the host cell's behaviour by inserting near to the cellular proto-oncogene, so that they either cause increased activity of the cellular gene or, possibly, induce a structural change in the gene. This is called **insertional mutagenesis**.

Transactivating viruses do not contain oncogenes but, in addition to the *gag*, *pol* and *env* genes, they have a fourth region which confers transforming properties. The human T cell leukaemia virus is in this group and its extra genes (*tat*) code for a variety of proteins, one of which activates the host's IL-2 and IL-2 receptor genes resulting in uncontrolled cell proliferation.

Oncogenic DNA viruses

Oncogenic DNA viruses contain genes which act early in infected cells to increase expression of a wide variety of genes. The purpose of this is to activate later viral genes concerned with replication and assembly. However, it can also have the effect of inducing excessive expression of host cell genes responsible for growth regulation. For example, the 'early genes' of the virus can produce proteins (e.g. T proteins of polyoma and SV40 viruses) that localise in the nucleus and alter the regulation of DNA synthesis. In some cases this is through binding to the p53 protein so that its half life is increased and DNA synthesis remains activated. Some 'growth enhancing' actions may actually result from inhibiting normal 'growth inhibiting' proteins.

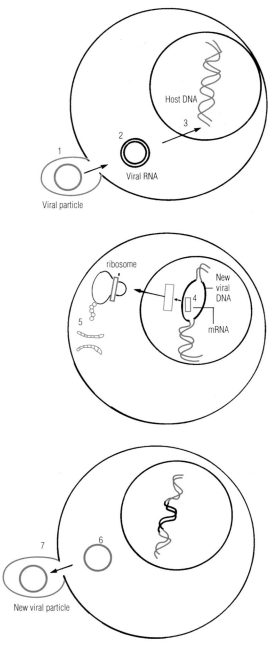

1 Virus attaches to cell surface receptor and injects viral RNA into cell
2 Reverse transcriptase catalyses formation of DNA copy
3 Viral DNA copy is incorporated into cell genome
4 Promotors & enhancers in the LTR sequences prompt transcription of viral D
5 Viral proteins are synthesised
6 Viral components are assembled at the cell membrane
7 A new viral particle buds off

Fig 5.18 Retroviral life cycle

DNA repair

DNA is usually copied accurately so that a genome of 3×10^9 base pairs will only change by 10–20 base pairs per year. This remarkable feat is achieved because there are a variety of DNA repair enzymes that continuously scan the DNA and repair any inaccuracies caused by replication or damage by environmental agents. The double-stranded nature of DNA is essential because the complementary information on the two strands allows the damaged piece to be rebuilt as Fig. 5.19 shows.

Any fault in this process will result in an increased number of mutations. This occurs in a number of rare human diseases where there is a failure of the repair systems. In xeroderma pigmentosa, there is a defect in the excision stage of repair. These patients are particularly susceptible to damage induced by ultraviolet radiation and have an increased risk of developing skin cancers. In Bloom's syndrome, there is a defect in one of the repair enzymes, DNA ligase I, and patients with this disorder have an increased risk of all forms of cancer. Ataxia telengectasia and Fanconi's anaemia are other examples with similar enzyme defects.

There is an old wives' saying: "Where god puts disease, He also puts a cure". Viruses undoubtedly cause infectious disease and can be one step on the road to cancer. However, they may also provide a possible cure for disease as they may be the ideal vehicle for altering the genetic code within human cells. Ultimately, it would be best if patients with single gene disorders could have their defective gene replaced by the correct gene. In theory, this is possible by using a retrovirus to introduce the gene, although in practice there are many problems to conquer. The most useful practical application of our rapidly expanding knowledge of the genes is in the manufacture of specific proteins.

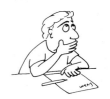

Discuss DNA damage

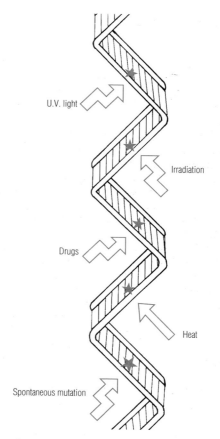

U.V. light

Irradiation

Drugs

Heat

Spontaneous mutation

Agents
Spontaneous mutation
U.V. light
Irradiation
Drugs
Heat

Change
Loss of base
Alteration of base
Bulk lesion
Alkylation

Recombinant DNA technology and therapeutics

Recombinant DNA involves inserting the relevant gene into a rapidly replicating organism, such as the bacterium *Escherichia coli* or a yeast. These organisms can be cultured continuously and large amounts of the protein are produced. First, the gene must be identified and, once a double-stranded cDNA has been prepared, it can be inserted via a plasmid.

In what way has production of these proteins been of use in therapeutics? The best established examples are hormones. Most people are aware that, until relatively recently, insulin was prepared from pig pancreas and that this method has problems related to the limited supply and

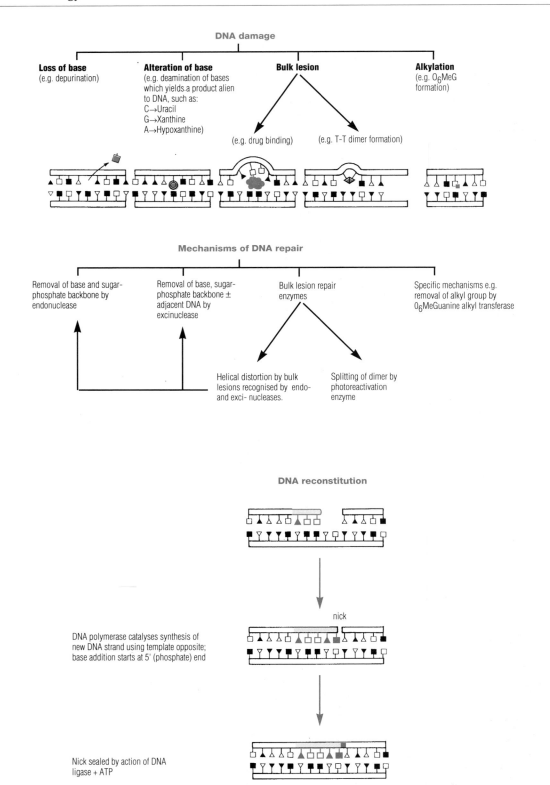

Fig 5.19 Types of DNA damage and examples of repair mechanisms

hypersensitivity reactions. Recombinant DNA technology has given us a method of producing this hormone synthetically and in unlimited quantities. The advantages of producing proteins this way are tremendous. We can produce vast quantities of the proteins and the risk of contamination with infectious agents is eliminated. This particular problem has been highlighted recently because of contamination of factor VIII by HIV. Now factor VIII can be produced by recombinant technology rather than through purification of human blood.

Does this new technology have a role in neoplasia? The answer is 'yes', although at present this is rather limited. Recombinant TNF and α-interferon are being tried in cancer chemotherapy (page 187) and growth stimulators, such as GM-CSF, may help to maintain the body's normal cells during chemotherapy and so minimise problems like neutropenia. With increasing understanding of the genes involved in cancer, maybe in time we will be able to direct treatment at the level of the abnormal gene. Alternatively, chemical mediators might be able to modify the expression of the mutant genes and hence the biological course of the disease.

Is there any more to know or have we come to the end of the road? Far from it! We are only just beginning to understand the intricate patterns that constitute life and we have only just embarked on the battle to conquer the genetic code. Our knowledge of the genes involved in disease forms a minuscule part of the whole genetic code. It is a bit like Columbus arriving in America and making a map of the port he had landed in. The discovery of that piece of land may indeed have been a great achievement, but it was only a small part of the continent, and that continent only a small part of the world. Just as it has been necessary to map out the whole of the world in order to gain an understanding of it, so it will be necessary to map out the whole of the genetic code before we can understand the complex interplay between all the different genes. This task is both necessary and immense, and it is a boring one! The paragraph below is an example of how a tiny part of it might read:

```
GGATTACCGTACCATAATTCCATGGGATTTACGTTAG
CAGTAGTTGATTACGTGCTGACGTACGTAGCTGACTG
TTGCAGTAAGGAGGATTACCGTACCATAATTCCATGG
GATTTACGTTAGCAGTGCGGATTACCGTACCATAATT
CCATGGGATTTACGTTAGCAGTAGTTGATTACGTGCT
GACGTACGTAGCTGACTGTTGCAGTAAGGAGGATTAC
CGTACCATAATTCCATGGGATTTACGTTAGCAGTGCG
GATTACCGTACCATAATTCCATGGGATTTACGTTAGC
AGTAGTTGATTACGTGCTGACGTACGTAGCTGACTGT
TGCAGTAAGGAGGATTACCGTACCATAATTCCATGGG
ATTTACGTTAGCAGTGCGGATTACCGTACCATAATTC
CATGGGATTTACGTTAGCAGTAGTTGATTACGTGCTG
ACGTACGTAGCTGACTGTTGCAGTAAGGAGGATTACC
GTACCATAATTCCATGGGATTTACGTTAGCAGTGCGG
```

```
ATTACCGTACCATAATTCCATGGGATTTACGTTAGCA
GTAGTTGATTACGTGCTGACGTACGTAGCTGACTGTT
GCAGTAAGGAGGATTACCGTACCATAATTCCATGGG
ATTTACGTTAGCAGTGCGGATTACCGTACCATAATTC
CATGGGATTTACGTTAGCAGTAGTTGATTACGTGCTG
ACGTACGTAGCTGACTGTTGCAGTAAGGAGGATTACC
GTACCATAATTCCATGGGATTTACGTTAGCAGTGCGG
ATTACCGTACCATAATTCCATGGGATTTACGTTAGCA
GTAGTTGATTACGTGCTGACGTACGTAGCTGACTGTT
GCAGTAAGGAGGATTACCGTACCATAATTCCATGGG
ATTTACGTTAGCAGTGC
```

Can you imagine a book in which every page looked like that, going on and on for 3,000,000,000 letters?! It would be one of the most tedious, but useful, books that any one can imagine. Still, we are in favour of the publication of such a book as it would provide a tremendous survival advantage for all pathology textbooks!

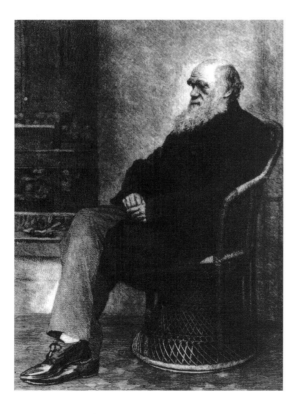

Fig 5.20 Charles Darwin was born at Shrewsbury on 12th February 1809. In 1825, he was sent to Edinburgh to study medicine; however, this was his father's choice and Darwin later chose to study classics at Cambridge. He joined the HMS Beagle which surveyed the coast of South America for five years. On this trip, Darwin pondered on the amazing diversity in nature. He was very religious and believed in the literal truth of the bible. Thus, he was reluctant to publish his heretical theory on evolution, preferring to direct his wife to publish it after his death. However, Alfred Russel Wallace had reached similar conclusions which he sent to Darwin in 1858. This resulted in both Darwin's and Wallace's ideas being presented to the Linnean Society in London that year followed in the next year by the Species by Means of Natural Selection, or the Preservation of Favoured Races in the Struggle for Life. Darwin died on 19th April 1882 and was buried at Westminster Abbey.

Further reading

J.M. Connor. (1992). Genetics and disease. Ch 2. *Muir's Textbook of Pathology*. Ed. R.N.M. MacSween & K. Whaley. 13th Edition. Edward Arnold. London.

R.S. Cotran, V. Kumar & S.L. Robbins. (1989). Genetic disorders. Ch 4. *Robbins Pathologic Basis of Disease*. 4th Edition. W.B. Saunders Company. Philadelphia.

B.A.J. Ponder. (1990). Inherited cancer syndromes. *Genes and Cancer*. Ed. D. Carney & K. Sikora. John Wiley & Sons. Chichester.

P.J. Talmud & S.E. Humphries. (1992). Molecular genetic analysis of coronary artery disease: an example of a multifactorial disease. Ch 2.7. *Oxford Textbook of Pathology*. Ed. J. McGee, P.G. Isaacson & N.A. Wright. Oxford University Press. Oxford.

A.E.H. Emery & D.L. Rimoin. (1990). *The Principles and Practice of Medical Genetics*. 2nd Edition. Churchill Livingstone. Edinburgh.

R. Dawkins. (1989). *The Selfish Gene*. 2nd Edition. Oxford University Press. Oxford.

Appendix

Bacon, Francis (1561–1626)

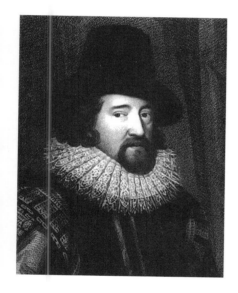

Francis Bacon was born on 22nd July 1561 at York House, off The Strand, in London. He was the second son of Sir Nicholas Bacon, Lord Keeper, and his second wife, Ann Cooke.

Francis Bacon, although recognised as an important figure in the history of thought, has not really been taken as a serious figure by philosophers. He is of course well known to students of literature for his sharp wisdom and clever writing. Besides literature, Francis Bacon also wrote about law, which was his profession, and about the history of the reign of Henry VII. His main works, *The Advancement of Learning* and *Novum Organum* (a presentation of a new method of logic), are, however, philosophical, and it is from his discourse on inductive reasoning that the quote at the beginning of Chapter 1 comes.

The Advancement of Learning

This consisted of two books, published in 1605. The first is essentially about the value of knowledge, which may seem a bit strange if you are unaware of the opposition to the acquisition of knowledge that existed at the time. The opposition was both religious and social and many believed that knowledge weakened action. It is not surprising therefore that Bacon felt inclined to provide a defence for knowledge.

The second book is about the classification of knowledge and is a reflection of his ordered mind. In Bacon's classification, all knowledge is divided according to the faculties of Memory ('history'),

Imagination ('poesy') and Reason ('philosophy'). Although he divided them into separate groups, he believed in the wholeness of knowledge. He did, however, have his own bias, as he put it, in the 'domain of philosophy and the sciences'.

It is true that Bacon has often been rejected and has been criticised for his lack of understanding of mathematics and the scientific advances that were being made at the time. In this there is an element of truth. What Bacon did, however, was to propagate the idea that it was possible to have a continuous growth of knowledge and that it was possible to find more knowledge. Until then, there was a pre-occupation with hanging on to the old knowledge in fear that it might disappear!

Novum Organum

In this book, the teaching was in the form of aphorisms. There are a group of three ideas: the need for a new logic, the attempt to discover the 'forms' of the simple natures, e.g. heat, and the collection of a comprehensive natural history. He believed that these three were tied in with natural history at the base, the laws of physics in the middle and logic as the crown.

A great deal has been written about the philosophical and scientific works of Francis Bacon and there is considerable literature about his personal and political life. He had a strong association with the Royalty and served in Parliament as a Member for Melcombe Regis in Dorset and later for Taunton and Liverpool. He fell out of favour in 1621 after admitting charges of bribery.

For those who are interested in reading more about the life of Francis Bacon, the *Encyclopedia Brittanica* is a good starting point. Oxford University Press also produce a series of '*Past Masters*' and the one on Bacon has been written by Anthony Quinton.

Gitanjali (1961–1977)

Gitanjali was born in Meerut, India on 12th June 1961. She died soon after her 16th birthday on 11th August 1977. That she died of cancer is not particularly remarkable in itself, many children and many adults do. What is remarkable is that born from a realisation of her own mortality, she left us with a record of her fears and worries and her faith and courage. Rabindranath Tagore, who is probably India's greatest poet, is best remembered for his poem entitled 'Gitanjali', which means 'song-offering'.

The first verse of Tagore's poem is as follows:

"Thou hast made me endless, such is thy pleasure. This frail vessel thou emptiest again and again, and fillest it ever with fresh life.

This little flute of a reed thou hast carried over the hills and dales, and hast breathed through it melodies eternally new.

At the immortal touch of thy hands my little heart loses it's limits in joy and gives birth to utterance ineffable.

Thy infinite gifts come to me only on these very small hands of mine. Ages pass, and still thou pourest, and still there is room to fill."

Gitanjali's wish was that she might live up to her name. She did. The publication of the poems in the form of a book is remarkable in itself. Gitanjali's mother had discovered the poems hidden around the house amongst her books and clothes. She tried in vain to get them published until having almost given up hope, she sent one to The Illustrated Weekly of India. They were so moved by it that they decided to publish it.

The book *Poems of Gitanjali* was first published by Oriel Press in 1982.

Harvey, William (1578–1657)

William Harvey was born in Folkestone on 1st April 1578. It may have been April Fools day, but this man provided Medicine with the boost it needed to get it out of stagnation. The value of his work is put into perspective when you realise that to be honoured as a Harveian Orator by the Royal College of Physicians is the greatest distinction that one can aspire to.

Harvey did his medical training at Caius College, Cambridge and later at Padua, Italy. In Padua, Harvey studied with Fabricius who had succeeded Fallopio (of Fallopian tube fame). Galileo was the Professor of Mathematics at Padua at the time but does not appear to have been influential in Harvey's developement.

Harvey was elected a full fellow of the College of Physicians in 1607 and soon afterwards became Assistant Physician to St. Bartholomew's Hospital. This helped to establish his private practice and, interestingly, his famous patients included James I, Charles I and the Lord Chancellor, Sir Francis Bacon! Although Bacon is given the credit for inductive thinking, it was Harvey who applied it to his investigations of the heart. Harvey, in fact, had very little respect for Bacon and had stated that Bacon "writes philosophy (science) like a Lord Chancellor; I have cured him of it".

The quote at the beginning of Chapter 2 is the first paragraph of Chapter 1 in his famous book, *De Motu Cordis*. The movements of the heart were so fast and complicated that he often despaired at ever being able to work out the sequence of each of the movements. *De Motu Cordis* evolved in two stages; initially it was an investigation into the heart beat and the arterial pulse and only later did he include the investigation of the circulation. Together, it forms one of the most important pieces of scientific work. The book is quite small, 72 pages, and would probably fit into a white coat pocket, but the few remaining copies of the original 1628 edition would set you back a cool £200,000! That is assuming anybody is willing to sell it. William Harvey died of a stroke on 30th June 1657. Much has been written about Harvey, and the Keynes translation of 1928 is believed to be the most accurate. Keynes has written a couple of books on Harvey. These are: *The Personality of William Harvey*, published by Cambridge University Press in 1949, and *The Life of William Harvey*, Oxford University Press, 1966.

Heisenberg, Werner Karl

Heisenberg, who is well known for his contribution to quantum mechanics, was born on 5th December, 1901, in Würzburg, Germany. He studied physics at the University of Munich. His doctoral thesis, which he presented in 1923, was on turbulence in fluid streams.

In 1927, Heisenberg published his 'uncertainty principle', which says that, in the subatomic world, it is not possible to know both the position and the momentum of a particle accurately. The better we know one variable, the less sure we can be of the other. The important point is that it is not the limitation of the technique of measurement that imposes this law, it is simply the limitation of the principle. What this means is that the uncertainty principle is a mathematical way of expressing the limitation of our classical models of looking at the world.

Our classical way of looking at the world is derived from gross appearances and we have a tendency to divide things into discrete units or, to put it another way, we perceive the world as being particulate. At the subatomic level, this particulate view is an idealisation without any meaning and it is not possible to describe anything without a reference to the whole. Hence 'entities' such as position and momentum are interrelated and cannot be defined precisely at the same time, since changes in one are tied in with changes in the other. These connections are of a statistical nature, i.e. probabilities rather than certainties.

This idea of interactions led to the proposal of the concept of the 'S matrix' which is a mathematical model for these interactions. It was this belief in the fundamental principles of a shift from objects to events that lead to the quotation at the end of Chapter 1. Just as in the subatomic world, the various events in the body are a manifestation of the many interactions between the various processes. They are not isolated events, but interact and combine in intricate ways in any given situation.

Heisenberg is mainly known for his achievements in physics, but he was also a philosopher trying to understand the relationships that are fundamental in nature. He was awarded the Nobel Prize in 1932.

Osler, William (1849–1919)

Many people believe that Sir William Osler was the most loved and the greatest physician of recent times. This was not for his scientific contribution but for his ability to fascinate young students and for completely transforming medical education and clinical medical training.

Osler was born at Bond Head, Ontario, Canada. His parents were English missionaries who had emigrated to Canada. He was the youngest of nine children. His initial intention was to follow his father into the church and he started his studies at Trinity College, Toronto. He changed his mind, however, and enrolled at the Toronto Medical School in 1868. He finished his medical education at McGill University. Having qualified, he spent the next two years travelling around Europe, the longest period being spent with Sir John Burdon-Sanderson at University College, London.

He returned to Canada with the intention of entering general practice but within a few months was appointed Lecturer in Medicine at McGill. He taught physiology and pathology to the medical students. The following year he was appointed Professor. After a decade in Montreal, he went as Professor of Medicine to Pennsylvania and in 1888, he accepted a post at the new Johns Hopkins Hospital in Baltimore. He was the second of the famous 'Hopkins four', the others being William Welch, Chief of Pathology, Howard Kelley, Chief of Obstetrics and Gynaecology and William Halstead, Chief of Surgery. It was with these three colleagues that Osler revolutionised the medical curriculum.

For the first four years at the Johns Hopkins, there were no medical students and Osler used these years to write *The Principles and Practice of Medicine*, first published in 1892.

In 1904, while visiting the UK, he was offered the Regius Chair of Medicine at Oxford. This was to succeed Burdon-Sanderson. Osler accepted and started his post in 1905.

Osler's name is associated with three medical conditions: Osler's nodes – tender, red swellings on the palms and fingers in bacterial endocarditis; Osler–Vaquez disease – polycythaemia rubra vera; and Rendu–Osler–Weber disease – recurrent haemorrhages from multiple telengectasias in skin and mucous membranes.

Osler has written a lot about almost everything, and especially so about the relationship between the teacher and student, teacher and teacher, and teacher and patient. The quotation at the end of Chapter 2 is from his book, *Counsels and Ideals from the Writings of Sir William Osler*, 1905.

Smithers, David Waldron

Sir David Smithers was the Director of Radiotherapy at the Royal Marsden Hospital and Institute of Cancer Research.

His schooling was at Boxgrove School in Guildford, Surrey, followed by Clare College, Cambridge. He qualified with MRCS LRCP from St. Thomas's Hospital in 1933 and obtained his MB BChir (Cantab) in 1934. He received his MD (Cantab) in 1937.

He has written extensively on various aspects of cancer and radiotherapy and the quote in Chapter 4 is from his writings in 1962. He is also the author of many books including *Hodgkin's Disease* (1973), *Castles in Kent* (1980), *Jane Austen in Kent* (1981) and *This Idle Trade* on doctors who were writers (1989).

Thomas, Lewis

Lewis Thomas is University Professor at the State University of New York at Stony Brook, and President Emeritus of the Memorial Sloan-Kettering Cancer Center in New York. The quotes come from essays that were first published in the New England Journal of Medicine, at the invitation of the editor Dr. F.J. Ingelfinger. The column was titled 'Notes of a Biology-Watcher'. These essays were first published in book form in two separate volumes, *The Lives of a Cell* (1974) and *The Medusa and the Snail* (1979), by the Viking Press. These are combined into one volume, *The Wonderful Mistake* and published by Oxford University Press (1988). His other books include *The Youngest Science* and *Late Night Thoughts*, also produced by Oxford Paperbacks.

Further reading

JS. Paget. (1897). *John Hunter. Man of Science and Surgeon.* Fisher Unwin. London.

P.J. Weimerskirch & G.W. Richter. (1979). Hunter and venereal disease. Lancet. 1: 503–504.

G. Pickering. (1964). William Harvey, physician and scientist. British Medical Journal. 2: 1615–1619.

L.J. Rather. (1957). Rudolf Virchow and scientific medicine. Archives of Internal Medicine. 100: 1007–1014.

J. Bamforth & G.R. Osborn. (1958). Diagnosis from cells. Journal of Clinical Pathology. 473-482.

A.J. Harding Rains. (1974). Edward Jenner and Vaccination. Priory Press London.

H.E. Sergerist. (1935). Great Doctors. A Biographical History of Medicine. George Allen & Unwin London.

S.B. Nuland. (1988). Doctors. The Biography of Medicine. Gryphon Editions. Birmingham, Alabama.

F. Capra. (1983). The Tao of Physics. 2nd Edition. Fontana Paperbacks. Glasgow.

Index _____